Hospital Leadership
& Accountability

Hospital Leadership & Accountability

An Anthology from
Hospital & Health Services Administration

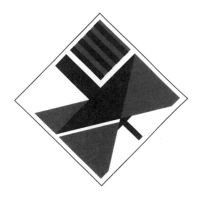

Samuel Levey
Editor

Health Administration Press
Ann Arbor, Michigan 1992

96   95   94   93   92   5   4   3   2   1

Library of Congress Cataloging-in-Publication Data

Hospital leadership & accountability / Samuel Levey, editor.
    p.   cm.
    "An anthology from Hospital & health services administration."
    Includes bibliographical references and index.
    ISBN 0-910701-84-9 (softbound : alk. paper)
    1. Hospitals—Administration.   I. Levey, Samuel.   II. Hospital & health services administration.
    [DNLM: 1. Hospital Administration—collected works.   2. Personnel Administration, Hospital—collected works.   3. Quality Assurance, Health Care—collected works.   WX 150 H8259]
RA971.H5936   1992   362.1'1'068—dc20
DNLM/DLC for Library of Congress   92-1523 CIP

Cover design by Barb Gunia
Adapted from an original painting by Samuel Levey

Health Administration Press
A division of the Foundation of the
   American College of Healthcare Executives
1021 East Huron Street
Ann Arbor, Michigan 48104-9990
(313) 764-1380

Contents

Contents

Foreword

The U.S. health care field faces profound challenges. Powerful and effective leadership is required to deal with problems such as limited access, the growing number of uninsured Americans, explosive rises in health spending, ever-increasing payment restrictions, and shrinking margins.

More than ever, it is imperative that health care executives fully understand the complexity of our field, and I am confident that the collected wisdom in the following pages of *Hospital Leadership & Accountability* will help them do just that.

I am especially pleased to be associated with the authors represented in this important body of work. For more than 37 years, *Hospital & Health Services Administration* has been the journal of choice for health care executives who want thoughtful commentary and significant insights into the turbulent, yet always rewarding, profession in which we serve.

As the official journal of the American College of Healthcare Executives, *Hospital & Health Services Administration* validates the College's responsibility as a professional society to expand the body of knowledge in the health care arena and to provide thought-provoking articles on the field it represents. This anthology of outstanding articles published in recent years in *Hospital & Health Services Administration* represents a significant contribution to our educational efforts.

From 1987 to 1991, *Hospital & Health Services Administration* was under the thoughtful editorial direction of Samuel Levey of the University of Iowa. As its first external editor, Sam Levey was instrumental in taking the Journal to a new level of editorial excellence. Today, we can again benefit from his work in this anthology of noteworthy articles.

This book is designed to meet two very important needs. As a collection of the best current articles on the pivotal themes of health care leadership, it should serve today's health care executives as a basis for serious reflection and considered action. In addition, I hope this work will become a useful educational resource for future health care executives, serving as a basic text for their development and training.

Hospital Leadership & Accountability explores six critical areas of health care leadership: governance, management, finance, quality, human resources, and ethics. The contributions to the literature in each subject area are impressive, and the introduction by Sam Levey is itself a major contribution to the literature. It offers many excellent examples of the current trends in the U.S. health care system and deals with vital issues in the hospital sector and the public interest, as well as the responsibility of health care executives to meet the leadership challenges that face them.

The American College of Healthcare Executives is grateful to Sam Levey for his work as editor of *Hospital & Health Services Administration* and for his compilation of this significant anthology. The College also gratefully acknowledges the enormous contributions of the authors included within this volume. They clearly represent some of the best thinking in the health care field today—these are individuals whose extensive research and perceptive commentaries have enlightened and inspired us for many years.

Thomas C. Dolan, FACHE
President
American College
of Healthcare Executives

Preface

My part in the production of this book began five years ago when I accepted the College's invitation to become editor of *Hospital & Health Services Administration*. At that time, I could not fully comprehend the extraordinary opportunities of editorship, nor could I fathom the range of responsibilities the assignment would entail.

Since then I have had the great pleasure of working with outstanding and dedicated authors from both the academic and practitioner worlds. In the past year, while sorting through dozens of articles for this project, I acquired an even deeper appreciation of the superb quality of thinking shown by our contributors. Unfortunately, in making the selection, I found that constraints of space and format made it impossible for me to include much that is excellent.

I am grateful to many others for their contributions. The Journal's referees deserve our thanks for their enthusiasm, hard work, and diligence. I would like to note in particular the critical importance of the Journal's publishing group in the overall production process. Here, several individuals who are associated with Health Administration Press in Ann Arbor, Michigan, deserve special acknowledgment. I would like to thank the Director of the Press, Daphne Grew, for her encouragement. The Journal's Managing Editor, Rebecca McDermott, and Associate Managing Editor, Kelly Sippell, assisted in many ways to bring this project to fruition. Working with them was both educational and enjoyable, and I very quickly came to depend on their capacity to dissolve difficulty with a few quick suggestions. On the production side of this enterprise, Edward Kobrinski, Acquisitions Editor, deserves credit for coaxing me when necessary; he and Associate Director Christina Bych moved the project forward in an expeditious fashion.

At the University of Iowa where the Journal's editorial officers were located, I am indebted to a sizable number of faculty, doctoral students, and research assistants, all of whom helped considerably in reviewing manuscripts and ensuring that the office ran smoothly. Special appreciation is due to my former secretary, Marilyn Simpson, as well as James Hill, Marcella Doderer, and Young-Joon Seo, who assisted in various phases of developing this anthology.

Of course, none of this would have happened if Tom Dolan had not persuaded me to accept an assignment that would become one of the highlights of my academic career, and I would like to underscore my debt of gratitude to the College and to him.

Introduction

Health Care in America

Many of today's commentaries on the condition of the American health care system begin with an implied question: How can anything so remarkable and expensive be so enigmatically flawed? At its best, our system is widely regarded as a marvel of technological innovation and progress. Its scientific achievements are esteemed around the world. Because of it most Americans receive better health care than any previous generation, and they can expect to lead longer and more productive lives.

In contrast to this dramatic picture of sophistication is the litany of problems we are exposed to virtually on a daily basis: an estimated 35–40 million individuals—one-third of whom are children—are without insurance coverage, and an additional 20–25 million are underinsured. The extent of this problem is underscored by the fact that the poor population grew 34 percent between 1978 and 1988, but the number of Medicaid recipients increased only 4 percent from 22 to 22.9 million (Health Insurance Association of America (HIAA) 1990). Over 200,000 Americans have the acquired immunodeficiency syndrome (AIDS) and as many as 1.5 million may be diagnosed with the human immuno virus (HIV) (American Hospital Association (AHA) 1991b). The burden of inappropriate or equivocal health care has been estimated at one-quarter to one-third of all care given to insured Americans (Brook 1991), and costs in administrative inefficiency and waste are said to run into the billions (Woolhandler and Himmelstein 1991). Our perception of the state of the American health care system becomes less glowing if we add to these figures a recent survey of 24 countries in the Organization for Economic Cooperation and Development that showed the U.S. infant mortality rate higher than that of 19 nations, and the life expectancy for men and women below that of countries such as Japan, Germany, and France (Schieber, Poullier, and Greenwald 1991). Taken together, these statistics can be viewed as a glaring failure of policy, political will, and public understanding and support. Is the American health care system in major crisis? Many believe that it is, but

1

in the view of McCarthy (1991), few think that a "total systemwide change is imminent."

A major source of discontent regarding health care is the seemingly unending escalation of expenditures. Since the implementation of Medicare in 1965, the national health bill has mushroomed from $42 billion to roughly $670 billion in 1990, an increase of 10.5 percent over the 1989 level (Health Care Financing Administration (HCFA) 1991). Annual rates of increase routinely exceed general economic inflation levels: from 1980 to 1989, medical care prices rose 8 percent while overall the consumer price index rose at a rate of 4.3 percent per year. The projected national health bill for 1991 is $740 billion, or over $2,800 per capita—more than any other nation spends on health care.

In the industrial sector, a recent survey of larger businesses found that between 1989 and 1990, average health care outlays rose 21.6 percent, with medical plan costs approximating $3,160 per employee (U.S. General Accounting Office 1991) and an astounding 100 percent of 1989 profits (Smith 1991). Federal programs accounted for 42 percent of national health expenditures in 1990, the largest proportion in U.S. history, perpetuating the dominant role of government in health care. Total health care expenditures are expected to reach over $1.6 trillion at the turn of the century, in excess of 16 percent of the gross national product.

Reasons advanced for the precipitous rises in health spending include increases in the volume and intensity of services, the proliferation of expensive technology, the practice of defensive medicine, soaring administrative expenses, cost shifting, demographic changes, and the rise in salary levels. Other factors include lack of provider accountability, an excess number of medical specialists, and the traditional and predominant driving forces of fee-for-service and third-party payment. Adding to the cost problem—or perhaps at the root of it—are uncompromising consumer expectations that lead to overuse. Consumers, however, believe that the main forces driving costs are predominantly moral, "factors such as greed, high salaries, corruption, waste and unnecessary testing" (Yankelovich and Immerwahr 1991).

Other surveys of the public's attitude toward our health care system are similarly critical. One opinion poll showed that only 10 percent of respondents agreed that the health care system as a whole works pretty well and requires only minor changes (Blendon et al. 1990). In a more recent study, researchers found that a majority of the public are satisfied with their health insurance and health care, but many are dissatisfied with the health care system and believe it is inefficient and wasteful (Blendon 1991). Another survey of public attitudes toward major institutions showed declining support of the health care system, ranking it behind business and industry, the public schools, and even the U.S. Congress (*Medical Benefits* 1991).

2

Beginning in the late 1960s, it appeared that the federal government was determined to come to grips with the need to advance provider accountability through cost containment. Since then, a number of cost-control measures have been introduced, including the Nixon administration freeze on wages and prices in the hospital industry in 1973, the creation of peer review organizations, the endorsement and sponsorship of health maintenance organizations (HMOs) and of managed care, and the introduction of the Medicare prospective payment system in 1983. This year the implementation of the resource-based relative value scale (RBRVS) will exert further effects on the Medicare bill and physician behavior. In the private sector as well, cost-control mechanisms have been introduced, including utilization management coupled with increased deductibles and copayments—a fast-growing trend. However, these "braking" measures have been largely ineffective in slowing down overall health care spending.

The 1980s also witnessed a loss of confidence in the ability of government to successfully attack elements of the problem of health care financial access, in addition to the cost spiral. It is accordingly not surprising that current prospects for developing workable cost-control strategies remain quite remote in the short term. This problem has been exacerbated by our patchwork system of health care and the limitations of the procompetitive approach. Indeed, some observers have noted the adverse effects of the competition model, including the erosion of trust and collaboration among providers, the reduction of health planning at the community level, the growing duplication of costly new technologies, and unprecedented levels of advertisement spending for health care products (Colloton 1991).

Proposals for health care reform now constitute a thicket of options.[1] One example of a proposal for achieving universal access that is now receiving national attention is the program of the National Leadership Coalition for Health Care Reform (1991): an "organization of organizations" made up of business, labor, health professionals, and consumers, the Coalition has recommended a blend of competitive and regulatory strategies that would yield guaranteed access to comprehensive benefits. Those not privately insured would receive coverage through a program that would incorporate the acute care part of Medicaid. The Coalition reports that under this plan total savings could exceed several hundred billion dollars per year by the turn of the century.

In 1990, median operating profit margins for all U.S. hospitals increased to about 4 percent—not an impressive performance. Under Medicare, however, margins have generally been negative. The median operating margin of hospitals with more than 400 beds was approximately 3 percent in 1990 while hospitals with 25–99 beds had a median operating margin of less than 1 percent. It is accordingly not surprising that the number of facilities confronted with serious economic distress is growing. One-quarter of Thomas R. Prince's sample of approximately 1,300 community hospitals (Chapter 12), for example, are facing financial distress. In the past decade, the total number of community hospitals has declined as a result of closures, mergers, and acquisitions. Between 1980 and 1990, the number of community hospitals in the United States dropped from 5,830 to 5,384, a decline of 7.7 percent, with the greatest losses in the New England and Pacific regions (American Hospital Association (AHA) 1991a)—recently, however, the rate of closures has slowed to 50 institutions in 1990, down from 65 in 1989 (*Medical Benefits* 1991). Reasons for the closures varied, but the primary causes were lack of profitability and large losses, poor operating margins, excessive costs per discharge, as well as high prices, low utilization, lack of investment in plant, deteriorating capital, eroding liquidity, and excessive long-term debt (Cleverley 1990). A study of rural hospitals indicated that mix of facilities and services is another important variable in risk of closure (Mullner 1990).

To be sure, chief executives of hospitals have shown considerable resilience and adaptability in their restructuring and reorganization approaches. In spite of pressures that have led to relatively high executive turnover rates in recent years, CEOs have adjusted remarkably well to the vicissitudes of an encroaching environment. One can argue that most voluntary hospitals seem to have acted pragmatically by embracing the rules of the competitive approach and adopting a more rigorous business orientation.

One obvious way for hospitals to address financial constraints is to become more efficient. Another option for survival and growth in a revenue-restricted environment is the pursuit of strategic initiatives—the creation and marketing of new services to attract more profitable patients. In the 1980s, under the pressures of reduced demand for acute care services and a reimbursement system that rewards the expeditious discharge of patients, many hospitals diversified into alternative delivery systems: prominent examples are HMOs, independent physician associations (IPAs), preferred provider organizations (PPOs), outpatient emergicenters, urgent care centers, surgicenters, and "expanded mission" services such as wellness, fitness, child care, long-term care, and retirement centers. Between 1985 and 1990, the number of community hospitals with outpatient departments jumped from over one-half to over three-quarters. Outpatient surgery grew 262.5 percent in the decade of the 1980s, from over 3 million to over 11 million procedures. At the same time, the number of long-term care units in community hospitals increased by over 80 percent (AHA 1991b). Among the possible benefits in pursuing these avenues are maintenance and expansion of market share, more effective competition, reduction of costs, enhancement of image, and extension of social responsibility.

Like other industries, the hospital sector has attempted to achieve operating efficiencies through mergers and consolidations. Indeed, hospital systems seem to have emerged as a sine qua non for political and economic survival, proliferating through both voluntary and for-profit auspices. Of the 311 multi-hospital systems reported by the AHA (1991a), 252 are not-for-profit, 54 are investor-owned, and 5 are federal. As Stephen M. Shortell and his colleagues point out in Chapter 11, however, hospital systems have not generated the benefits that had been anticipated. Moreover, some observers fear that the expansion of systems will weaken the traditional responsiveness and sense of obligation of hospitals to their local stakeholders (Gray 1991). The extent of such effects, however, cannot be verified without further empirical study.

Unfortunately, we have a Congress that seems to walk in circles on the issue of health care reform, finding reasons to confound or reject steps leading to substantive legislation. Moreover, we have an administration in Washington that is willing to wait and see if "micromanagement" in the private sector will succeed in resolving our health care dilemmas, and that is once again seeking recommendations for means to extend access and control costs. In an October 1991 press release, Louis Sullivan, M.D., Secretary of the Department of Health and Human Services (DHHS)—who has not been in favor of comprehensive reform—observed that "we need to slow the growth of health care costs without reducing the quality of care, and we need an active partnership of business, medical professionals, government, the insurance industry, and private citizens to achieve these goals." At this writing, a weak economy and the results of the off-year senatorial election in Pennsylvania have moved health care reform to the forefront, but it remains to be seen whether consensus among the principals will be achieved. According to Senate Republican leader Robert Dole, health care will be the number-one issue in the 1992 presidential campaign (Pear 1991).

The Hospital Sector and the Public Interest

In the view of Rosemary A. Stevens (Chapter 1), America has fostered "an amazing system of hospitals in the twentieth century: huge, disorganized, nervous, ebullient, dedicated, wasteful, technically innovative, luxurious, inegalitarian, daring, competitive, pluralistic, self-contained, and conflict-ridden." Can a chief executive officer—one who is expected to function as the "personification, strategist, coordinator, and spokesman of the hospital" (Kinzer 1987)—ever hope to understand, much less manage, so complex and unwieldy a creation?

As John R. Griffith indicates in Chapter 6, today's hospital leaders find themselves embattled by the most demanding environment in over half a century. Because their organizations are highly visible focal points for health

5

services delivery and consume roughly 38 percent of total health care expenditures—$256 billion in 1990, a figure projected to grow to $620 billion in the year 2000 (HCFA 1991)—they have been subjected to increasing scrutiny and criticism. The 1980s saw the onset of diagnosis-related groups, "partial" competition, and ambulatory care—three of the most far-reaching developments of the past 25 years. Combined with the forces mentioned earlier, these developments encouraged a shift in the central concerns of hospital executives toward survival-oriented management and planning strategies. According to Kinzer (1987), "When a CEO is trying to cope with a declining census, a rebelling medical staff, and a fragile and unpredictable revenue base, and when a neighboring hospital is bent on making off with his or her market share, there is often little enough time or energy left for community and social issues."

The entrepreneurial element in health care is not entirely new, however. Although the subject heading "Marketing of Health Services" first appeared in the *Hospital Literature Index* in 1979 and "Economic Competition" appeared in 1982, the competitive and commercial aspects of health care have, in fact, long been with us. Yet the rapid expansion of for-profit health care enterprises, including the growth of for-profit subsidiaries in the voluntary sector, has never been more intense than in the past decade, with health care becoming increasingly commercialized and competitive. According to Gray (1991), "The most basic element that all the changes share is simply that health care has become oriented more toward economic performance."

Misgivings over the ascendancy of the entrepreneurial ethos in health care began about a decade ago with the (then) editor of the *New England Journal of Medicine*, Arnold Relman (1980), describing the metamorphosis of the "new medical-industrial complex"—the enormous aggregation of for-profit organizations providing health services. At the same time, Starr (1982) described the "rise of a corporate ethos" and Ginzberg (1984) called attention to the "monetarization" of health care. In a recent Shattuck lecture, Relman (1991) described the continuing commercialization of health care, observing that "altruistic motives that formerly guided the decision of voluntary hospital management are giving way in many institutions to a primary concern for the bottom line."

These misgivings led to questions about the tax-exempt status of the hospital. In this era of bottom-line emphasis, it has become increasingly difficult to differentiate not-for-profit hospitals from investor-owned institutions, both in terms of organizational mission and commitment to community. Recent judicial and political debates have generated questions regarding the tax-exempt status for voluntary institutions, and a report from the U.S. General Accounting Office (1989) has suggested that Congress should consider changing the present liberal rules for qualification as charitable entities. Whether or not such concerns boil over from local sanctions into nationwide demands and impositions remains to be seen.

One could argue that ever since the introduction of the competitive model in health care, pressures to compromise have grown enormously. Whether hospital executives pursue financial goals or take balanced leadership approaches toward their social responsibilities will largely depend on the values and managerial philosophy of the CEO, as well as those of governing board members and professional staff, particularly physicians. It is clear that the old "soft" models of hospital governance and organization are becoming obsolete, and that improved measurement, evaluation, and accountability must be championed, implemented, and monitored in order to enhance prospects for the economic and human service missions.

Doing Well and Doing Good

Today's hospital leaders must "do well" while "doing good" (see James W. Summers, Chapter 22) without succumbing to the stresses and strains of conflicting objectives. Serving both imperatives now involves a complex weave of forces and steps: institutional as well as community interests, access for the needy and uninsured, cost containment, and management of a service-driven ethic with a central focus on quality. The "fiducial" exchange that the hospital shares with society has been undergoing considerable revision, especially in the last decade, and aspects of it are distressingly at risk. In their discussion of ethics in health services management (Chapter 23), Kurt Darr, Beaufort B. Longest, Jr., and Jonathon S. Rakich identify "fiduciary duty" as a fundamental principle of management. "Fiduciary" is often used to characterize a legal arrangement involving a trust and has been frequently invoked to describe the special relationship between physician and patient; trust and implicit obligation are at the heart of the term.

Where the voluntary hospital is concerned, however, a term that more accurately represents the spirit of public trust is "fiducial" since it bears the implication of religious belief as opposed to intellectual knowledge. The modern American hospital, as Rosenberg (1987) points out, was conceived out of the eleemosynary spirit of charity and framed by the "responsibilities of Christian stewardship." Hence, "fiducial" expresses more of the original raison d'être.

The origin of this fiducial norm is the deontological social responsibility fostered by our Judeo-Christian heritage. Its history is as old as our religious roots; its visible form is the monastic medicine of the Middle Ages, the almshouse of the seventeenth century, and the charity hospital of the nineteenth.

According to Rosner (1988), in the nineteenth century "most of the [hospitals] that developed were small, urban, locally sponsored charity facilities almost exclusively serving working class and poor." From the community almshouse, the voluntary hospital evolved incrementally, with the growth of technology and the health professions, maintaining its roots in charity while branching out into profit-based enterprises. The latter development, as mentioned earlier, is viewed with disquiet in certain quarters. According to Starr (1982), for example, the "extension of the voluntary hospital into profit-making businesses and the penetration of other corporations into the hospital signal the breakdown of the traditional boundaries of voluntarism."

Of course, this does mean the eventual extinction of voluntarism. In the view of Stevens (Chapter 1), there has been no single trajectory of change in hospital history over the course of the twentieth century, no linear trends from which to project an obvious future. In her essay she reviews several aspects of the history of hospitals in this century, reading them as keys to the present. Concluding that American hospitals are characterized by "oscillation and flexibility," she sees the nation as "coming out of the cycle of competition as defined in the 1980s into a cycle in which public goals will be expressed." In her scheme, hospitals will have to sell themselves as "quasi-public institutions." This movement from private interest to public purpose may be a part of a wider movement, perhaps ushered in by a new cycle of American political history.

Whatever the direction, executive leadership accountability will become much more prominent in the future, far different from that which applied in the early years of the profession. In the mid-twentieth century, managerial accountability for hospital executives evolved into fairly loose agreements regarding task definition, delegation of authority, and performance. Ultimately, it was a relationship of trust and expediency among concerned parties: patients, physicians, and executives. A powerful element of trust on the part of the community and a strong sense of obligation on the part of each hospital were largely responsible for keeping health care outside the public sector. In the past decade, however, the weakening bond between the institution and society has been seen as an erosion of the fiducial aspect of those exchanges, and with it public trust.

Fiducial accountability is not easily enforceable, however. As Gray (1991) points out, health care providers are not "held accountable for failures to meet societal needs in the same way they are held accountable for individual patients." Today, the measures of accountability for hospital executives are institution- and communitywide, revolving around specific task obligations. Such a pattern lends itself more readily to institutional performance indicators than to general estimations of responsiveness to social need.

Fiducial Accountability

Hospital executives participate in the fiducial ethic of the health professions. The tools of their work are business skills, yet the nature of their profession and a tradition of public trust give that ethos a focus different from that guiding business. According to Starr (1982), "In justifying the public's trust, professionals have set higher standards for themselves than the minimal rules governing the marketplace and maintained that they can be judged under those standards by each other, not by laymen."

That trust can be strained under certain conditions, of course. Just as physicians may experience a conflict of interest in being both medical professionals and entrepreneurs, hospital CEOs have the difficult assignment of serving two distinct and often conflicting missions: make the organization a consistently better provider of community service, and give it a sound business underpinning. Increasingly, skeptics question whether these missions can be reconciled within the spirit of a not-for-profit organization—which Vladeck (1992) points out "exists not for its own benefit, or the benefit of any stockholders or employees, but for the benefit of a broader community or public purpose." While this special kind of public trust may raise the fiducial duty of the hospital CEO above other considerations, it is clear that it should not mean the provision of benefits at any cost.

Whether a CEO can be held accountable for the fulfillment of this duty is an issue that should be approached through an understanding of terms. "Accountability" does not submit to a single definition, but is often used interchangeably—and incorrectly—with "responsibility" to mean duty or conscientious self-discipline in carrying out one's obligations. Accountability is, of course, closely related to responsibility. It "follows" responsibility (i.e., duty and performance) in two respects: (1) responsiveness to a higher authority in giving an account of performance and (2) willingness to accept the consequences if responsibility is shirked or performance is lacking. In a sense, then, accountability is the counterpoint of responsibility: its usage is rarely neutral but is usually shaded with an implied threat of retribution. In other words, accountability can be conceptualized as normative and critical, whereas responsibility is often regarded as positive and proactive: like traffic police at an intersection, accountability ensures the orderly flow in an organization, guaranteeing that all personnel follow the stated terms of duty, procedure, and law. Where leadership is concerned, it proceeds from the assumption that individuals are more likely to carry out the full scope of their responsibilities if they are made aware of the requirement incumbent upon them to be answerable for their behavior, as well as the duty to be an example for others.

Accountability can, therefore, be viewed as a moral trust with other individuals and society-at-large, and it is this perspective that dovetails with the conception of true fiducial accountability presented here. This connection becomes clearer if we view accountability as deriving from two sources, objective and subjective, or formal/legal and moral. One finds an illustration of these bases in the segment of the American College of Healthcare Executives (ACHE) Code of Ethics that deals with accountability. For example, the formal/legal base of hospital managers' accountability is seen in the externally imposed controls of their role in the institution: patients, governing board, physicians, and professional staff hold managers responsible for the fulfillment of specific responsibilities. The moral base of the ACHE Code is evident in the internally imposed, subjective demands—for example, in exhortations to promote a supportive working environment and to practice strict personal integrity. Fiducial duty is an implied aspect of the moral base.

To strengthen the formal/legal base of accountability, one adds more "police" at institutional, state, and national levels—monitoring mechanisms from internal audits to regulatory requirements. To fortify the moral base with "internal police," however, is far more problematic. Afterall, one can no more internalize a code of ethics and fiducial obligation to community than one can become profoundly ethical by taking a course in ethics. Strengthening the moral base of accountability requires the development of fiducial leadership.

Fiducial Leadership: Performance and Vision

To begin to understand the concept of fiducial leadership, we must define what it is we mean by leadership. To be sure, the term has long been a focus of interest among managers, politicians, and scholars. In recent years, we have witnessed an avalanche of publications on leadership from both the "real" and academic worlds. From slender collections of epigrams by famous figures to more substantial, thought-provoking expositions, the production of literature continues at a brisk pace. In 1974, when the first edition of Stogdill's definitive *Handbook of Leadership* was published, some 3,000 studies of leadership were cited; the 1990 edition boasts approximately 8,000 entries.

Despite this vast expenditure of effort, the concept remains hazy, with hundreds of competing definitions as numerous as leaders themselves. Academics, for their part, having created an industry of theory and empirical studies, appear to be desperately trying to discover a way out of the maze. The "schools" of leadership they have generated range from trait theories popular until the postwar years, to behavioral approaches that became popular in the

1950s and 1960s, to the contingency models in the 1970s, to the current interest in transformational empowerment rather than transactional exchange. Practitioners in the public and private sectors are beset by different preoccupations: they continue to worry about enhancing the quality of products and services as well as improving productivity and economic performance—an endless quest.

Approaching the concept, one may wonder that empirical studies could apply to so broad and shifting a term. For example, kinds of leaders may extend from organizational to public; types may range from autocratic to democratic. The functions of leadership may overlap with those of management to such a degree that any distinction between the two terms is lost.

One distinction between management and leadership seems to always arise: while a manager is expected to be in possession of a certain fund of knowledge and workaday skills, a leader must have "vision," a special power or capacity. In spite of its frequent invocation, however, the term lacks a clear referent, a fact that causes some contemporary leaders to discount its importance (recall President Bush's disdain for the "vision thing"). Such leaders see themselves as doers rather than ivory tower visionaries far removed from the hurly-burly of production.

In the hospital sector a successful leader combines performance with vision, the former essentially effectiveness and efficiency—the sine qua non of the manager—and the latter breadth and depth of understanding and force of imagination in protecting and promoting the community service ethic. How does one cultivate a vision that will promote the fiducial aspect of hospital leadership? To begin, vision is not the power of the unschooled and sedentary mind, but of one that has spent considerable effort reading, observing, and gathering information, and that is able, as a consequence, to marshall a depth of learning in the synthesis of new ideas. The basis of vision for the hospital executive would seem to grow out of a liberal education, with a heightened emphasis on fostering the interdisciplinary frame of mind, and a set of values consistent with the highest ideals of the health professions. Above all, it demands a level of "literacy" considerably beyond what is generally gained in the skill and tool courses of health management curricula. In my view, there can be a "literacy" for hospital leadership that promotes a philosophy of management based on performance within the institution and fiducial obligation to community.

From the establishment of the first graduate program in hospital management in 1934 at the University of Chicago, literacy has been generally understood as the mastery of economic and business theory and skills, as well as knowledge of general management and health care organization. Variation on the Chicago prototype was common across the field, of course, though most

11

programs tended to adjust curricula in accordance with recommendations that followed periodic reviews of the status of graduate programs (for example, those by the 1948 Joint Commission on Education, the 1953 Olsen Commission, and the Dixon Commission of the 1970s). Since 1968, most programs have necessarily followed the curriculum recommendations of the Accrediting Commission on Education for Health Services Administration.

Today, literacy in health management and policy recognizes that the surge of competition among health care organizations means an ever greater need for both a broad knowledge base in organization and management and the latest and most sophisticated business skills and analytic methods; however, general knowledge of the health industry and of changing societal expectations concerning the role of the hospital may be considered by some as less important for survival than concentration in functional areas such as finance or human resources.

Literacy in hospital and health care management will continue to be judged primarily as competence in state-of-the-art business skills and up-to-date knowledge of social and health organizations. For now, educators could try to encourage a more broad-based literacy by regularly reviewing curriculum requirements and by introducing innovations on an experimental basis that are based on changing expectations of employers. Ideally, each student would embark on graduate education with a solid base in the liberal arts to serve as the foundation for the high, yet narrow literacy of specialized coursework and the ensuing esoterica of practice and continuing education. Obviously, a systematic study of the history of hospital affairs and health policy is an important part of graduate work and a vital element in the promotion of a literacy leading to fiducial vision. In the view of Etzioni (1975), "Every program should make it one of its cardinal commitments to develop the normative backbone of the health administrators it trains."

I would urge that health care leaders engage in sober reflection on their mission, that they examine and affirm the fiducial foundations of health care values, and that they develop within themselves a philosophy of management that is rooted in both performance and social responsibility. If the formal/legal and moral bases of accountability are to be enhanced, such efforts are essential.

Conclusion: Looking Ahead

Among the prominent issues hospital managers will confront in the 1990s are: (1) further pressures toward cost-containment, efficiency, and access for the under- and uninsured; (2) declines in operating margins in many facilities that will force an increased rate of closure; (3) a new round of reorganization efforts, including flatter organizational hierarchies, and emphasis on organizational leadership; (4) reexamination of the role and status of systems and of the freestanding hospital; (5) acceleration of technology development fueled by infusions of venture capital; (6) greater reliance on ambulatory care; (7) more attention to quality management and auditing of patient care outcomes, with emphasis on practice guideline refinement; (8) caring for the special needs of the elderly population; (9) a revitalized emphasis on the health needs of mothers and children; and (10) AIDS and Alzheimer's disease.

In addressing these issues, can a hospital executive exercise a balance of performance and fiducial accountabilities at institutional and community levels —and for leaders of exceptional ability, at the state and national levels as well? Several years ago, David Kinzer (1986) questioned the need for "balancing" accountabilities at the institutional level. He argued that humanitarianism must remain the priority value. In his view, it is "impossible to 'balance'. . . business ethics with the traditional humanitarian and community service ethics of our nonprofit hospital world. . . . In fact, going back in our country's hospital history, there has never been a time when economics has not imposed some degree of constraint on altruism. What is relatively new in our situation is the expectation that CEOs also exhibit 'businesslike' behavior." Priority rather than "balance" is essential where fiducial accountability is concerned.

Recently, another prominent observer of our health care system commented on accountability at the patient care level that is out of balance. According to Bruce Vladeck (1992), health care leaders, generally, have addressed only a narrow range of accountabilities: "As enormous and powerful forces of change have swirled all around them, leaders in the health care community have too often been preoccupied with narrow and parochial interests, misunderstanding the significance to their organizations' long-term well-being of efforts to change the broader environment."

Clearly, a leadership comprised of performance guided by fiducial vision is required if the hospital executive is to address the full range of accountabilities and pursue the work of "doing well" while "doing good." In the words of Stevens, "Hospitals are more than just factories for treatment. They are social institutions through which the moral values of America are expressed. What [health care leaders] do in the next decade will help to delineate how the United States sees itself as a nation." The direction taken on health care reform, whether toward "managed competition" or enhanced public interest agendas, will have a profound effect on the vitality of fiducial accountability in our nation's hospitals.

How can we fashion a hospital leadership with a philosophy of management based on balanced accountabilities of performance within the institution and fiducial obligation to society? Perhaps we could begin to answer this question

13

with Dimock's (1958) use of "philosophy" in the sense of "trying to discover the principles of human action and conduct that promote institution vitality and the good life." In short a revitalized philosophy of fiducial accountability should take maximum advantage of sound plans aimed at promoting organizational excellence and high-performing service objectives without sacrificing the high ground essential to the eleemosynary enterprise. Whether this philosophy can be realized and promulgated in a competition-driven reimbursement climate, however, is very much in question.

The basic principles that promote "institutional vitality" can be seen as deriving from six critical areas that when integrated into effective strategies form the core of a renegotiated service ethos: governance, management, financial strategies, quality management, human resources management, and managerial ethics. The articles in this collection have been selected because they underscore the importance of each of these areas and will assist the executive in the understanding of the stages that must be undertaken to achieve organizational excellence and fiducial responsibility.

Note

1. Blendon (1991) has listed a representative 13 proposals in four categories: (1) those that are "compulsory, employer-based private insurance programs, with the government insuring nonworkers and the poor" include the Pepper Commission proposal and that of the American Medical Association; (2) an example of those that "require employers to provide their employees with health insurance or pay a tax" is the Enthoven and Kronick "consumer-choice health plan"; (3) an example of a program of "income-related tax credits for individuals, independent of their employers, for the purchase of private insurance" is that proposed by the Heritage Foundation; and finally (4) an example of those programs that advocate an "all-government insurance system" is that offered by the Physicians for a National Health Program.

References

American Hospital Association. *Guide to the Health Care Field.* Chicago: The Association, 1991a.

——. *Hospital Statistics, 1991–92.* Chicago: The Association, 1991b.

Blendon, R. J. "Caring for the Uninsured: Choices for Reform." *Journal of the American Medical Association* 265, no. 19 (15 May 1991): 2563.

Blendon, R. J., R. Leitman, I. Morrison, and K. Donelan. "Satisfaction with Health Systems in Ten Nations." *Health Affairs* (Summer 1990): 185–92.

Brook, R. H. "Health, Health Insurance, and the Uninsured." *Journal of the American Medical Association* 265, no. 22 (12 June 1991): 2998–3002.

Cleverley, W. O. "After the Fall: Reasons Behind 1989 Hospital Closings." *Healthcare Financial Management* 4 (July 1990): 22–24.

Colloton, J. W. "The Impact of Federal Health Legislation on the State of Iowa's Community Hospitals and the University of Iowa Hospitals and Clinics." Presentation to the Iowa Chapter of the American College of Surgeons. Des Moines, 6 April 1991.

Dimock, M. E. *A Philosophy of Administration: Toward Creative Growth.* New York: Harper & Brothers, 1958.

Etzioni, A. "Epilogue: Alternative Conceptions of Accountability." In *Accountability In Health Facilities*, edited by H. I. Greenfield. New York: Praeger Publishers, 1975.

Ginzberg, E. "The Monetarization of Medical Care." *New England Journal of Medicine* 310 (3 May 1984): 1162–66.

Gray, B. H. *The Profit Motive and Patient Care: The Changing Accountability of Doctors and Hospitals.* Cambridge, MA: Harvard University Press, 1991.

Health Care Financing Administration. *National Health Expenditures for Selected Calendar Years 1960–90.* Washington, DC: Office of National Health Statistics, 1991.

Health Insurance Association of America. *Health Trends Chart Book.* Washington, DC: The Association, 1990.

Kinzer, D. M. "Commentary." *Journal of Health Administration Education* 4, no. 2 (1986): 2440.

———. "Where Is Hospital Leadership Coming From?" *Frontiers of Health Services Management* 3, no. 2 (1987): 3–26.

McCarthy, C. M. "Executive Office Activity: What Is Going on in Executive Offices?" In *Revisiting the Three–Legged Stool: Striking A New Balance Among Trustees, Administrators, and Physicians*, edited by B. J. Jaeger, 1–6. Durham, NC: Duke University Department of Health Administration, 1991

Medical Benefits. "Disgruntled Consumers Want Reform Soon." 8 (15 April 1991): 6, 7.

Mullner, R. M. "Rural Hospital Survival: An Analysis of Facilities and Services Correlated with Risk of Closure." *Hospital and Health Services Administration* 35, no. 1 (Spring 1990): 121–37.

National Leadership Coalition for Health Care Reform. *Excellent Health Care for All Americans at a Reasonable Cost.* Washington, DC: The Coalition, 1991.

Pear, R. "Heeding Elections, Lawmakers Offer Health-Care Ideas." *New York Times*, 8 September 1991, A1, 10.

Relman, A. S. "The New Medical-Industrial Complex." *New England Journal of Medicine* 303 (23 October 1980): 963–70.

———. "Shattuck Lecture—The Health Care Industry: Where Is It Taking Us?" *New England Journal of Medicine* 325 (19 September 1991): 854–59.

Rosenberg, C. E. *The Care of Strangers: The Rise of America's Hospital System.* New York: Basic Books, 1987.

Rosner, D. "Heterogeneity and Uniformity: Historical Perspectives on the Voluntary Hospital." In *In Sickness and In Health: The Mission of Voluntary Health Care Institutions*, edited by J. D. Seay and B. C. Vladeck. New York: McGraw-Hill, 1988.

Schieber, G. J., J. Poullier, and L. M. Greenwald. "Health Care Systems in Twenty-Four Countries." *Health Affairs* 10, no. 3 (Fall 1991): 22–38.

Shortell, S. M., E. M. Morrison, and B. Friedman. *Strategic Choices for America's Hospitals: Managing Change in Turbulent Times*. San Francisco: Jossey-Bass, 1990.

Smith, L. "A Cure for What Ails Medical Care." *Fortune* (1 July 1991): 44–49.

Starr, P. *The Social Transformation of American Medicine*. New York: Basic Books, 1982.

Sullivan, L. W. "Health and Human Services News Release." Washington, DC: U.S. Department of Health and Human Services, 2 October 1991.

U.S. General Accounting Office. *Nonprofit Hospitals: Better Standards Needed for Tax Exemption*. Report to the Chairman, Select Committee on Aging, House of Representatives. Washington, DC, May 1989.

―――. *U.S. Health Care Spending: Trends, Contributing Factors, and Proposals for Reform*. Report to the Chairman, Committee on Ways and Means, House of Representatives. Washington, DC, June 1991.

Vladeck, B. C. "Health Care Leadership in the Public Interest." *Frontiers of Health Services Management* 8 (Spring 1992): 3–26.

Woolhandler, S., and D. U. Himmelstein. "The Deteriorating Administrative Efficiency of the U.S. Health Care System." *New England Journal of Medicine* 324 (2 May 1991): 1253–57.

Yankelovich, D., and J. Immerwahr. "A Perception Gap." *Health Management Quarterly* 13, no. 3 (1991): 11–14.

Part I

Leadership and Governance

The turbulent and demanding health care environment has exerted significant influence on hospital board composition and the perspectives and behavior of individual members. In most cases, hospital planning has evolved into a strategic process involving "working" boards, senior and middle management, and medical and health professionals. The accountability of the governing board extends from its formal agreements with multiple stakeholders to informal fiducial responsibility to the community. Today, important issues for board members include the prodigious time requirement, as well as questions regarding the mechanisms for strengthening relationships with communities. Additional concerns regarding board members include criteria for appointment and evaluation, as well as tenure.

In discussing the hospital as a social institution, Rosemary A. Stevens (Chapter 1) notes that while American hospitals are overwhelmingly nonfederal, they are subject to more detailed national regulation than any other hospital system in the world. She argues that by tracing the history of American hospitals one can visualize more clearly what we want hospitals to be in the 1990s and beyond.

John R. Griffith (Chapter 2) charges that many of the criticisms leveled at the hospital industry, such as pricing structures, costs, and productivity, are really judgments of governing board failures. He argues that boards cannot solve all difficulties, but they can accept a mandate to guarantee quality and act more effectively to control costs. He suggests that opportunities to improve quality are "clearer and more promising than the cost-saving possibilities." At the same time, Griffith emphasizes the complexity of the relationships among quality, cost, and efficiency.

Richard J. Umbdenstock, Winifred M. Hageman, and Bruce Amundson (Chapter 3) believe that voluntary boards have become increasingly nervous, which makes managerial decision making more arduous. They ask for a new approach to governance of not-for-profit institutions that would be based on: (1) a common working definition of "governance"; (2) a clearly defined mission with specific goals and objectives; (3) a well-planned decision-making process; (4) a board structure tailored to the priorities at hand; and (5) an information, reporting, and communication system that keeps the priorities clearly in focus. Ways to link the board's work directly to the strategic plan are suggested.

John D. Blair and Carlton J. Whitehead (Chapter 4) maintain that effective management of stakeholders is mandatory for hospital managers in an era of environmental uncertainty and confusion. The stakeholder approach helps integrate managerial concerns normally considered separately, such as strategic management, marketing, human resource management, organizational politics, and social responsibility. The authors discuss strategy development for handling conflicting demands for effectiveness and efficiency from various stakeholders. Four generic strategies are detailed and an overarching strategy for hospital managers is presented.

Proposing cooperation—as opposed to competition—as a means to survive and prosper appears radical in today's environment. Stephen E. Foreman and Robert D. Roberts (Chapter 5) develop a case for the formation of health care value-adding partnerships as a viable, if not preferred, alternative to the integrated health care system owned and controlled by a single entity. The article addresses the conceptual and the practical aspects of obtaining voluntary cooperation and presents examples of successful value-adding partnerships.

Chapter 1

The Hospital as a Social Institution, New-Fashioned for the 1990s

Rosemary A. Stevens

Rosemary A. Stevens is Dean and Thomas S. Gates Professor of the School of Arts and Sciences at the University of Pennsylvania, Philadelphia. She is the author of six books, including the award-winning *In Sickness and In Wealth: American Hospitals in the Twentieth Century.*

This article, the Parker B. Francis Management Lecture delivered at the American Hospital Association Annual Meeting in July 1990, was published in *Hospital & Health Services Administration* 36, no. 2 (Summer 1991).

Hospitals, remarked a speaker to the American Hospital Association in 1917, are "human repair shops, without which the cities would be choked with human scrap heaps and the whole social fabric would deteriorate" (Greene 1917). We might not describe hospitals in quite the same way today—as human repair shops and vacuum cleaners for the messiness of human ills. Or would we? This is the question: What broad social functions do hospitals serve? This lecture begins with two premises. First, we cannot plan adequately for the future without assessing the assumptions and values built into the system as it now is, and second, the best way to do this is to understand its history. We need a better set of ideas of what we want for hospitals in the 1990s, and the past can be useful as we think ahead.

From the outside, American hospitals may seem to send clear messages. Former Prime Minister Margaret Thatcher looked to America for a mythical model of "competition" as a base for tinkering with the British National Health Service. Meanwhile we, confused, are reassessing the various meanings of competition—and look at Britain as a system that has managed, at least, to provide basic services to all its citizens.

The United States has, in fact, created an amazing system of hospitals in the twentieth century: huge, disorganized, nervous, ebullient, dedicated, wasteful, technically innovative, luxurious, inegalitarian, daring, competitive, pluralistic, self-contained, and conflict-ridden. Hospitals are organizational chameleons. They can be viewed as both charities *and* businesses, as saviors and profligates, heroes and villains, technological successes and social failures. American hospitals are overwhelmingly nonfederal, but they are subject to more detailed national regulation—micromanagement—than any other hospital system in the world. Yet the hospitals express, too, the all-American virtues of voluntarism and community—vague, patriotic, and flexible as these may be in terms of showing what hospitals do. We are living in a jungle of ideas about what kind of an enterprise this system is. In this invented jungle the payers and regulators keep redesigning the fruits and berries; that is, the incentives and constraints. Managers respond with a single-minded purpose, leaping toward the fruits that seem most juicy.

How do we move ahead to conceive, more clearly, the idea of what we want hospitals to be in the 1990s—and beyond? Political ideologies have never really been of much use in describing the social values that are reified in the American hospital system. "Capitalism" and the "free market" were not entirely helpful as organizing ideologies for hospitals in the 1980s, or for that matter in earlier decades. Quite apart from the increasing accompaniment of government regulation and the arguments that medical care is not, strictly, a "commodity," capitalism is not so much an organizing philosophy as a statement of intent or rhetoric. Hence the paradox that well before Medicare and the other

Great Society programs of the 1960s, the United States could be described as a "welfare state that has acquired a universal reputation as arch-defender of the free enterprise system" (Krieger 1963). The United States spends four or five times as much on its government health programs as does Britain with its National Health Service, and is not too far apart in terms of the proportion of gross national product (GNP) devoted to this purpose. The United Kingdom allocated 5.2 percent of GNP to government health expenditures in 1987; we spent 4.6 percent (Organization for Economic Cooperation and Development 1990).

But the U.S. system cannot be usefully understood by being recast as "socialistic," either. (Although, interestingly, the phrase "socialized medicine" is gaining social respectability in the 1990s, it no longer carries the sense of ominous threat it once did.) Despite the heavy involvement of government in health care in the United States, especially since Medicare, American hospitals have never represented the dogma of the welfare state. And, in any event, welfare states are under attack or breaking down in all directions, east and west; it would make little sense to reinvent them now. A Swedish observer recently described Medicare as "market socialism," with hospitals competing against a set of predetermined prices (diagnosis-related groups (DRGs)). Undoubtedly there will be many more ways to explain the American system as an expression of political theory in the next few years. But such attempts, while interesting, will do more to describe what the system expresses through its actions and operation rather than its underlying values and assumptions. Who would have guessed in 1965 the relations between hospitals and Medicare today? Inevitably we come back to the underpinnings of history, in trying to understand the dynamics of the system.

In my book, *In Sickness and In Wealth* (1990), I trace the history of U.S. hospitals, the major institutions of health care in this country, from 1900 to the present. One major conclusion is that there is no single trajectory of change in hospital history over the century, no linear trends from which to project an obvious future. If anything, the pattern is one of oscillation. Hospitals are not inevitable institutions. They are constantly negotiated and renegotiated in response to immediate crisis and the practicalities of change.

A second, related conclusion is that American hospitals are remarkably adaptive and flexible institutions, able to shift gears rapidly with changes in the environment: fiscal, regulatory, political, professional. The wide range of ideas attached to hospitals in the United States has made apparent changes in philosophy remarkably easy. The Veterans Administration (VA) hospital system, for example, a system of "socialized medicine" par excellence, was designed after World War I as a progressive and reasonable solution to the lack of interest and skills in rehabilitation, tuberculosis, and neuropsychiatric condi-

21

tions in civilian hospitals at the time, and the inability of Congress to conceive a different system—socialist philosophy had nothing to do with it.

Over the decades hospitals have appeared as relatively more "public" or more "private," with major changes in direction as opportunity beckons (what Mrs. Thatcher calls U-turns). In the 1920s, for example, short-term hospitals were enthusiastic consumer institutions. Massive hospital-building programs were geared toward private patients, small rooms, and technical spaces; hospitals concentrated on obstetrics, T and A's, appendectomies, and other conditions with an obvious and happy outcome, avoiding the complexities of long-term care. The short-term hospital was an upbeat, clean and happy place, welcoming streams of visitors. The journal *Modern Hospital* led the successful campaign for an annual Hospital Day, which celebrated the hospitals' successes, and sought publicity, donations, and community understanding of any remaining problems or difficulties. In line with the expansion of credit as a means of mass consumption in other spheres of life, hospitals invented various forms of credit so that you could finance a surgical operation as easily as an automobile or refrigerator. Hospitalization, too, could be conceived as a mass consumption service, not unlike the provision of electricity, with hospitals the providers, and patients, consumers.

But then how swift was the change toward a more "public" stance in the depression years of the 1930s. Voluntary hospitals now saw themselves as a distinct "nonprofit" sector, more closely allied with government; they dissociated themselves from the many small, for-profit hospitals that were the major casualties of the depression. How urgent, now, the problems of hospital access, availability and distribution, problems generated by the marketing successes of the 1920s. Hence the beginnings of the Blue Cross movement, a truly radical undertaking, hewing to the theme of community (not governmental) responsibility. Hence, too, the politicization of the major hospital associations, which sought a place in New Deal funding, and learned how to be effective lobbyists in the search for federal funds.

In the 1940s and 1950s, however, in response to changing times, the hospitals presented themselves primarily as "community" institutions, autonomous in their local centers, an autonomy encouraged by the success of the federal Hill-Burton program. Each hospital, however small, provided a range of as many specialties as it could, and intensive care became the rage. In the 1960s, in another see-saw of presentation, the public agenda received more play. Hospitals now represented the "mainstream" of medicine, which should, it was held, be available to everyone. But in turn, the 1970s brought rapid reappraisals, setting the stage for the last decade or so: competition and private markets, managerialism, and massive federal regulation. And still the play and counterplay continues.

In the 1980s, hospitals were pushed via federal policy to become competitive and profit-oriented. How admirably they rushed to conform to the message of the day! Virtually overnight, it seemed, there were the posters marketing the excessive kindness of different institutions; there were vice presidents for finance hawking the creative possibilities of huge new debts; the helicopters buzzing dramatically toward roofs and parking lots, clearly showing the hospitals' names in their descent; the far-flung ventures in prosperous suburbs; the stalking of medicine's "fat cats," who might bring their inpatients to Hospital Y, leaving quite a gap, perhaps (too bad!) at Hospital X; the strange manipulations of DRGs. Everyone seemed to be playing games, or more accurately everyone was "gaming the system." Success was to prosper under adverse conditions. Whether the patient improved or not—or even who the patient was—seemed curiously irrelevant. Administratively, a lot of this was fun; it was also valued behavior in the system. Administrators became presidents, sometimes of several boards at once, in the rush for corporate restructuring and diversification; and their salaries rose to the levels prevailing in the business sector. But did the other ideas about hospitals really go away? I think not. There they were—there they *are*—in the hospital's own cultural bank for reconsideration.

There is no reason to think that these characteristics of oscillation and flexibility will not continue. I think we are coming out of the cycle of "competition" as defined in the 1980s into a cycle in which public goals will be expressed. Indeed the only way to avoid the excesses of regulation, including the overstandardization of clinical practice, is to come up with sensible, decentralized alternatives within the system. To do this, hospitals and health care systems will need to "sell" themselves as responsible quasi-public institutions.

As the era of ruthless managerialism draws to an end, we also need to think about what kinds of skills will be called for next. At the very least, the new managers of the 1990s will require more delicate, manipulative skills: bonding together alienated, busy, perhaps truculent physicians; striking allegiances with third party payers and with employers; persuading bewildered board members, emotionally committed to the hospital as is, that a merger is the next best step; and working with the press, lobbyists, and local groups. (It goes without saying that the budget remains in watchful view.) Hospitals need more than ever the skills of communication, the art of persuasion, the science of listening, the director's ability to create a buoyant sense of purpose in a changing, perhaps shrinking organization.

The broader point I am making here, though, is that with no single trajectory of change in U.S. hospital history as a whole, no consistent underpinning of political values, the ideas attached to hospitals and their policies may fluctuate widely between generations—and sometimes between hospitals as well. Hospitals do not necessarily have to choose, once and for all, whether to be "public" or "private," profit-oriented or with a primary community mission. All of these ideas exist in many institutions simultaneously. They are, as it were, a bank to be drawn on as conditions change; this is what I mean by describing hospitals as chameleons. The future is more open to change than we might think.

A third conclusion drawn from the hospitals' history is that we are hampered by assumptions and expectations about hospitals as "technological" institutions that are now long out-of-date. Hospitals are stuck in a conceptual groove, holding on to ideas of a much earlier period—holding, for example, to the importance of inpatient care as the central function of the institution (Why should all hospitals have acute care beds?), concentrating on getting patients in and out of hospital rather than on a total period of illness, and rarely using the social authority vested in the institution as a force for health in the community as a whole. Our fundamental ideas about the hospital are still products of its formative period, the period from 1870 to 1920. To say that this makes no sense is an understatement.

As a medical treatment center the hospital was virtually a new institution in the early twentieth century, with a heavy concentration on surgery. X-rays and laboratories were dazzling symbols of medicine's ability to probe and to explain what happens within the human frame. The hospital was a "hygienic machine," a modernistic factory for treatment. Its images joined other ultramodern images of the day: department stores, resorts, production lines, luxury hotels. Medicine was a glorious form of warfare, battling disease with modern tools. Surgeons cut through tissue with the enthusiasm of contemporary mining engineers. As a multifaceted, multipurpose institution, the new hospitals carried reassuring messages to diverse constituencies. To the physician the hospital was the doctor's workshop—and there are still trailing expectations that this is what it is today, together with the lingering, dangerous assumption that hospitals and doctors are natural enemies rather than allies, even in the very different environment of the present.

But the prospect of a new hospital appealed, too, to leaders of (and aspirants to) social class elites and sectional groups in the burgeoning towns and cities, swelling with immigrants. Hence the large number of hospitals, even in one city, each with its own adherents and names like Baptist Hospital, Swedish, Beth Israel, or St. Mary's. The conjunction of scientific, humanitarian, and social purposes in the hospital before 1920 made it a quintessentially American institution.

It was also rapidly successful. By 1930 hospitals had attained the dubious distinction of being one of the largest enterprises in the nation, outstripped only by iron and steel, textiles, the chemical and food industries. This was a nation that was proud to be sick. A steady stream of income flowed in from members of a society that tended to link quality with the amount spent. Hospital construction costs in the United States in the 1920s were three times those in Germany, and American hospital visitors to hospitals in Britain spoke disparagingly of their "appalling poverty" and lack of amenities (Frank 1928).

Critics of hospital policy tend to explain the dissonance between what hospitals do best and the population's general health by concentrating on the pattern of financial incentives. These are said to be "perverse," drawing hospitals (reluctantly, innocently, eagerly, or just blindly?) in socially unproductive directions. But history suggests a more complex tale, for hospitals as a group have been successful in pushing their own agendas, and in helping to mold their conditions of work. The technological image of hospitals that we still have 70 years later is based on the medical and demographic conditions and on social expectations that existed prior to 1920.

We urgently need a new set of ideas about what the "technology" of hospitals should be. I use the word advisedly, for we have narrowed and subverted its meaning in the past decades, so that the very word "technology" conjures up pictures of machines.

Hospital technology should include *all* medical knowledge that can usefully be applied to health and illness. To update the image of the hospital to the demographic, social, and medical environment of the 1990s, we should be taking pride, for example, in the technologies of disability and chronic illness. A high-technology hospital is, ideally, one that does the most good for the health and happiness of individuals who come into contact with its members, and can demonstrate that this is so through research and through the judicious presentation of statistics.

The word "technology" should indeed encompass data systems too, for hospitals are natural organizers and repositories of patient care and community health information, for the benefit of the individual patient and clinician, and for research into effectiveness and need. Incidentally, it's now almost *80 years* since the noted, now rediscovered outcomes expert, Ernest Amory Codman (1914), challenged hospital staffs to accept responsibility for "the quality of the Product which their Hospital factories give to the Public."

Well before World War I there were critics of the narrow function of the hospital, of its aloofness from general community concerns, and of its apparently mercantilist goals. The patient was seen only in terms of his or her disease, complained one critic, not as a "social unit"; hospitals should be centers for education and for social reform, committed to care of the population in a defined local district (Goldstein 1907). Others saw the move toward comprehensive care as preordained. A well-known insurance expert, Frederick Hoffman, confidently told the American Hospital Association in 1916 that

25

hospitals were "only at the beginning of their field of broad public usefulness." He predicted: "They will soon be used far more for the treatment of the half-sick and to-be-sick than for the already sick and the half-dead. We should have hospitals where people may go at the beginning rather than the end of the sickness." Such ideas remain as possibilities today, together with other assumptions about hospitals as *public* institutions, as *moral* institutions, and as *community* institutions, ideas that have continued through the last decade or so of "competition."

Cynics and economic realists as we now are, we may no longer buy into the claims of an earlier generation that the "real hospital" is an idea of transcendent social virtue. The concept of the hospital, the editors of *Modern Hospital Yearbook* once claimed (in 1919), excludes bickerings and unworthy aims, provides the energy to drive the nation forward for the "betterment of human race," demands an "uplifting vision of service," and encourages a cooperative community spirit. "To work, to fight, to die if need be to make the vision come true—that is the hospital idea," wrote the editors. Such phrases now appear quaint, amusing, and naive. Nevertheless, we have not abandoned these notions entirely. Roman Catholic hospitals are looking for their "Catholic" mission. Jewish hospitals seek to preserve some special Jewish identity when they merge. Voluntarism is not dead. Indeed we may want to ask ourselves why hospitals still have, in the main, hospital trustees rather than corporate boards. The project to develop "community hospital benefit standards" now being run out of New York University is more than a ploy to allow some hospitals to game their way out of local property taxes by claiming they deserve tax exemption for demonstrated public service—although it may well have this effect for some. The Foster McGaw Prize is a matter of pride. There is still a strong streak of moral purpose in the hospital community, a sense that part of the mission of hospitals is to care about what happens in society as a whole, particularly at the local level. "Community" is a fundamental American idea—even though it is just as difficult to operationalize as it has been at other periods.

Words are organizing concepts around which actions can be taken and programs built. The word "community," like "technology," offers promise for refurbishing in the 1990s. New views of what a hospital's "community" is are beginning to be created across the United States, by necessity in some cases as hospitals in different areas contemplate merging. I spent the summer in the Shenandoah Valley of Virginia where the attempts to merge King's Daughters' Hospital in Staunton with Waynesboro Community Hospital by creating a new hospital in neither place, but instead in Fisherville, are an issue of almost daily news in the local press; community as an idea is intensely political.

Mergers and networks make practical sense for the 1990s—not just as a response to fiscal and organizational problems in existing hospitals, but also in terms of community redefinition and community betterment (to revive a nice old-fashioned phrase); in plain English, the potential to design a better system of care. Mergers often do not make it plain exactly what they will do better.

Through the years of expansion in hospital service, conflict has often been avoided by allowing something for everyone as far as possible. Paradoxically the constrictions to be faced in the 1990s may bring new opportunities for innovation—provided that the major vested interests in hospitals are willing and able to work together, and to work where necessary with their counterparts in sister institutions: physicians, managers, trustees. Acceptance of the possibilities of downsizing, limited funds, mergers, survival even, are not, then, necessarily bad news to those of us working in the field.

In the cities, managers, boards, and their associated physicians have a promising opportunity, not yet firmly grasped in any metropolis, to work with each other, with employers, political leaders and others, to consider how hospital "technology" could be optimally designed for the "community" at the citywide level. The governing principle here is not "rationing" with its overtones of bureaucratic control and service limitations, but sharing skills as a matter of common sense, in order to raise the quality of services throughout the system. Trustees need to be mobilized to consider multihospital rather than single-hospital strategies on grounds of quality of care, even without the crisis of a pending merger; and managers are the most likely force to do this. Given sufficient good-faith action across the country, antitrust constraints could be renegotiated, for they, too, are not cast in stone.

Where are we then in 1990? At the end of two cycles, one short and one long: entering, that is, the period to follow the decade or so of "competition," while also struggling to redefine old, comfortable notions of the hospital's "technology" and its "community." Refashioning assumptions about what hospitals are for—and who they are for—is a fundamental next step. Are hospitals to stand for more than workshops for bodily repair and repositories for the ravages of civilization? If so, this country may only need a relatively small number, their functions concentrated, not necessarily based on a particular community. The country could be covered, instead, by an airborne fleet and sophisticated systems of communications. It is only by redefining the ideas of hospital technology and community for the 1990s that local hospitals make any sense. This message will come through increasingly loud and clear.

To whom does the responsibility of planning, implementing, and—most of all—of *conceiving* the hospitals of the next few years devolve? Federal health policy and the "market" may well determine the nature of these strange social institutions, with community interests and values assuming a secondary or lesser importance. Much of what hospitals have learned to do recently is to react to incentives, new payment systems, and regulations; to be adversarial and opportunistic; and to be expert at playing fiscal games. But the history of hospital management also shows the ability to achieve rapid change. In the United States, hospital service is still local and idiosyncratic; we are wary of big government, and with reason. Acceptable ideas for hospitals have to be negotiated, consciously or unconsciously, at the local, regional, or metropolitan area. Although power games are being played here too, particularly with Medicaid—for example, give us another $13 million or we will close our emergency room—there has to be a better way.

Managers have a critical role as the conscience of the enterprise like it or not, for good or ill. But one hospital can do little by itself. The direction has to be toward more alliances between hospitals, between doctors and hospitals, and among power structures inside and outside the hospitals themselves. Managers, working with their boards and medical representatives and through their own local, state, and national networks, are the obvious catalysts for change: the experts, the professionals, the agents in place.

But whose agents? Representatives of a profit-oriented trade, or the spokesmen and women of all of us? Given the vacuum in leadership in health policy in the United States, managers serve, willy-nilly, as proxies of the general public. For as long as the United States avoids a wholly public system, chief executive officers, together with trustees and medical staff, carry an essential public burden.

In the climate of ideas in which we live, the future of hospitals is in some ways a self-fulfilling prophesy: we may well get what we expect. The present mood of the "hospital industry" suggests a dangerous indecision about what hospitals should be. Yet it is certainly possible to design modern community service systems, not necessarily the same from place to place, that offer Americans health care technology with the same efficiency that they are offered electricity.

If hospitals do not show industrial leadership, major changes may be imposed by outside agencies. Look what has happened to another set of trusted community service agencies, local banks for savings and loans. They too played games. I'm not suggesting that hospitals are engaging in similarly irresponsible behavior—we are unlikely to see a Desperado General Hospital crisis of the nature and scope of Silverado—but there are some instructive parallels here.

I want to leave you both challenged and uneasy. The new watchwords are mobilization, consolidation, common sense, imagination. But these are more than catch-phrases replacing (or redefining) the rhetoric of competition. For hospitals are more than just factories for treatment. They are social institutions through which the moral values of America are expressed. What all of us here do in the next decade will help to delineate how the United States sees itself as a nation: self-serving, perhaps, rigid and money-oriented; or technologically innovative in service provision. It is a great time to be working in this field.

References

Codman, E. A. *A Study in Hospital Efficiency as Demonstrated by the Case Report of the First Two Years of a Private Hospital.* Published privately, 1914.

Frank, L. J. "What I Found in the Hospitals of Europe—Part I." *Modern Hospital* 30 (February 1928): 67–74.

Goldstein, S. E. "The Social Function of the Hospital." *Charities and the Commons* 18 (4 May 1907): 161.

Greene, F. D. "Publicity as a Means of Education." *Transactions of the American Hospital Association* 19 (1917): 77.

Hoffman, F. Quoted in "The Fifth Hospital Year." *Modern Hospital* 3 (October 1916): 28.

Kreiger, L. "The Idea of a Welfare State in Europe and the United States." *Journal of the History of Ideas* 24 (1963): 556.

Modern Hospital Yearbook. "The Hospital and the Community It Serves." 1919.

Organization for Economic Cooperation and Development. *Health Care Systems in Transition: The Search for Efficiency.* Social Policy Studies No. 7. Paris: The Organization, 1990.

Stevens, Rosemary A. *In Sickness and In Wealth.* New York: Basic Books, 1990.

Chapter 2

Voluntary Hospitals: Are Trustees the Solution?

John R. Griffith

John R. Griffith is Andrew Pattullo Collegiate Professor, Department of Health Services Management and Policy, School of Public Health, The University of Michigan, Ann Arbor. He is a Fellow of the College.

This article was published in *Hospital & Health Services Administration* 33, no. 3 (Fall 1988).

The nation's hospital system is the most prominent example of voluntarism in America. Thirty-three hundred voluntary hospitals consume nearly three quarters of the $180 billion annual expenditure for acute hospital care (American Hospital Association 1986).[1] Many of them are religious sponsored; all operate with a substantial contribution of volunteer labor, including their trustees, who usually perform the governing board or directors' functions without compensation. The voluntary model is unusual among nations, but historically important and deeply rooted in the United States. It appears in education, research, social services, and religion as well as health care (Weisbrod 1977). Many voluntary organizations, including most hospitals, have been granted the privilege of tax exemption in return for charitable and socially important services that might otherwise be the responsibility of government. Voluntary organizations also serve as an important mechanism for relieving tensions between church and state. Hospitals are an exception. For example, religious-sponsored hospitals may decline to provide services unacceptable to their beliefs, such as artificial fertilization and abortion (Southwick 1978).

Hospitals are also arguably the most troublesome example of voluntarism. Critics of voluntary hospitals are ever-present and highly vocal. Although the critics differ in their conclusions, with some recommending more for-profit enterprise and others more governmental control, they have generally argued that the voluntary organization fails at the level of complexity of the modern hospital and is unable to control costs (e.g., Vladeck 1981; Brown 1981), quality (Sullivan 1987a, 1987b), or efficiency of production (Rossett 1984; Herzlinger and Krasker 1987). The allegations have included self-interest (Ehrenreich and Ehrenreich 1970), lack of willpower (Citrin 1985), unnecessary freedom from market discipline (Herzlinger and Krasker 1987), and exploitation of tax exemption (Stark 1987).

Implicitly or explicitly, critics have blamed the central governance structure of voluntary hospitals, that is, the directors (generally called trustees) and the chief executive. Many of the decisions they question—expansion, pricing, borrowing, costs, and productivity—lie at the basis of directorial obligations. The charge of poor quality, only now beginning to be heard but likely to become more prominent in the near future, is also the obligation of hospital trustees. Although the medical staff has important self-governance rights and obligations, trustees legally appoint the staff, approve the bylaws under which they work, and limit the privileges of individual physicians.

The critics may be incorrect; there are several important counterclaims and defenses.[2] But no one would argue that voluntary hospitals are blameless. These criticisms are an important source to identify weaknesses that can be corrected. What are the possibilities that stronger governance in voluntary hospitals would significantly improve costs, quality, and contribution to the commonweal? This broad question can be examined under two subheadings:

Can hospitals under any form of governance control health care costs and quality?

How does the moral and wise trustee respond to the complex pressures?

Can hospitals under any form of governance control health care costs and quality?

The answer to this question is, "Yes, but only to the extent that the society as a whole permits." Hospitals are obviously only part of the whole social system, which includes patients, doctors, insurers, and buyers as well. Although insurers and buyers want cost control, patients and doctors have a different agenda that tends to emphasize convenience, technology, and high cost. Patient behavior and doctor decisions determine much of the cost and the outcome of care. Patients and doctors cannot be coerced by hospitals because they control each hospital's revenue through their market decisions. The health care system of the United States is deliberately designed so that both patients and doctors have extensive freedom to vote with their feet. Hospitals have very high fixed costs that make them more sensitive to patient and doctor demands. As a result, the trustee's desire to take a leadership position on quality and cost must be tempered by the response of the ultimate customers as well as the insurers and buyers.

The Quality Perspective

The trustees' opportunity to improve quality is clearer and more promising than the cost-saving possibilities. There is rapidly growing public concern, reflected in several sectors. Business has become sensitive to the importance of sound care in reducing health insurance premiums (e.g., National Leadership Commission on Health Care 1987; Wyden 1986; *Business and Health* 1986; National Health Council 1986). Government agencies feel the issue is an important aspect of public health (Sullivan 1987). The growth of malpractice awards indicates, among other things, a view that injury is an unacceptable result of the health care process (U.S. General Accounting Office 1986). Organized medicine and the provider-backed Joint Commission on Accreditation of Healthcare Organizations have spoken quite clearly on the need to improve quality, particularly as measured by outcomes of care (Bowen 1987; O'Leary 1987).

Management technology is also in the trustees' favor in improving quality of hospital care. Although the subject remains abstract and complex, important components of quality are much easier to measure than they were before computers. Treatment has improved so that there are now many situations where death or serious disability is simply not an acceptable outcome. Counts of these

33

adverse outcomes are available and meaningful as evidence of quality, if carefully used. Advances have been made in diagnosis, coding of diagnosis, specification of treatment, data capture, and data processing, which remove much of the ambiguity about process measures of care, that is, about what was done and what should have been done. Sampling and polling techniques make it possible to measure patient satisfaction to supplement the medical record. As a result, specific questions about quality of care can now replace what formerly was philosophical general discussion. A given case, or more realistically a set of consecutive cases,[3] can now be judged "good" or "bad" more reliably than ever before. In addition to analyzing unfavorable outcomes, the process of care can be evaluated in an ongoing effort to improve. Long strings of highly technical but unarguable process questions can now be asked about most cases. They deal with whether a diagnosis and a plan for care exist and whether these are consistent with the clincial evidence and accepted practice.

The goal of Sir William Osler (1905) and E. A. Codman (1920), two turn-of-the-century physician advocates of self-review and peer-review, is more achievable than ever. The trustee needs to see that the questions are asked, that appropriate professionals (obviously not just physicians) study actual performance and act on the findings. This can be done by requiring explicit and widely circulated reporting of important quantifiable outcomes including death rates, complication rates, and patient satisfaction. Trustees should expect an overall trend toward better results. They must encourage physicians and other health professionals to set, achieve, and raise goals on these measures, while avoiding setting such goals themselves.[4] Steady improvement is achievable, if the trustees begin by hiring a competent executive and develop a strategy with him or her to improve quality measurement and quality review processes. The results of the strategy will change future recruitment processes, patterns of care, capital requirements, and of course, costs.

The relationship of quality, efficiency, and cost is complex. Although conventional wisdom in our society holds that quality costs money, many sophisticated observers believe that the search for quality and the search for economy are similar; an organization that seeks quality can, if it desires, find economy in the process.[5] Certainly economical health care systems exist that are noted for both quality and economy.[6] Low utilization of a facility may be an attribute of both high cost and poor quality (Kelly and Hellinger 1986; Luft, Hunt, and Maerki 1987). On the other hand, Shortell and Hughes (1988) have noted that severe regulation or competition is associated with significantly reduced survival. Thus one route to increase quality may be to encourage a more extravagant pattern of treatment, resulting in increased costs. A key obligation of trustees may be to see that this route is rejected and the goal of low cost and high quality is established.

The Cost Control Perspective

The trustee's opportunity to control costs is considerably more limited because the public consensus is far less clear. The current vogue is procompetitive both in the marketplace and the government. But competition leads to lower prices only when the customers prefer lower prices. The evidence that Americans are seeking price competition in health care is not wholly convincing. If they are actually seeking some of the other benefits of a hospital, such as physician recruitment, convenient technology, local employment, and the luxury of cure instead of prevention, competition may be the most important part of our health care cost problem. A U.S. hospital that tried to achieve cost containment in defiance of these goals would not be applauded; it would be bankrupted and plausibly might be sued. The grounds would be gross negligence in interpreting the marketplace, failing to take advantage of federal programs offering substantial revenue to the community, and willfully reducing the community's attractiveness to potential new doctors, employers, and taxpayers.

Hospital expenditures are stimulated by a wide variety of public subsidies over and above the basic exemption from income tax on profits. Federal programs include Medicare, Medicaid, direct and indirect support for health professions education, the National Institutes of Health (which pay for virtually all health care research except drug development), tax deductions to encourage the purchase of health insurance, and tax subsidies for hospital capital (in the form of tax-exempt bonds). The states assist with Medicaid and sales tax exemption, and local governments forego property taxes. These programs all stimulate growth, and growth in hospitals increases costs. Perhaps even more important, these programs are enduring expressions of popular will. They have been established by duly elected bodies over several decades and have proven politically immune to repeated attack (Blendon 1985). Thus the governmental buyers of health care equivocate: despite the prospective payment system (PPS) and a flood of rhetoric, there are numerous green lights on the road to higher costs.

On the private side, health insurance is a highly prized employment benefit, carried over into retirement to supplement Medicare. The record of the major industrial unions has been to press for steady expansion of health insurance benefits, and until recently, management offered little objection. How serious management is remains to be seen (Altman, Greene, and Sapolski 1982). As for the unorganized citizenry, there is plenty of evidence of their enthusiasm for hospitals. Two billion dollars of donations are received by hospitals each year (Waldo, Levit, and Lazenby 1986), and about 800 million hours of volunteer time (Hodgkinson and Weitzman 1986).

An additional point deserves emphasis: the result of the incentives is a flow of outside funds into each local community and a source of support for an investment with extrinsic value beyond health care. A hospital that has typical

Medicare and Medicaid patient loads will receive 40 percent of its revenue from the federal government and five percent from the state. If, in addition, its private insurance is paid by a distant corporation, more money comes from outside. (The stockholders and customers pay the insurance bill.) The multiplier is estimated at two to one (Smith and Wheeler 1986). A relatively small hospital represents $10 million in revenue and about 250 jobs. About $5 million—depending on the source of private insurance—comes from outside. Including the multiplier, the hospital earns for the community its full cash requirement in external subsidies. In addition, the hospital is almost essential to recruiting doctors, is important to bringing new industry to town, provides an expression of community pride and Samaritan motives, and offers convenient care of the sick (Griffith 1987).

The hospitals and doctors are at the point of use in this funding chain, not the point of decision. It is Congress, state legislatures, unions, businesses, consumer groups, and insurance buyers who determine how much will be spent on health care. No hospital holds a gun at the heads of the decision makers; they can always invest less in high-technology research, cut back the tax subsidies, fund more economical health insurance benefits, or divert their efforts to smoking and alcohol use reduction (worth more than $100 billion a year in health care avoidance) (Rice, Hodgson, and Sinsheimer 1986; Harwood et al. 1984).

The underlying political truth is that subsidy for expansion and growth of a convenient, high-tech hospital system was enormously popular from 1965 to 1983. Despite thorough discussion in debating the Tax Reform Act of 1986, only limited and modest efforts have been made to curtail the incentives. It appears that Congress correctly reads the views of the electorate: the popular enthusiasm for economizing is limited. Community business and political leaders—even *Fortune* 100 executives who have spoken strongly on the subject—have substantial ambivalence that comes out when the decision alternatives are clear in a local context (Altman, Greene, and Sapolski 1982). The wise trustee must, like Congress, recognize the profound ambivalence the American people have for cost control.

How does the moral and wise trustee respond to the complex pressures?

Despite the pervasive ambiguity on costs, trustees must also recognize that like the national debt, hospital costs cannot grow indefinitely. Hospital quality is intrinsically a moral obligation. In today's environment, the trustees' mandate is to improve prudently both quality and cost. Carrying out the mandate requires both a stronger will to achieve community goals and a more professional approach to management than has been common to date.

Will is the commitment to make difficult decisions in the absence of obvious reward and is the more difficult of the two requirements. Fortunately, there are a great many charitably inclined and morally committed individuals who are willing to accept the limited public recognition and other intangible rewards offered by hosptial trusteeship. Their will to do what needs to be done must be encouraged by careful selection, systematic education, planned personal development with increasing responsibility, and an atmosphere of mutual suport in difficult decisions. Moral firmness requires intellectual security and personal self-confidence. Trustees must understand the importance and contribution of the hospital to the community, well beyond the superficial notions of a place for the sick or a workshop for doctors. They also must understand the processes of governance and its sources of influence, including important lessons of what cannot be delegated and what must be delegated. Only then can they aggressively pursue the obligations of the role.

Understanding the Contribution
of the Hospital to the Community

Sound governance decisions are cost/benefit judgments, and the problem in health care is that the benefits are more difficult to assess than in many other endeavors. Health as a measure is elusive and the choices are morally as well as intellectually taxing. Does one invest, for example, in the comfort of the aged through rehabilitation and restorative surgery, in the prolongation of the end of life through high technology, in prevention and health promotion among adults, or in the prevention of unwanted babies and disability among children? Hospital trustees face practical applications of such questions monthly. When they act, they affect not only the hospital, but the entire health care system because their actions influence both the number, type, and quality of physicians who will practice in a community and the future pattern of disease.

Despite the complexity of these issues, methods to handle them can be taught systematically to new trustees and reinforced among older ones. One method of educating is to increase feedback of empirical evidence of contribution and to use it routinely in the decision process. Sound trusteeship begins with the best possible measures of the hospital's contribution to the community:

- Objective surveys of patient, buyer, and physician satisfaction
- Quantitative reports summarizing outcomes, quality measures, and improvement against current goals
- Measures of market share and the competitive status of the hospital in the community's health care system

- Measures of the contribution of the hospital to the local economy and the cost burden imposed on local industry.

These measures assume that a good product begets satisfied customers, a growing market share, and as a result, increased contribution to community goals. At present, few hospital governing boards have many of them routinely reported. The focus of most board information is on the financial status of the hospital as an enterprise, not the implications of its operation on community satisfaction, health, and economic well-being.

Improving the Board Decision Process

The processes that hospital governing boards follow in debate and decision, the use of subcommittees, the reliance on staff work, and the management of the agenda needs to be quite rigorous both to match the complexity of the problems and to make clear to doctors and employees how the institution decides critical questions. Most serious of these is the efficient management of the agenda. Governing boards can do anything they desire, but there are five specific tasks that, if delegated, constitute abdication and, if left undone, invite disaster (Kovner 1985).

The five nondelegable duties are the establishment of the hospital's mission, the appointment and support of the chief executive, the approval of a long range plan, the annual reappointment of the medical staff, and the approval of the annual budget (Griffith 1987). These actions, properly carried out, define the cost, quality, scope, location, and acceptable level of performance of any community hospital. Although they all rely on a fact base and a reporting system, they are all heavily prospective in character. They are the essential direction-setting that imposes the will of the local community on what is otherwise a self-governing professional guild.

More Explicit Mission Setting

The mission serves as a test of most board decisions, particularly those embodied in the long-range plan. The question "Is this consistent with our mission?" is essential to evaluate any proposal, and the mission should be clear enough to provide an answer in most applications without laborious investigation and debate. It guides not only the trustees, but also management and the medical staff. Clearly written, the mission stimulates consensus and speeds decision making; vague, it encourges self-interest and dissent.

A complete mission statement has three parts.[7] One defines the product, the second the market, and the third the limits on cost and quality that make the mission practical. Because of its explicit identification of a marketplace, the mission requires detailed study to write correctly (Griffith 1987). Few hospital mission statements now realistically specify the community receiving care, and even fewer constrain costs to the needs of the market and its ability to pay. Such a constraint is essential if hospital costs are to be curtailed by hospitals themselves. Open-ended missions lead to open-ended cost increases.

Better Relations with
the Chief Executive Officer

A governing board, sitting as a board, cannot implement. Just as important, without an executive the board has no staff and no source of data. Therefore, from one perspective, selecting the chief executive is more important than setting the mission. More practically, most hospitals already have a CEO, and the question is how to use him or her more effectively. The key to this is the separation of duties, leaving to the CEO all those things the CEO can do, preserving precious board time and wisdom for those things the board *must* do. Separation works because the other four essential duties are well-handled. Clear mission, plans, medical staff relations, and budgets permit an executive to support a board.

More Reliance on a
Formal Planning Process

A modern corporation has an integrated set of plans, including at least financial, facilities, information systems, and human resources components. In hospitals, an additional component covers medical staff planning. These are highly dynamic, adapting constantly to external changes and requiring at least annual updating. The majority of the work on these plans is done by doctors and employees, rather than by the board, for two reasons: they have more time and better knowledge, and they must be committed to the result to implement it effectively. The board's role, simply stated, is to approve the plans as appropriate to the mission. They serve as arbiters on the possibilities, judging them in the light of their knowledge not of the hospital but of the community and in particular, bringing the community's values to a process that is otherwise an exercise of professionals. They also reward ideas that are in the community's interest and thereby encourage more such ideas.

In an appropriately disciplined planning process, the board comments on revision of the plans at the beginning, where it establishes general directions, and the end, where it selects the specifics from a rank-ordered list of opportunities. These two jobs require extensive knowledge of the environment, supplementing the board's inherent grasp of the community with health care industry details such as trends in disease and treatment, new technology, and the position of competitors. The missing knowledge must be supplied by the executive.

Even so, contributions to the planning process require a significant portion of the annual schedule of the governing board.

More Collaborative Medical Staff Relations

The relationship between hospitals and doctors is extraordinarily symbiotic. Hospitals simply cannot exist without doctors, and very few doctors can practice medicine that is both economically and professionally satisfying without hospitals. Given such interdependence, conflict is probably inevitable, but the assumption of incessant adversarial or antagonistic relations that appears occasionally in the literature is self-defeating (Johnson 1986). To assure quality and make progress on costs, the bond between hospitals and doctors, and between doctors and other health care professions, must be strengthened. Hospitals must help doctors affiliate more closely. To do this they must act in ways that provide their physicians with competitive income, economic security, professional support, and rewards for contribution to the community needs.

Many wise physicians fear that closer hospital affiliation will mark the bureaucratization of medicine and potentially the destruction of personal moral commitment to patient care. Their fears are not unfounded, but the risk must be faced and overcome rather than avoided. It is less and less possible for a doctor to treat patients comprehensively and continuously without help. The health care system maintains the health of an aging population by a complex variety of technologies requiring corporate-scale investments and bureaucratic-scale management. The doctor-patient relationship is fundamental to success, but unaided it is no longer adequate to the task.

The job of the trustee is to lead doctors, executives, and other hospital professionals to a sound solution that is not yet clear. There is sufficient evidence to move unhesitatingly on two parts of the problem. First, the strong scientific empiricism that has carried medicine to its present achievements can be used to resolve the current dilemma. Facts and numbers should drive the search for more cost-effective medical organizations. Wise trustees must invest heavily in the systems of trained personnel and computers that collect, analyze, and display these facts for doctors to use in their own development of new solutions. Second, trustees must ensure that the integrity of the individual doctor is encouraged at every step. There is no room for adversarial behavior toward physicians, and the current heavy emphasis on punishment that pervades such existing systems as malpractice trials, prospective insurance approval, and professional review organizations must be replaced by rewards. The system that is required will use personal, professional, and financial rewards to encourage physicians both to retain their individual dedication and to contribute to the collective good through the staff organization. Among the rewards will be increased opportunity to participate in the meaningful decisions of the hospital. The trustee's power will be enhanced by delegation, not by concentration (Likert 1961).

More Reliance on Budget Cycle
The fifth opportunity trustees have to improve their contribution is through more aggressive management of the budget cycle. Given the inseparability of cost and quality goals, the annual budget development exercise must become a forum to explore the possible improvements in both, evaluating them in the light of the priorities of the community. This demands a process that is more extensive, more fact-based, and more sophisticated than most hospitals appear to have at present. Again the board role is at the beginning and the end. The board must set the community's priorities at the outset, amplifying and quantifying the concepts of the plans. These can be incorporated in the traditional budget guidelines that, when approved by the board, establish acceptable cost, prices, profits, and by identifying problems most needful of correction, quality (Berman, Weeks, Kukla 1986). The programs for the coming year, including the financial budget, should then be developed by the staff, including of course the medical staff. Ideally, the decisions required of the board will be consistent with the guidelines and pro-forma, although the board may be asked to resolve debates or make selections between key competing programs (Griffith 1987).

The board's budget decisions are much more structural than programmatic: Does the mission need adjustment? Is the level of profitability consistent with the financial needs? What price increase or decrease does the community require? Are there pressing quality problems that must take precedence? Are there issues of growth or change within the community that must be addressed by the hospital? Is the final proposal consistent with the mission, the plan, and the budget guidelines? Is the fact base for making these decisions adequate? Until recently, hospital boards have rarely operated at this level of abstraction or discipline. It is unfortunately fun to vote yes seriatim on ill-developed proposals for curing the ills of the world and taxing to consider competing arguments with long-term and far-ranging implications within a framework where the executive and the medical staff deliberately argue the concrete in terms of the abstract. Yet this precisely is what only the board can do.

Improving Board Processes

Obviously, boards differ in their ability to deal with these decisions. It is likely that selection of board members must change to gain improvement in board and hospital performance, but such changes have occurred in the past (Perrow 1963). Trustees have been selected for their tangible contributions, their influence in the community, and their ability to represent specific viewpoints (Kovner 1985). What is now required is acumen or wisdom, the moral, emotional, and intellectual preparation to deal with complex abstract questions. The best source of this is experience, suggesting that service that begins at a token or honorific level and increases in difficulty over several years is the key (Griffith 1987). An interested board member can move to more demanding tasks with experience, honorably retire when the demands are too great, and, in a few instances, culminate a career with service on the executive committee or as an officer. In the process, he or she can learn and be evaluated upon the necessary skills in an environment that is suitably discreet and respectful of the contribution made even at beginning levels.

Can trustees save the voluntary system?

The agenda for trustees is unsettling in its difficulty. In an idealized, absolute sense, the agenda may be beyond reach of the typical American community. But the opportunity for trustees is comparative, not absolute. The question is whether voluntary trusteeship can be improved to a point where it has a clearer margin over alternatives such as for-profit structures or government ownership. I believe that it can. The record to date is better than the critics allege. From 1945 to 1983, society requested and received rapid growth, high technology, and great convenience. Society's demands for universal coverage, outcomes quality, prevention, and cost control have been much more sporadic, and often have been minority rather than majority concerns. A consensus is now developing for these goals; there is reason to think that voluntary hospitals can respond as well as any other structure.

The principal cost of abandoning the voluntary system is the loss of a highly visible community statement for Samaritanism: tarnished though it might be, the voluntary hospital is a statement of love for fellow man, freely given, not mandated; for the benefit of all, not the stockholder. This statement in almost every community of our land is an important part of our civilization. To improve it (and improvement is certainly possible) is to enrich our national estate.

Notes

1. There are also several hundred smaller hospitals run by local governments that differ from the voluntary structure only in name.

2. The most frequent countercriticism is that other systems do not work any better. Regulation of planning and costs has been no panacea (e.g., Melnick, Wheeler, and Feldstein 1981; U.S. General Accounting Office 1981). Neither government nor for-profit health care organizations are free of similar criticisms on quality (e.g., the Bethesda Naval Hospital record in the trial of Commander Donald Billig, M.D. (Boffey 1986), or Vladeck 1980). While discipline is a virtue, especially in board rooms, the

alleged power of the equities marketplace may be more of a shibboleth than a reality. A prominent health care economist, Uwe Reinhardt of Princeton, described the Herzlinger and Krasker work as "a truly shoddy statistical analysis" (Lewin 1987). More objective efforts such as the National Institute of Medicine study (Gray 1986) fail to find any pronounced advantage for for-profit hospitals.

3.   Quality control in medical care depends heavily on the central limit theorem of statistics, which implies that residual random errors or variations in judgment about several cases will be reduced by grouping them together (Griffith 1972).

4.   Cf. W. E. Deming (1982). The lauded American consultant to Japanese industry during the World War II recovery, makes the point that the workers themselves must identify the goals and causes. The point is more relevant to hospitals than to industry; we must have doctors, not managers, treating patients.

5.   The published views in the health care field apparently do not recognize the opportunity (Deming 1982; Skinner 1986; cf. Aaron and Schwartz 1985).

6.   Rochester, New York, and Rochester, Minnesota, are outstanding examples (e.g., McClure 1982).

7.   There is a style that states the mission in the broadest possible terms and uses subordinate statements of greater length to specify the particulars. I prefer a succinct mission covering the specifics so that several hundred trustees, employees, and doctors can bring it quickly to mind.

References

Aaron, H. J., and W. B. Schwartz. "Hospital Cost Control: A Bitter Pill to Swallow." *Harvard Business Review* 63 (March–April 1985): 160–67.

Altman, D., R. Greene, and H. M. Sapolski. *Health Planning and Regulation: The Decision-Making Process.* Washington, DC: AUPHA Press, 1982.

American Hospital Association. *Hospital Statistics, 1986.* Chicago: American Hospital Association, 1986.

Berman, H., L. E. Weeks, and S. F. Kukla. *Financial Management of Hospitals,* 6th ed. Ann Arbor, MI: Health Administration Press, 1986.

Blendon, R. J. "Policy Choices for the 1990's: An Uncertain Look into America's Future." In *The U.S. Health Care System: A Look to the 1990's,* edited by Ginsburg. Totowa, NJ: Roman & Allanheld, 1985.

Boffey, P. M. "Officer Asserts Efforts at Inquiry on Top Surgeon Were Thwarted." *New York Times.* 16 January 1986.

Bowen, O. R. "Congressional Testimony on Senate Bill S. 1804." *Journal of the American Medical Association* 257 (13 February 1987): 816–20.

Brown, L. D. "Competition and Health Cost Containment: Cautions and Conjectures." *Milbank Memorial Fund Quarterly* 59 (Spring 1981): 145–89.

Business and Health. Various authors. 3 (June 1986): 7–28.

Citrin, T. "Trustees at the Focal Point." *New England Journal of Medicine* 313 (7 November 1985): 1223–26.

Codman, E. A. *A Study in Hospital Efficiency*. Boston: Privately published ca. 1920. Available from the Yale Medical Library, inter alia.

Deming, W. E. *Quality, Productivity, and Competitive Position*. Cambridge, MA: Massachusetts Institute of Technology, Center for Advanced Engineering Study, 1982.

Ehrenreich, B., and J. Ehrenreich. *The American Health Empire, Power, Profits, and Politics*. New York: Random House, 1970.

Gray, B., ed. *For-Profit Enterprise in Health Care*. Institute of Medicine. Washington, DC: National Academy Press, 1986.

Griffith, J. R. *Quantitative Techniques for Hospital Planning and Control*. Lexington, MA: Lexington Books, 1972.

————. *The Well-Managed Community Hospital*. Ann Arbor, MI: Health Administration Press, 1987.

Harwood, H., D. M. Napolitan, P. L. Kristiansen, and J. J. Collins. *Economic Costs to Society of Alcoholism, Drug Abuse, and Mental Illness, 1980*. Research Triangle Park, NC: Research Triangle Park Institute, 1984.

Herzlinger, R. E., and W. S. Krasker. "Who Profits from Non-Profits?" *Harvard Business Review* 65 (January–February 1987): 93–106.

Hodgkinson, V. A., and M. S. Weitzman. *Dimensions of the Independent Sector: A Statistical Profile*. Washington, DC: Independent Sector, 1986.

Johnson, R. L. "Hospitals, Medical Staffs Will Be in Adversarial Roles under PPS." *Modern Healthcare* 16 (14 February 1986): 69–70.

Kelly, J. V., and F. Hellinger. "Physician and Hospital Factors Associated with Mortality of Surgical Patients." *Medical Care* 24 (September 1986): 785–800.

Kovner, A. R. "Issues in the Structure and Process of Hospital Governance." *Frontiers of Health Services Management* 2 (August 1985): 4–34.

Lewin, T. "A Sharp Debate on Hospitals." *New York Times*. 2 April 1987.

Likert, R. *New Patterns of Management*. New York: McGraw-Hill, 1961.

Luft, H. S., S. S. Hunt, and S. C. Maerki. "The Volume-Outcome Relationship: Practice Makes Perfect or Selective Referral Patterns." *Health Services Research* 22 (June 1987): 157–82.

McClure, W. "Toward the Development and Application of a Qualitative Theory of Hospital Utilization." *Inquiry* 19 (Summer 1982): 117–35.

Melnick, G., J. R. C. Wheeler, and P. J. Feldstein. "Effects of Rate Regulation on Selected Components of Hospital Expenses." *Inquiry* 23 (Fall 1981): 240–46.

National Health Council. *Preserving the Quality of Health Care in a Changing Environment.* New York: The Council, 1986.

National Leadership Commission on Health Care. Washington, DC: The Commission, 23 June 1987.

O'Leary, D. "The Joint Commission Looks to the Future." *Journal of the American Medical Association* 258 (21 August 1987): 951–52.

Osler, Sir William. Valedictory address to the students at McGill University, 1905. Reprinted in *A Way of Life.* New York: Dover Publications, 1951.

Perrow, D. "Goals and Power Structure." In *The Hospital Modern Society,* edited by E. Freidson. Glencoe, IL: The Free Press, 1963.

Rice, D. P., T. A. Hodgson, and P. Sinsheimer. "The Economic Costs of the Health Effects of Smoking." *Milbank Memorial Fund Quarterly* 64 (Fall 1986): 489–547.

Rossett, R. N. "Doing Well by Doing Good: Investor-Owned Hospitals." *Frontiers of Health Services Management* 1 (September 1984): 2–9.

Shortell, S. M., and E. F. X. Hughes. "The Effects of Regulation, Competition, and Ownership on Mortality Rates Among Hospital Inpatients." *New England Journal of Medicine* 318 (23 April 1988): 1100–07.

Skinner, W. "The Productivity Paradox." *Harvard Business Review* 64 (June–July 1986): 55–59.

Smith, D., and J. R. C. Wheeler. "Multiplier Estimates for Local Economic Impact Analysis." *Journal of Business Forecasting Methods and Systems* 5 (Spring 1986): 20–21.

Southwick, A. F. *The Law of Hospital and Health Care Administration.* Ann Arbor, MI: Health Administration Press, 1978.

Stark, F. H. Quoted in R. Pear, "Tax Exemption Status Questioned for Nonprofit Hospitals." *New York Times.* 15 July 1987.

Sullivan, R. "New York Doctors Face Tighter Reviews." *New York Times.* 8 April 1987a.

———. "Inadequate Care Blamed for 43 Hospital Deaths." *New York Times.* 21 April 1987b.

U.S. General Accounting Office. *Health Systems Plans: A Poor Framework for Promoting Health Care Improvements.* Gaithersburg, MD: U.S. General Accounting Office, 1981

————. *Medical Malpractice: No Agreement on Problems or Solutions.* Gaithersburg, MD: U.S. General Accounting Office, 1986.

Vladeck, B. C. "The Market vs. Regulation: The Case for Regulation." *Milbank Memorial Fund Quarterly* 59 (Spring 1981): 209–23.

————. *Unloving Care: The Nursing Home Tragedy.* New York: Basic Books, 1980.

Waldo, D., K. Levit, and H. Lazenby. "National Health Expenditures 1985." *Health Care Financing Review* 8 (Fall 1986): 20.

Weisbrod, B. A. *The Voluntary Nonprofit Sector, an Economic Analysis.* Lexington, MA: Heath Lexington Books, 1977.

Wyden, R. "A Crusade for Access to Health Care Data." *Business and Health* 4 (December 1986): 35–38.

Chapter 3

The Five Critical Areas for Effective Governance of Not-for-Profit Hospitals

Richard J. Umbdenstock
Winifred M. Hageman
Bruce Amundson

Richard J. Umbdenstock and Winifred M. Hageman are Associates in the Umbdenstock–Hageman Partnership, Spokane and Seattle, Washington. Bruce Amundson, M.D., is Senior Scientist, Fred Hutchinson Cancer Research Center, and rural health consultant, Seattle, Washington.

This article was published in *Hospital & Health Services Administration* 35, no. 4 (Winter 1990).

The effective governance of a not-for-profit health care corporation is a challenging venture for both the board and executive management. The pressures on hospitals continue to mount, whether they are one of several providers in a populated area or struggling to survive on their own in a small community. It comes as no surprise that voluntary board members increasingly are nervous about their ability to help determine what needs to be done, making management's task of guiding the board and building board confidence in management's approach to critical issues all the more difficult.

Traditionally, voluntary community hospitals have had boards composed of trustees with widely differing organizational and management experiences. The belief that voluntary boards generally should be "representative" of the community, and the trustees' generally low level of first-hand experience in health care policy and practices, makes it difficult for management to focus the board's attention on a fluid strategic planning process. The result is a "catch-22" for governance: time spent "educating" the board means less time for the board to carry out its work; less time spent bringing the trustees up to speed means increasing the risk for the executive who moves ahead without them. Nowhere is this more clear than in the smaller organization, having more limited staff resources, and in those rural settings where few volunteers might have had the opportunity to manage an organization as complex and resource-intensive as a hospital.

We believe the environment demands a new approach to the process of not-for-profit institutional governance. The Rural Hospital Project (RHP), funded by the W. K. Kellogg Foundation through the University of Washington Department of Family Medicine, offered an opportunity to assess the strength of governance in selected community hospitals. The project staff, during the early process of community interviews, observed a lack of appreciation for the relationship between the function of governance and the process of strategic planning in a challenging environment. An opportunity existed, therefore, to assess the weaknesses in the traditional approach to governance and to fashion one better suited to a dynamic, and difficult, environment.

Are Voluntary Boards No Longer Viable?

When many in the field are questioning whether the time has come for wholesale change in the role of voluntary boards, or whether they already may be obsolete, we believe the answer is "no." As Cyril Houle (1989) states, "A board is a far from simple mechanism, and nobody outside it can fully understand its complexities. . . .Inherent in its very nature are several seeming contradictions; delicate balances must constantly be achieved if it is to succeed. They might seem unworkable if it were not for the fact that they are at work everywhere."

The volunteer board model has worked very well, and it only needs to be adapted to the changed environment. What must occur is the development of a much more direct link between the function of institutional governance and the priorities identified through the strategic planning process. In other words, voluntary boards must behave much more like the well-organized, but off-site, owner of a business enterprise that is in a dynamic marketplace. In this image, the owner's opportunities to check in with resident management will be infrequent, thus requiring that both the owner and the manager have a common assessment of the environment and the priorities of the organization, and that an effective communications process exists for continually focusing on these priorities and the targeted results.

Boards and chief executive officers (CEOs) often have asked us, "How can we plan, manage the organization, address special objectives, and still have time for other things like board education, committee meetings, board-medical staff functions, self-evaluation, and all the extra activities expected of a part-time, volunteer governance structure?"

Our response is that the key to solving the dilemma is found in the words "other" and "extra." After all, every successful organization must plan, manage, and evaluate—how the voluntary governance process is organized around, linked to, and driven by the mission, goals, and objectives of the hospital will be the key to the board's understanding and successful fulfillment of its responsibilities. Or, as Peter Drucker (1989) suggested recently, "The key to making a board effective. . .is not to talk about its function but to organize its work."

Defining Institutional Governance

Governance has suffered as a discipline due to the lack of a common working definition of it. People commonly refer to the "board's role and responsibilities," an approach that tends to define the entity and its activities, but not the function of governance itself. This would be like using the term "management" only to define the administrative entity (management) and not the process of operating an organization (management).

The commonly used definition of governance as "setting policy," as distinguished from that of management as "implementing policy," is too simplistic. What is "policy"? Policies about what? Doesn't management have a role in "setting policy"? Another definition being offered is that governance is "the making of important decisions" (Kovner 1990). While the decisions made by a governing board certainly should be important to the organization, this definition fails to supply the foundation of the board's right (or responsibility) to make these decisions and leaves a void in the delineation of functional areas of responsibility in which the issues for decision will be found.

Brian O'Connell (1985), President of the Independent Sector, refers to boards as being "ultimately accountable" and elaborates by saying that "the board has the principal responsibility for fulfillment of the organization's mission and the legal accountability for its operations." This is true, but again, the rationale for placing these responsibilities in the board is not readily apparent to those who are not experienced as directors or as students of boards.

Our approach to improving the process of governance is rooted in what we feel is a clear, concise definition of the function. We define "governance," in the context of the not-for-profit community-based organization, as "the fulfillment of responsible ownership on behalf of the community" (Umbdenstock 1987). This definition provides two critical understandings: (1) it recognizes the board's primary responsibility for protecting and enhancing the corporation (as the entrusted "owner"), and (2) it acknowledges the fact that the board's final accountability is to the community (the "stakeholders") that the organization was established to serve.[1]

The concept of "responsible ownership" builds on the private ownership model, the model we have found to be most familiar among volunteers, regardless of their background or previous service. It also leads easily to the identification of areas of functional responsibility of the board, such as

- Mission and values identification
- Policy (operating parameters) determination
- Plan development
- Financial viability
- Quality assessment and improvement
- Legal and regulatory compliance
- Effective customer relations.

All of these functions are quickly associated with "owner" responsibility. Last, the "owner" concept clarifies the relationship to management. The CEO who is not a voting trustee does not share the ultimate responsibilities of "ownership"; the CEO with a vote becomes more of a "managing partner," in this business analogy. Thus, the "board as owner" concept identifies the need for clear delegation of responsibility to the CEO and established methods of accountability from management back to the board.

50

This definition also helps to sort out the relationships within multi-unit corporations or systems—a common organizational model in health care today. In this case, confusion often exists over what board at what level is allowed to perform which activities. In fact, it really is misleading even to call some groups in a multileveled organization "boards" without some sort of qualifier, such as "delegate board." In any event, understanding that "responsible ownership" and "ultimate accountability" can reside at only one level makes it clear that other, lower organizational levels are answerable to that highest organizational level and serve at its pleasure.

Five Factors to Improve Board Effectiveness

Through our consulting experiences, and in particular those gained in the community-based RHP planning project, we have identified five factors that organize the work of the board and distinguish effective boards from those that are struggling to comprehend and address the priorities of their hospital. It is our belief that these five critical areas of governance are fundamental to all hospital boards and apply across the spectrum of voluntary agencies with which hospitals must collaborate if health care delivery is to be coordinated effectively. The balance of this article explores these five critical areas and their appropriate relationship to common board functions.

Governance can be most effective when it is designed to meet specific challenges. It is least effective when organized through a traditional, or stereotypical, structure in which no refinements are made in response to changes in the organization's needs, strategies, or objectives. It has been our observation that truly effective boards have the following critical areas clearly in focus within the board and between the board and senior management:

1. A common working definition of *governance* and what it means for the leadership roles, responsibilities, and relationships within a particular organization
2. A clearly defined *mission* with specific *goals* and *objectives* for the organization that drive virtually everything the board does
3. A well-planned *decision-making process*, based on the specified priorities and ongoing responsibilities of the board, and supported by a continuing education process that prepares the board for critical decisions it knows it must make in the future
4. A *board structure* that is tailored to the priorities at hand and enables the efficient accomplishment of the board's work

5. An *information, reporting, and communication system* that keeps the priorities clearly in focus and utilizes formats to help the board ascertain progress toward the accomplishment of its goals.

Furthermore, boards must build coordinated, ongoing processes around these factors. Individual activities such as trustee recruitment, board orientation, and the design of committee structures all can and should be linked directly back to the mission and strategic priorities of the organization. In this way, board activities, and the all-important relationships among the board, administration, and medical staff cannot be viewed as "other" or "extra." They become integral to strategic direction and success.

As a result of addressing these critical points, voluntary boards will find they have

- A common orientation to the responsibilities of governance and a clarification of the roles that must be played by each component of the organization's leadership
- A common "game plan," directly related to the organization's mission, around which governance and management activities are identified, planned, and conducted
- A strategic rationale for designing the board's structure and work methods
- A common context within which to base board self-evaluation and CEO performance evaluation
- An ongoing agenda for the organization that provides guidance when considering changes in board structure or composition
- Improved understanding of the board's need for specific, concise, and useful information on the results of strategic initiatives
- Improved methods of communication
- Increased opportunities for board education that are related directly to the organization's strategic objectives.

Without a clear focus on the five critical areas, board organization, strategic planning, and organizational evaluations are isolated functions, not fully integrated into the leadership function of the organization. They become functions for which no one feels any accountability.

An examination of each of these factors and ways to better organize the board's work follow.

What Is Governance?

When voluntary hospital boards find themselves divided, or in "turf" struggles with management or the medical staff, most often it is because there is no common understanding of what governance is and how it will be carried out in that particular organization.

As we have said, the board must define what it believes "responsible ownership on behalf of the community" to be, and to be comfortable in its accepted role and responsibilities. The delegated responsibilities to management and medical staff to assist the board in fulfilling these responsibilities also must be clear and accepted.

The usual rub here is that the hospital's management and medical staff undoubtedly are better prepared to operate the entity than is the board; in this sense, the board is more like a relatively passive "investor-owner" who delegates heavily to the professionals brought in to operate the company. This investor-owner is no less responsible for the entity than an owner-operator, but the distance between the investor-owner and the daily operations of the company necessitates different relationships and interactions with management than does the owner who is on-site everyday.

To fulfill the role of "owner" with technical and experiential "distance" from the hospital, the board has to establish clear definitions of authority and accountability for management and medical staff so that the potential for turf wars within the board, or between the board and its delegates, is minimized.

A Clearly Defined Mission with Specific Goals and Objectives

Peter Drucker (1989) commented recently that the mission "focuses the organization on action. It defines the specific strategies needed to attain the crucial goals. It creates a disciplined organization. It alone can prevent the most common degenerative disease of organizations. . .splintering their always limited resources. . . ."

Effective governance requires the existence of a clearly written statement of mission, one that is specific enough to identify the purpose and, if applicable, the sponsoring philosophy of the organization; the values of the organization; its primary services (nature, level, and locations of, etc.); its intended customers or service populations; the geographic scope of its service area; and, a statement of why the sum of these elements will enable the organization to make the community a better place to live. Some organizations go on to elaborate in a "vision statement" what it is the organization is aspiring to be in five to ten years.

53

From the major features of this statement stem the goals of the organization. From each goal must stem annual objectives, the priorities for that particular year, that, if addressed and achieved, will move the organization closer to its goals and the fulfillment of its mission.

It is impossible to build any coherent organizational process, whether governance or management, in the absence of these documents. Yet, many health care organizations either do not have them or do not live by them, alleging there has not been time to put them together or to update them. With these directives in hand, a hospital board has the primary tools it needs to map out a "common game plan" for effective governance and for the assessment of managerial effectiveness. What needs to be done now is to *use* these priorities as the ongoing agenda for the board's work and that of its committees, for guidance to management, and for targeting and measuring organizational performance. Finally, they serve as the continuing education agenda for the "think tank" of the organization, namely, the combined leadership of the board, senior management, and the executive committee of the medical staff.

A Well-Planned Decision-Making Process

With specific objectives for the year, along with an approximate time frame for each, and with the identification of the routine annual functions the board must perform (such as election of new members/officers, approval of budget and the audit, reappointment of medical staff members, etc.), a calendar of board meeting agendas can be developed. From such a calendar, or work plan, many important steps can be taken.

- Board meetings can be planned well in advance and each agenda organized by priority.
- The meeting schedule can be tailored to the level of work to be done, and not simply continued on the usual basis of whether an action agenda exists or not.
- Educational needs can be determined and appropriate sessions included in the board meetings leading up to key decision dates.
- Delegation of authority to committees and/or management can be made so that the board, when meeting as a whole, is able to focus mostly on strategic issues.
- Board and management evaluations can be based on how well the priority work plan was accomplished, or why the work plan had to be modified to accommodate unforeseeable developments.

A Board Structure Tailored to the Priorities

In recent years, many hospitals have been advised by various sources that changes should be made in board structures because they are seen as unwieldy and ineffective. These sources usually recommend that not-for-profit boards change to be more like corporate boards. We've never seen a responsible corporate board change in order to be more like some other group, but we certainly are aware that successful corporate boards will change readily *if the purpose and priorities of the organization require such change for the sake of successfully achieving their goals!*

We suggest, once again, that the best source for guidance in determining the proper board structure for a given organization is its mission, goals, and objectives. From these documents, and the resulting work plan of the board, many determinations can be made.

- The size and general composition of the board can be decided, including a determination of what constituencies, if any, should be tapped for linkage at the board level.
- Trustee recruitment and replacement can be directed toward those individuals whose expertise can help address specific priorities of the board and its committees.
- Committee structures can be redesigned and/or committee charges rewritten to address the priorities of the board's work plan.

Once the structure has been determined, changes can be made in the bylaws to accommodate these adjustments.

An Information, Reporting, and Communication System

Boards and their executives must appreciate the need to support the decision-making process and the board structure with an effective communication system that takes every opportunity to highlight and reinforce the stated priorities and performance targets. Communication can take many forms and should not be limited only to packets prepared for board meetings.

Both trustees and executives complain about the burden of producing and digesting large board packets every month. These complaints have led us to utilize different combinations of remedies, such as

- Weekly or biweekly one- to two-page briefings from the CEO on priority issues and general developments of interest

- Three- to four-page issue papers, discussing the nature and consequences of a given issue or objective, including questions the board will have to consider in making a decision in the near future

- Using what ordinarily would have been the time set aside for a monthly board meeting to have study sessions once a quarter to examine in detail the subject of an upcoming key decision by the board (the issue paper may be used as the primer for this session)

- Using more graphics and simplified formats in reporting to the board on the progress toward specific objectives and performance targets in the financial and service utilization areas

- Informing all trustees of committee meeting dates and agenda items so that interested trustees not on a particular committee can attend and obtain helpful background information prior to board meetings

- Utilizing one or two board meetings each year as retreat sessions to assess progress on all aspects of the strategic plan, the institution's overall performance, the board's structure and performance, or the relationships among the board, management, and medical staff.

Viewing the board, senior management, and medical staff leadership as the "think tank" of the organization will lead to better use of time when they are together, more selectivity in the information generated and distributed, more focus on strategic issues in board meetings, and a general inclination toward more thinking and questioning as a group.

Application of These Critical Factors

Under the sponsorship of the RHP, the critical factors were utilized by hospitals in the project as a framework for assessing their respective approaches to governance and reorganizing them as appropriate. One hospital utilized the authors to help them through the process and the outcomes of that process follow.

- All board members and the CEO were interviewed, and a good deal of confusion was exhibited over the board's role and responsibilities, particularly regarding the hospital's relationship to the city, which approved its budget and covered its employees in a pension fund. The new trustee orientation process was revised to address the important points that surfaced in these discussions.

- The mission of the hospital was assessed and later revised. The limited resources of this rural community demanded a more coordinated approach to the community's health care delivery system. A task force representative of all providers (hospital, mental health service, nursing home, pharmacy, private practitioners, etc.) determined that the hospital could serve best as the "hub" of this system, and the mission statement was revised to reflect this mandate as catalyst and leader in the community system.

- Stemming from the new mission statement, six corporate goals were adopted, specific objectives to pursue each goal were formulated, and an annual board calendar for tracking the accomplishment of the objectives was developed and used by the board and management.

- The board's committee structure was reviewed, resulting in recommendations that the board's work be consolidated into a planning committee, finance committee, quality review committee, and an executive committee. Committee memberships were recomposed to reflect the broader community mandate and need for involvement. Two inactive directors were asked to resign and new members were recruited through the development and use of a board profile and constituency mapping process that attempted to provide better linkages to the other providers in the area.

- The changes that were made were used for a period of time to assure their appropriateness and then the necessary changes in the bylaws were made.

- The need for regular evaluations of board performance and CEO performance were recognized, and the responsibility to develop these processes was assigned to the new executive committee.

- The mission statement, goals, and objectives will be reviewed on an annual basis to ensure that the priorities of the hospital are clear and that the board's structure and methods of addressing them are tailored to these priorities.

Conclusion

There are many models from which to select when determining the governance system for a voluntary hospital or organization. Depending on the purpose and priorities of the organization, the variables to choose from can include: the size and composition of the board; the relationship of the board to management; the frequency and nature of board meetings; the organization of the board (committees vs. committee-of-the-whole, etc.); the chosen methods of communication to, from, and within the board; and other such factors as determined by state law regarding the responsibilities of the particular board. Based on how boards define their governance responsibilities and select their organizational features from among these variables, widely divergent approaches to governance can be designed.

The question then becomes, "What is more important?" Determining whether a large board is more or less efficient than a smaller board? Whether meetings should be held once a month or quarterly? Or, as an alternative, determining what the group's working definition of governance really is and then designing a structure with a process that is effective for carrying out that definition in the environment facing the organization? We are firmly convinced it is the latter and believe our approach demonstrates that an orderly, integrated process can be designed to link directly the work of voluntary boards to the pursuit of their hospital's mission and the performance expectations they set for it.

Note

1. Technically, the corporation "owns" the typical not-for-profit hospital and a mechanism is determined for selecting the group (board) to govern it (Griffith 1987). Because many boards are self-perpetuating, and because most "associations" or "corporations" function each year only to ratify the selection of board members, we feel comfortable using the loose analogy of "board as owner" for the sake of clarifying the level of responsibility the board has for the corporation.

References

Drucker, Peter F. "What Business Can Learn From Nonprofits." *Harvard Business Review* 67 (July–August 1989): 91.

Griffith, John. *The Well-Managed Community Hospital.* Ann Arbor, MI: Health Administration Press, 1987.

Houle, Cyril O. *Governing Boards.* San Francisco: Jossey-Bass Publishers, 1989.

Kovner, Anthony R. "Improving Hospital Board Effectiveness: An Update." *Frontiers of Health Services Management* 6 (Spring 1990): 3–27.

O'Connell, Brian. *The Board Member's Book.* New York: The Foundation Center, 1985.

Umbdenstock, Richard J. "The Role of the Board and its Trustees." In *Health Care Administration: Principles and Practices,* edited by Lawrence F. Wolper and Jesus J. Peña. Rockville, MD: Aspen Publishers, 1987.

Chapter 4

Too Many on the Seesaw: Stakeholder Diagnosis and Management for Hospitals

John D. Blair
Carlton J. Whitehead

John D. Blair is Professor of Management and Director, Graduate Program in Health Organization Management (College of Business Administration); Associate Chair, Department of Health Organization Management (School of Medicine); and Director of the Research Program in Health Organization Management, Institute for Management and Leadership Research, Texas Tech University, Lubbock. Carlton J. Whitehead is Professor and Coordinator, Area of Management (College of Business Administration) and Professor of Health Organization Management (School of Medicine), Texas Tech University, Lubbock. Both are Faculty Associates of the College.

This article was published in *Hospital & Health Services Administration* 33, no. 2 (Summer 1988).

Health care is changing from a relatively sheltered, noncompetitive, high-growth industry to a low-growth, competitive one (Smith and Reid 1986). These changes pose numerous problems for the industry, especially for the traditional, stand-alone, community-supported general hospitals. These problems have been compounded by Medicare's shift to the prospective payment system and its emulation by other third party payers to contain escalating costs (Smith and Fottler 1985). In short, the health care industry is experiencing fundamental, turbulent, and revolutionary changes (Johnson and Johnson 1982, 1986). And although their environmental munificence varies, many hospitals are confronting hostile contexts (Whitehead and Blair 1987).

The concept of organizational stakeholders is becoming increasingly important to the analysis of the forces affecting organizations and their managers (Mason and Mitroff 1981; Mitroff 1983; Freeman 1984; Blair et al. 1986). Stakeholders are those individuals, groups, and organizations who have an interest in the actions of an organization and the ability to influence it (Carper and Litschert 1983). Because hospitals affect stakeholders through policy and action, they must become better able to manage their relationships with relevant stakeholders.

Most stakeholders are either internal or external to the hospital. Internal stakeholders, for example, include staff employees as well as clinical managers; external stakeholders include the federal government and other hospitals. Some key stakeholders, however, are neither clearly internal nor external but reside on the interface between the hospital and its environment. For instance, the hospital's governing board and medical staff typify these interface stakeholders. Each of these stakeholders has expectations for the hospital and its managers and can oppose or support any of its actions (Fottler 1987).

The analogy of the seesaw with too many on it, used in the title of this article, seems particularly appropriate for hospital executives who attempt daily to balance conflicting stakeholder demands and pressures. This balancing is becoming a problem because the number of stakeholders and their influence on hospital executives is increasing. For example, patients as consumers were passive stakeholders until this decade. Low competition and relatively abundant resources allowed physicians to make most of the key decisions regarding patient care. Now the consumer is a major stakeholder, and marketing programs are directed at the individual consumer, employer, and physician. Likewise, many states now have hospital rate-setting commissions with varying degrees of control over hospital pricing policy. Twenty years ago, such stakeholders were practically nonexistent.

Organizations in the health care industry have to rethink their strategies and operations as they face increasingly conflicting demands from internal, external, and interface stakeholders. For example, the public—an external stakeholder—

sees health care as a right. It expects both the quality and the access to medical care to increase. Many health care professionals support the public's expectations for increased organizational effectiveness. Physicians, nurses, therapists, and other internal and interface stakeholders believe they should do everything possible to improve the health of as many people as possible using every available means (Flood and Scott 1978). On the other hand, external stakeholders such as federal and state governments, insurance companies, and employers expect health care administrators to contain the costs of providing health care (Egdahl 1978). Here, the key demand is for organizational efficiency.

Although much of the health care management literature focuses on how to enhance efficiency and effectiveness, effective managers do *not* try either to minimize costs nor to maximize quality for *all* stakeholders. Rather, they *minimally* satisfy the needs of *marginal* stakeholders while they *maximally* satisfy the needs of *key* stakeholders.

A Diagnostic Framework for Hospital Stakeholders

Stakeholder management integrates in a systematic way what managers often deal with separately: strategic management, marketing, human resource management, public relations, organizational politics, and social responsibility. This integrative perspective assumes that an organization requires some degree of consensus among key stakeholders about what it should be doing and how it should be done.

To manage stakeholders, health care managers must be involved in a continuous process of internal and external scanning when making strategic decisions. They must go beyond the traditional issues in strategic management, such as the likely actions of competitors or the attractiveness of different markets. They must also look for those external, internal, and interface stakeholders who are likely to influence the hospital's decisions. Managers must then make two critical assessments about these stakeholders: (1) their potential to threaten the organization and (2) their potential to cooperate with it (Freeman 1984).

Diagnosing Potential Stakeholder Threat

Hostility or threat appears as a key variable in several formulations of organization-environment-strategy relationships (Miller and Friesen 1978). Physicians, for example, are sometimes explicitly identified as potential threats to effective strategic management by hospitals (Sheldon and Windham 1984). Looking at

61

the potential threat of stakeholders is similar to developing a "worst case" scenario and protects managers from unpleasant surprises.

The stakeholder's relative power and its relevance to any particular issue confronting the hospital's managers determines the stakeholder's potential for threat. Power is primarily a function of the dependence of the hospital on the stakeholder (Pfeffer and Salancik 1978; Korukonda and Blair 1986). Generally, the more dependent the hospital, the more powerful the stakeholder. For example, the power of staff physicians is a function of the hospital's dependence on those physicians for patients, the use of hospital beds, and the provision of hospital services.

Diagnosing Stakeholder
Potential for Cooperation

Because stakeholder analyses emphasize the type and magnitude of threats that stakeholders pose for the organization, the second dimension of potential for cooperation is often ignored. It should be equally emphasized, since it allows stakeholder management strategies to go beyond the merely defensive or offensive. Hospitals should find the potential for cooperation particularly relevant because it may allow them to join forces with other stakeholders and better manage their respective environments.

Assessing the potential for cooperation is also similar to scenario development, here a "best case" one. The stakeholder's dependence on the hospital and its relevance to any particular issue facing the hospital determine its potential for cooperation. Generally, the more dependent the stakeholder on the hospital, the higher the potential for cooperation with the hospital. Often, however, the hospital and the stakeholder may be very interdependent. For example, in a small town with a limited number of physicians and one hospital, the hospital and the physicians usually have high levels of mutual dependence. Although the hospital may encounter threats from some physicians who send patients to another hospital in a larger city, it may also have cooperation from most other physicians who want to keep the patients in the community.

Factors Affecting Potential
for Threat and Cooperation

Besides power, there are other factors that affect the stakeholder's potential for threat or cooperation. In Table 1, a list of stakeholder characteristics that hospital managers should examine when diagnosing the potential for threat or cooperation is provided. Also, whether the presence of particular factors might

Table 1
Factors Affecting Stakeholder Potential for Threat and Cooperation

	Potential for Threat	Potential for Cooperation
Stakeholder controls key resources (needed by hospital)	Increases	Increases
Stakeholder does not control key resources	Decreases	Either
Stakeholder more powerful than hospital	Increases	Either
Stakeholder as powerful as hospital	Either	Either
Stakeholder less powerful than hospital	Decreases	Increases
Stakeholder likely to take action (supportive of the hospital)	Decreases	Increases
Stakeholder likely to take nonsupportive action	Increases	Decreases
Stakeholder unlikely to take any action	Decreases	Decreases
Stakeholder likely to form coalition with other stakeholders	Increases	Either
Stakeholder likely to form coalition with hospital	Decreases	Increases
Stakeholder unlikely to form coalition	Decreases	Decreases

increase, decrease, or *either* increase or decrease each type of potential is indicated.

Some of the factors in the table are concerned with the relative power of the stakeholder vis-à-vis the hospital, in general, or with specific power resulting from control over key resources (Mintzberg 1983). Other factors concentrate on the kind of action the stakeholder might take. Is that action likely to be supportive or counteractive? Is the stakeholder likely to form a coalition with other stakeholders or, instead, with the hospital?

Exactly how a factor will affect the potential for threat or cooperation depends on the specific context and history of the hospital's relations with that stakeholder and with other key stakeholders influencing the hospital. For example, a manager may only be able to assess the cooperation or threat potential of the medical staff in the context of how competing hospitals manage their medical staffs *and* of how the hospital has treated its medical staff in the past. By carefully considering the factors in Table 1, hospital executives can fine-tune their analyses of stakeholders.

Types of Stakeholder

The two dimensions—potential for threat and potential for cooperation—map the stakeholders of a hospital into a diagnostic framework. Using these two dimensions of classification, we can characterize four types of hospital stakeholder as shown in Figure 1.

Figure 1
Diagnostic Typology of Hospital Stakeholders

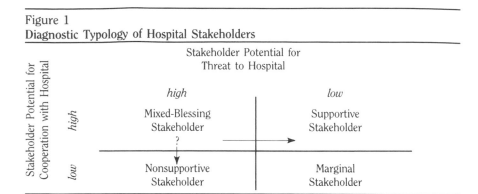

The Supportive Stakeholder

The ideal stakeholder is one who supports the hospital's goals and actions. Such a stakeholder rates low on potential threat and high on potential for cooperation. For a well-managed hospital, its board of trustees, managers, staff employees, parent company, local community, and nursing homes are usually of this type.

The Marginal Stakeholder

Marginal stakeholders are high on neither threat nor cooperative potential. Although they potentially have a stake in the hospital and its decisions, they are generally not relevant for most issues. For a well-run hospital, stakeholders of this kind may include special interest groups, stockholders or taxpayers, and professional associations for employees. However, certain issues, such as cost containment, could activate one or more of these stakeholders, causing their potential for either threat or cooperation to increase.

The Nonsupportive Stakeholder

Stakeholders of this type are the most distressing for a hospital and its managers. They rate high on potential for threat and low on potential for cooperation. Typical nonsupportive stakeholders include competing hospitals, freestanding alternatives such as urgi- or surgicenters, employees unions, the federal and local government, indigent patients, the news media, and employers.

The Mixed-Blessing Stakeholder

The mixed-blessing stakeholder plays a particularly key role. Here, the hospital manager is facing a situation where the stakeholder is high on both types of potential threat and cooperation. Generally, in a well-managed hospital, stakeholders of this type include not only the medical staff but other physicians not on the staff, insurance companies, insured patients, and hospitals with noncompeting, complementary services. Physicians are probably the clearest example of this type of stakeholder. Although they can do much for a hospital, they can also threaten it because of their general control over admissions, the utilization and provision of different services, and the quality of care.

In Figure 1, there is a question mark as well as two arrows under the mixed-blessing stakeholder type. One arrow is directed toward the supportive stakeholder. The other is pointed at the nonsupportive stakeholder. These arrows imply that a mixed-blessing stakeholder could become either more or less supportive. Later, in looking at appropriate stakeholder management strategies for each type of stakeholder, how to manage a mixed-blessing stakeholder most effectively will be emphasized.

Issue-Specific
Stakeholder Diagnosis

Not everyone will agree with the set of stakeholders we have used here as examples for each type. There is good reason to be uncomfortable with such global classifications of particular stakeholders. Of all the possible stakeholders for a hospital, the ones who will be relevant to the hospital's managers depend on the particular issue. If the issue is cost containment, the stakeholders who are concerned will be different than if the issue is access to health care. The diagnosis of the relevant stakeholders in terms of the four stakeholder types will probably be different on these two issues as well.

This issue specificity suggests that stakeholder diagnosis should be an ongoing activity for hospital managers. Managers cannot assume that a stakeholder who is supportive on one issue will be supportive on every issue, nor that a stakeholder who is nonsupportive on one issue will be nonsupportive on another. Both opportunity and danger await the hospital in the form of stakeholders, especially the mixed-blessing type.

Moreover, whatever the classification of a particular stakeholder on a specific issue, managers should explicitly classify stakeholders to surface managerial biases. For example, if a manager identifies all stakeholders for any particular issue as nonsupportive, then the manager should critically examine his or her assessment of the relationship between the hospital and its stakeholders.

Generic Strategies for Hospital Stakeholder Management

Stakeholder diagnosis as attempted in Figure 1 suggests some generic strategies for managing stakeholders with different levels of potential for threat and for cooperation. In Figure 2, a fourfold typology of such strategies is presented.

Involve the Supportive Stakeholder

Hospital executives can maximize supportive stakeholders' cooperation potential by involving them in relevant issues. Because these stakeholders have little threat potential, they are likely to be ignored as stakeholders to be managed, and their cooperative potential may be ignored as well.

Hospital managers can involve these stakeholders by using participative management techniques (Counte, Barhyte, and Christman 1987), by decentralizing authority to clinical managers, or by engaging in other tactics to increase the decision-making participation of these stakeholders. For example, hospital executives might invite clinical managers to participate in the analysis and planning for the elimination of redundant programs. The clinical managers will more likely become committed to achieving such an organizational objective than if they had not been involved in establishing it. A key requirement for the

Figure 2
Generic Hospital Stakeholder Management Strategies

		Stakeholder Potential for Threat to Hospital	
		high	*low*
Stakeholder's Potential for Cooperation with Hospital	*high*	Collaborate with the Mixed-Blessing Stakeholder	Involve the Supportive Stakeholder
	low	Defend against the Nonsupportive Stakeholder	Monitor the Marginal Stakeholder

success of this type of strategy is the ability of the managers to enlarge their vision of ways to further involve supportive stakeholders in higher levels of cooperation.

Nonmanagerial professional and support employees represent another class of stakeholder belonging in this category. Employees generally do not pose a great deal of direct threat to an organization, although union activism or human resource shortages can make their continued service problematic under certain circumstances. However, their cooperative potential may not have been fully tapped. Quality circles represent a straightforward example of the involvement strategy, presenting a means of managing employee relations and improving productivity which more closely links the employee to the organization and its objectives (Cornell 1984; McKinney 1984).

Monitor the Marginal Stakeholder

Monitoring helps to manage those marginal stakeholders whose potential for either threat or cooperation is low. For example, special interest groups may be opposed to certain procedures such as abortion or artificial implants or concerned about certain patient groups such as the aged. Typically, these special interest groups have only a marginal stake in the activities of the hospital, affecting operations indirectly by advocating a moral or ethical standpoint. Other marginal stakeholders are taxpayers and stockholders. They are unlikely to be either much help or much hindrance unless the hospital takes actions that activate them.

The underlying philosophy for managing marginal stakeholders is maintaining the status quo, with finances and management time kept to a minimum. Hospital executives address issues on an ad hoc basis. The general thrust of this approach is to "let sleeping dogs lie." Keeping them asleep, however, may require ongoing public relations activities and sensitivity to issues that could activate these groups.

Defend against the
Nonsupportive Stakeholder

Stakeholders who pose a high threat but whose potential for cooperation is low are best managed using a defensive strategy. The federal government and indigent patients are good examples of this nonsupportive stakeholder group. In terms of Kotter's (1979) framework on external dependence, the defense strategy tries to reduce the dependence that forms the basis for the stakeholders' interest in the organization. However, health care executives should not attempt to eliminate totally their dependence on nonsupportive stakeholders. Such efforts are either doomed to failure or may result in a negative image for the organization. For example, trying to sever all ties with the federal government is counterproductive if a hospital hopes to market to older patients. A public hospital that tries to deny access to all indigent patients will surely be viewed negatively by the public and the local government.

Let us consider an example of this defense strategy in action, using the federal government's regulatory agencies as the stakeholder. Given the regulations hospitals face, their most appropriate tactic is to explore ways of complying with the demands imposed by the federal government at the least possible cost. Diagnosis-related groups (DRGs) that produce a surplus for the hospitals define areas of distinctive competence. Hence, hospital executives might adopt a case-mix approach to the delivery of health care, modifying the services they offer based on cost and process accounting.

This generic strategy could also take the form of driving out or reducing competition. A hospital might drive out competition by securing a monopoly over a particular market segment through preferred provider organization (PPO) contracting. On the other hand, to reduce competition with urgi- or surgicenters, a hospital could build new ambulatory facilities or restructure existing facilities. In these examples of the defense strategy, the connection of stakeholder management to broader strategic management is very clear, involving many traditional marketing and strategic methods for handling competitors.

However, other nonsupportive stakeholders, such as the news media and employers from other industries, are not traditionally examined in strategic management. Nonetheless, the investigative media can be defended against through careful monitoring of organizational information, good external relations, and clinical managers trained in how to talk to the media. Employers can be appeased through PPOs.

Collaborate with the Mixed-Blessing Stakeholder

The mixed-blessing stakeholder, both a potential threat and a potential ally, may best be managed through collaboration. If hospital executives seek to collaborate with them, these potentially threatening stakeholders will find it more difficult to oppose the hospital. A variety of joint ventures or other collaborative efforts up to and including mergers is possible (Marcino 1984; Snook and Kaye 1986).

For example, a hospital might form a joint venture with a group of its medical staff to build a freestanding surgicenter or imaging center. Such collaboration stops the physicians from building a center themselves and thus competing with hospital-based surgery or diagnostic procedures. The hospital can contribute its name and capital resources while the physicians will presumably send their patients to the hospital when inpatient services are needed. Both the hospital and the physicians will benefit.

In the case of insurance companies, the value of a collaborative strategy seems to be well recognized. For example, the recent joint venture between Aetna Insurance and the Voluntary Hospitals of America—called "Partners"—involves the insurance company, the hospital, and the medical staff in a nationally marketed, collaborative PPO (Coddington and Moore 1987). Such a PPO may even help a participating hospital manage a normally nonsupportive stakeholder such as an employer.

For the mixed-blessing stakeholder, effective collaboration may well determine the long-term stakeholder/hospital relationship. In other words, if this type of stakeholder is not properly managed using a collaborative strategy, it could become a nonsupportive stakeholder.

An Overarching Stakeholder Management Strategy

In addition to using the four strategies specifically tailored for stakeholders who are classified into one of the four diagnostic categories, health care executives may also employ an overarching strategy. This overarching strategy moves the stakeholder from a less favorable category to a more favorable one. Then, the stakeholder can be managed using the generic strategy most appropriate for that "new" diagnostic category.

For example, rather than simply defend against the news media as a nonsupportive stakeholder, a hospital could implement an aggressive program of external relations with openness to the media. If successful, the program would move the news media to a less threatening category as a marginal stakeholder, allowing it to be managed through a monitoring strategy (Fitzgerald and Wahl 1987).

As another example, a hospital could involve an employee union in a quality of work life program of productivity enhancement combined with gain sharing to union members. Such an effort could succeed in moving the employee union from the least favorable stakeholder category (nonsupportive) to the most favorable (supportive).

Of course, stakeholders generally will not just sit still and be managed. Stakeholders who are powerful, and hence threatening, are just as likely to try to manage hospitals. Many hospitals and their stakeholders continuously engage in management and countermanagement strategies, often leading to direct negotiations (Blair, Savage, and Whitehead 1989). The full range of the negotiations between organizations and their stakeholders cannot be discussed here. (See also, for example, the results of the Harvard Negotiation Project [Fisher and Ury 1981].) Nonetheless, to manage these stakeholders effectively, hospital executives should continuously assess stakeholders and match their diagnosis with appropriate strategies.

69

Conclusion

To survive the turbulent and revolutionary changes facing the health care industry, hospital executives must better manage internal, external, and interface stakeholders. Hospitals need to rethink their strategies and operations as they face increasing, potentially conflicting demands for effectiveness and efficiency from these stakeholders. In short, hospital executives must minimally satisfy the needs of marginal stakeholders while they maximally satisfy the needs of key stakeholders.

Hospital executives need to do more than merely identify stakeholders or react to stakeholder demands. They must proactively develop or enhance their hospitals' capacity for strategic stakeholder management rather than concentrating only on effectively dealing with a particular stakeholder on a specific issue. Hospitals should establish goals for their relationships with current and potential stakeholders as part of an effective strategic management process (Shortell 1985).

To aid hospital executives in this endeavor, future health care management research and practice should focus on (1) analyzing stakeholders' stakes and power, (2) identifying stakeholders' critical dimensions, (3) finding ways to facilitate hospital managers' abilities to challenge their own assumptions, (4) examining how hospital managers may negotiate effectively with stakeholders, and (5) creating and assessing strategies to enhance cooperation with stakeholders.

Many other topics and issues also need to be addressed (Fottler 1987). Unresolved issues include how stakeholder management varies by type of hospital, by autonomy, by stage in the organizational life cycle (Quinn and Cameron 1983), and by type of external environment (Whitehead and Blair 1987). We encourage others to address these issues so as to extend the stakeholder diagnostic model and strategies we have presented here. Such future research is critical for a better understanding of the processes and strategies involved in effective stakeholder management.

References

Blair, J., G. Savage, and C. Whitehead. "A Strategic Approach for Negotiating with Hospital Stakeholders." *Health Care Management Review* 14 (Winter 1989): 13–23.

Blair, J. D., B. R. Baliga, C. J. Whitehead, and A. R. Korukonda. "Stakeholder Management Strategies for Health Care Organizations." Paper presented at the annual meeting of the Health Care Administration Division of the Academy of Management, Chicago, August 1986.

Carper, W. B., and R. J. Litschert. "Strategic Power Relationships in Contemporary Profit and Nonprofit Hospitals." *Academy of Management Journal* 26(1983): 311–20.

Coddington, D., and K. Moore. *Market-Driven Strategies in Health Care*. San Francisco, CA: Jossey-Bass, 1987.

Cornell, L. "Quality Circles: A New Cure for Hospital Dysfunctions?" *Hospital & Health Services Administration* 29(September/October 1984): 88–93.

Counte, M. A., D. Y. Barhyte, and L. P. Christman. "Participative Management among Staff Nurses." *Hospital & Health Services Administration* 32(February 1987): 97–108.

Egdahl, R. H. "Should We Shrink the Health Care System?" *Harvard Business Review* 62(January-February 1978): 125–32.

Fisher, R., and W. Ury. *Getting to Yes; Negotiating Agreement Without Giving In*. Boston, MA: Houghton Mifflin, 1981.

Fitzgerald, P. E., and L. E. Wahl. "Media Relations: Clues for Improvement." *Hospital & Health Services Administration* 32(February 1987): 39–47.

Flood, A. B., and W. R. Scott. "Professional Power and Professional Effectiveness: The Power of the Surgical Staff and the Quality of Surgical Care in Hospitals." *Journal of Health and Social Behavior* 19(September 1978): 240–54.

Fottler, M. "Health Care Organizational Performance: Present and Future Research." In the *1987 Yearly Review of Management* of the *Journal of Management*, edited by J. D. Blair and J. G. Hunt. 13(Summer 1987): 179–203.

Freeman, R. E. *Strategic Management: A Stakeholder Approach*. Marshfield, MA: Pitman Publishing, 1984.

Johnson, E., and R. Johnson. *Hospitals in Transition*. Rockville, MD: Aspen Systems, 1982.

Johnson, E., and R. Johnson. *Hospitals under Fire: Strategies for Survival*. Rockville, MD: Aspen Systems, 1986.

Korukonda, A. R., and J. D. Blair, "Resource Dependence and Stakeholder Management: Strategies for Managers of Today's Health Care Organizations." *Proceedings* of the Southern Management Association (November 1986): 97–99.

Kotter, J. P. "Managing External Dependence." *Academy of Management Review* 4(January 1979): 87–92.

Marcino, D. "Hospital-Physician Joint Ventures: Some Crucial Considerations." *Hospital Progress* 65(1984): 30–35.

Mason, R. O., and I. I. Mitroff. *Challenging Strategic Planning Assumptions*. New York, NY: Wiley, 1981.

McKinney, M. M. "The Newest Miracle Drug: Quality Circles in Hospitals." *Hospital & Health Services Administration* 29(September/October 1984): 74–87.

Miller, D., and P. Friesen. "Archetypes of Strategy Formulation." *Management Science* 24(May 1978): 921–33.

Mintzberg, H. *Power In and Around Organizations.* Englewood Cliffs, NJ: Prentice-Hall, 1983.

Mitroff, I. I. *Stakeholders of the Organizational Mind.* San Francisco, CA: Jossey-Bass, 1983.

Pfeffer, J., and G. Salancik. *The External Control of Organizations: A Resource Dependence Perspective.* New York, NY: Harper and Row, 1978.

Quinn, R., and K. Cameron. "Organizational Life Cycles and the Criteria of Effectiveness." *Management Science* 29(January 1983): 33–51.

Sheldon, A., and S. Windham. *Competitive Strategy for Health Care Organizations.* Homewood, IL: Dow–Jones Irwin, 1984.

Shortell, S. M. "High Performing Healthcare Organizations: Guidelines for the Pursuit of Excellence." *Hospital & Health Services Administration* 30(July/August 1985): 7–35.

Smith, H., and M. Fottler. *Prospective Payment: Managing for Operational Effectiveness.* Rockville, MD: Aspen Systems, 1985.

Smith, H., and R. Reid. *Competitive Hospitals.* Rockville, MD: Aspen Systems, 1986.

Snook, I., Jr., and E. Kaye. *A Guide to Health Care Joint Ventures.* Rockville, MD: Aspen Systems, 1986.

Whitehead, C., and J. Blair. "Environmental Munificence and Organizational Response: Implications for Managing Hospitals." Paper presented at the annual meeting of the Health Care Administration Division of the Academy of Management, New Orleans, August 1987.

Chapter 5

The Power of Health Care Value-Adding Partnerships: Meeting Competition through Cooperation

Stephen E. Foreman
Robert D. Roberts

Stephen E. Foreman is a health care attorney and consultant. Robert D. Roberts is a certified public accountant and independent health care consultant, Sonoma, California.

This article was published in *Hospital & Health Services Administration* 36, no. 2 (Summer 1991).

Competition

The Evolution of Price Competition

During the 1980s the U.S. health care delivery system witnessed an escalation of price competition and turbulence. Previously, the industry climate might have been termed an era of "cooperation" (Starr 1982). By cooperation, we mean that there was little or no competition for patient revenue on the basis of price even though there was often intense competition in the delivery of service.

The cooperative era encouraged economic "inefficiency." Payment philosophies encouraged providers to generate excess capacity, to duplicate services, and to emphasize service without regard to cost (Fuchs 1986). However, during the last decade payers began to use providers' fear, mistrust, and surplus capacity to extract price discounts (Goldsmith 1981).

Hospitals have traditionally competed with one another to attract patients on the basis of service (usually through medical staff recruitment). However, competition for patients intensified dramatically, indeed changed, with the advent of price discounts. Providers now attempt to increase revenue by seeking exclusive relationships with payers and by offering services theretofore reserved to other providers. The reaction was predictable: a counterattack by those threatened. For example, physicians began to offer services previously provided by hospitals (Cowan 1984).

What has been the result? Increased levels of price and service competition between and among hospitals, physicians, and other providers, which we believe can reasonably be expected to continue and to escalate so long as there is excess capacity in the health care system and so long as health care providers remain fragmented.[1] Accordingly, there is some risk that the health care world of the future may be characterized by even more price discounting, curtailments in service, uncertainty, stress, facility closures, and change. How can health care providers survive, indeed succeed in such a world? Strange as it may seem, those providers who learn to cooperate may have the best opportunity. Value-adding partnerships are one way that cooperation can evolve in such a world.

Surviving Competition

In a classic study, Robert Axelrod (1984) has shown that in the midst of a hypercompetitive environment, cooperation (tempering self-interest by working together) can be a powerful strategy, even when it is practiced by only a few (see also Sugden 1986). Axelrod considered the "prisoner's dilemma"[2] a situation where two parties have a choice whether to cooperate or to compete. If both cooperate, both are moderately successful. If both compete, both are moderately unsuccessful. If one cooperates while the other competes, the cooperating party loses and the competing party wins, as shown in Figure 1.

Superficially, strategy is clear: a party who seeks to gain by cooperating is completely at the mercy of an opponent who competes. A competitor at least has the chance to win if an opponent is naive. Therefore, a "sophisticated" player must compete. Even where the parties can communicate and both agree to cooperate, without a penalty for "cheating" or "defecting," the parties may not be able to agree to cooperate because the incentive to defect is so strong. Both must continue to compete to avoid disaster.

How, then, can cooperation evolve? Axelrod (1984) demonstrated that when the relationship extends over time, a simple "tit for tat" strategy can provide a strong basis for cooperation. Players who were able to cooperate using such a strategy substantially outperformed those whose strategy was based on pure competition. Why?

The party (1) who is willing to be the first to cooperate, (2) who punishes an opponent's "defections," (3) who is "forgiving" (returns to cooperation after the punishment), and (4) who *communicates* this strategy, is the most effective participant. Both players come to understand that where they cooperate they can both win. Competition will doom them both to future losses because the party who is the victim of the first defection will then "punish" the defector. The party playing "tit for tat" shows the other the best strategy for both, as shown in Figure 2.

The concept has intuitive appeal in the competitive health care environment. In essence, health care is an extended prisoner's dilemma. Hospitals

---

Figure 1
The Prisoner's Dilemma: An Illustrative Matrix

		Player #1	
		Cooperate	Compete
Player #2	Cooperate	Win / Win	Large win / Large loss
	Compete	Large loss / Large win	Lose / Lose

Figure 2
The Prisoner's Dilemma: "Tit For Tat" Strategy

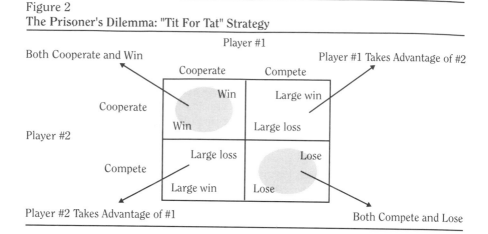

compete with other hospitals. Doctors compete. Long-term care facilities compete. Payers and providers compete. Naturally, a provider must avoid becoming a "victim"; "nice guys finish last." However, this approach will inevitably lead to continued fragmentation and greater competition. Health care providers will "lose," ostensibly at the expense of payers.[3] As was shown by Axelrod (1984), those health care providers who are able to establish a basis for cooperation cannot only survive, they can succeed.

How can this work? It can even at a simple level: a hospital and its medical staff learn to work together and to trust one another, to "cooperate," and they have an advantage over hospitals and medical staffs that are mutually distrustful, fearful, and greedy. The same holds true for a hospital and its employees.

On a broader level, those health care providers who become part of effective "linkages" will be in a stronger position to negotiate with payers, to reduce costs through economies of scale, and to react to changes. A single, stand-alone provider is in the most vulnerable position because without "allies," it must compete and may lose to those entities that build effective alliances.

The concept holds true even at a macrolevel. If competition destroys the health care delivery system, payers also lose. If escalating costs destroy payers, providers lose as well. If providers and payers learn that it is important to balance cooperation with competition, the health care delivery system may be enhanced. In short, those health care industry participants who can learn when and how to cooperate will have an advantage over those who cannot.

Cooperation through Value-Adding Partnerships

Given the obvious importance of cooperation in a hypercompetitive environment, how can it begin? Cooperation can be mandated (in the form of government-granted monopoly or total corporate integration in the form of a conglomerate) or it can take place voluntarily (through devices like the value-adding partnership). Observation of the effectiveness of various providers leads to the conclusion that voluntary cooperation is a much more powerful force (Deutsch 1973; Kriesberg 1982).

One form of mandatory cooperation is evidenced by fully integrated health care conglomerates. The components of such an enterprise can be forced to cooperate because the enterprise operates under single ownership and control. However, this form of cooperation provides little motivation for the entity's constituent parts to be efficient. Companies that are integrated through ownership are usually managed with a single management style. However, the style that works for some divisions or subsidiaries does not always work for others. Accordingly, divisions or subsidiaries are often not as responsive to one another as they would be if they were independently owned and operated enterprises.[4] Witness how many hospitals encountered economic disaster by owning nursing homes and urgent care centers. Many health care conglomerates have struggled during the 1980s as a direct result of the economic and management problems of the fully integrated enterprise.

What does this suggest? In effect, cooperation that is mandated may be better than outright competition but it still has substantial drawbacks. It would be far better if there were a way to accomplish cooperation on a voluntary basis. Fortunately, value-adding partnerships are an effective approach to achieve this.

A value-adding partnership (VAP) is a group of autonomous enterprises, each of which performs one or more services or functions in a "value-adding chain." Each partner coordinates its activities with the rest of the chain's participants (Johnston and Lawrence 1988).

The concept of the value-adding chain is an outgrowth of the business system concept in which the firm is seen as a series of functions—what Michael Porter (1985) calls a collection of activities performed to design, produce, market, deliver, and support a product. (Porter evaluates the value-adding chain in terms of the firm.) The concept applies equally well to an industry (like health care) where service is offered in a continuum. The health care continuum extends from primary care (physicians), to ambulatory care (surgery centers, imaging centers), acute care (hospitals), long-term care (skilled nursing facilities), and home care (home health and hospice), as shown in Figure 3. The value-adding chain includes support activities as well as direct provision of services and supplies.

A good example of a VAP in a related industry is the McKesson Corporation and its drug distribution network. How is this VAP organized? In the continuum that makes up the drug industry (manufacturer to distributor to retailer), McKesson is a distributor. At a time when large drug chains were forming integrated networks through the acquisition of independently owned drug stores, they threatened the existence of McKesson and its independent drug store customers (the retailers) because the chains enjoyed the advantages of the economies of scale produced through volume purchasing. In response, McKesson designed an order entry computer system that permitted it and its drug store customers to look and to perform like the chains. As a result, McKesson could negotiate volume purchasing arrangements with drug manufacturers on behalf of its customers.

The McKesson VAP thus acts and looks like the drug chains from the standpoint of distribution and supply, but each part of the system remains independently owned and operated (Johnston and Lawrence 1988). While there are supply contracts, there is little or no need for the parties to enter into a formal "partnership" agreement. The partnership is maintained by self-inter-

Figure 3
The Health Care Value-Adding Chain

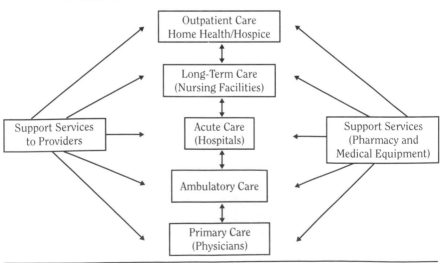

est, but each firm in the partnership acts in its own interest. So long as there is external competition from the chains, the concept of self-interest extends to concern for the well-being of the other partners. The McKesson system is, therefore, a VAP since each participant makes its own contribution to the enterprise and derives value by cooperating with the others. Each partner gains as other partners become stronger. Competition is not eliminated, it is actually enhanced. Accordingly, the McKesson system competes effectively with the chains. A McKesson partner who is not efficient or competitive can and must be replaced.

There are also examples of VAPs in other industries. The construction industry is built on this concept. Rarely is the general contractor more than a coordinator. Independent subcontractors supply electrical work, plumbing, heating, ventilating, air conditioning, elevators, tile and flooring, steel work, paneling, and so on. The airline industry is a particularly interesting example since, like health care, it is experiencing the novelty of a competitive marketplace. Some airlines have tried to own and operate a full-service travel firm and have encountered some difficulty. Others have formed VAPs (primarily through joint marketing programs) that include national carriers and regional carriers, travel agents (tied in through computer systems), automobile rental companies, hotels, and so forth. For example, many travel companies now include a host of travel partners in their frequent flier or frequent traveler bonus programs.

Some commentators have pointed out that to survive in a competitive environment a firm must either offer a full range of services or a few "boutique" services where it can enjoy a competitive advantage. Another way of looking at the VAP is that it provides a means for its participants to offer "full industry service" (either on a local or a national level) without the capital investment requirements and management challenges that stem from owning and operating each segment of the value-added chain. Partners offer those services in the value chain that lie within their areas of expertise, which may be why some VAPs like McKesson's drug distribution network, the construction industry, and the travel industry may seem to evolve naturally.

The power of the VAP arises from the fact that each participant or partner maintains its own identity and control and is responsible for operating its business as efficiently as it knows how. Participants are valued for their expertise and efficiency. In the construction industry, subcontractors are experts in the engineering and construction services they provide. A general contractor gains little by owning the subcontractor and risks a "fall off" in expertise and efficiency when it owns the subcontractor. The partnership emphasizes network coordination and information sharing. Partners realize that each participant must be financially sound, efficient, and market wise if the enterprise is to remain competitive. Accordingly, systematic, close cooperation becomes a governing maxim (Johnston and Lawrence 1988).

In an integrated company, there is usually a single focus. For example, companies often emphasize low-cost or high-quality service. They are rarely able to emphasize both. Further, components of integrated companies have difficulty responding to the rest of the firm in the same way that an independent enterprise would respond to its customers. Conversely, each VAP participant focuses on a portion of the value-adding chain. It can thereby tailor its organization to narrower tasks, such as improving focus. This sense of focus translates into lower overhead, leaner staff, and fewer middle-level managers. Marketing orientation develops naturally (Johnston and Lawrence 1988).

The VAP sidesteps many of the disadvantages of the wholly owned or controlled corporation but maintains the advantages of "integration." The vertical nature of the partnership emphasizes information sharing and coordination and control. The partners can share those activities that produce economies of scale (joint purchasing, research and development, education, marketing, etc.). Properly conceived and executed, the VAP can achieve the best aspects of vertical integration without the attendant disadvantages of common ownership.

What then, should be the contents of a "partnership" agreement for a VAP? A VAP can take a tremendous variety of forms and provide an infinite variety of services, so any definitive how-to list would be quite impossible to structure. We can make a few general observations, however. The agreement should contain few rules and should be as simple as possible. Value-adding partnerships stay together because it is in the best interests of the partners to do so, not because the partnership agreement commands it. The agreement should, however, spell out the goals and objectives of the partnership, not in any legal sense, but to give the partners a common basis of understanding.

The agreement should also specify in some detail the relationships between and among the partners. What is each partner expected to contribute? What standards attach to the provision of service? Are the partners expected (or permitted) to compete with or among one another? Can the partners engage in new or different services? How are new partners admitted? How will the partnership find or develop partners to provide additional services? How will prices be established for each partner's service? Will the other partners have any input?

Inevitably there will be attempts to violate the agreement or to defect. How are defections to be dealt with? What sanctions are provided to limit the temptation to defect? As in Axelrod's (1984) prisoner's dilemma, how can the partnership agreement reinforce each partner's recognition that mutual cooperation is in every partner's best interest?

Health Care as Ideal Focus for VAPs

Given the competitive health care industry of the last few years, proposing cooperation may appear to be radical. However, the health care value-adding partnership (HCVAP) may provide the best alternative available to health care providers. The HCVAP has a history that providers can understand—it permits providers to obtain the advantages of integration while continuing to emphasize their autonomy, and it allows health care providers to avoid the pitfalls encountered in integration through single ownership and control.

HCVAPs Are Not Really New

The traditional health care industry is a model for the VAP. In a sense, formation of HCVAPs represents no more than a return to traditional values. For example, the traditional relationship between hospitals and their medical staffs is a VAP, rather than ownership and control. Physicians provide "hands-on" health care. Hospitals generally provide beds and support service. These areas of expertise are different and, by and large, complementary. The hospitals that work best are those that enjoy the most effective partnership between the hospital and the medical staff.

On a more general level, the last major crisis that threatened the financial viability of hospitals and physicians occurred during the 1930s. In the midst of the Great Depression patients often had no resources to pay for health care. Hospitals and physicians responded by forming Blue Cross and Blue Shield plans that were, in effect, VAPs. Hospitals and physicians remained autonomous yet cooperated. The success of the plans over a 40-year period is testimony to their effectiveness.

Are HCVAPs the Best Way to Compete?

Rediscovery of the VAP may be a solution to the dilemma of finding an effective way to organize to meet the challenges of the current environment without loss of autonomy. Properly accomplished, health care providers can form partnerships that permit each partner to work with others in an integrated fashion while maintaining each partner's existing ownership, identity, and control. This is the essence of an HCVAP.

The HCVAP can avoid the pitfalls encountered in mandatory cooperative relationships. Each HCVAP partner is responsible for operating its organization as effectively as it can in a competitive environment. Each partner has an incentive to keep costs down by staffing efficiently and by making its services desirable. Evidence of success or failure is direct. If one of the partners is unable to provide efficient service, the other partners must find a way to help the weaker partner become strong or the HCVAP will have to find a stronger partner.

The HCVAP may represent the only way many health care providers can become "integrated." Health care providers who find a way to forge cooperative linkages in an environment characterized by uncontrolled competition will have an advantage. There are essentially two ways to cooperate—by common ownership and control and through the HCVAP. Health care providers must integrate in order to provide a continuum of services and to use limited resources more effectively. Indeed, for many who cannot become part of wholly owned systems (politically or economically), an HCVAP offers the only real alternative and in many cases, a better alternative, to a wholly owned enterprise.

Examples of an HCVAP

One of the best examples of an HCVAP is still the relationship between the hospital and its medical staff. The hospital and the medical staff each have specific areas of expertise. Effective care is provided to patients when both the hospital and the medical staff are strong and viable. Where one or the other is dominant, the service provided by the dominated party can deteriorate. A good HCVAP project might well focus on ways to strengthen the relationship between a hospital and its medical staff. Hospital/physician joint ventures have received increasing attention for this reason. Beyond this, there are a great number of services that hospitals might provide for their physicians as a way of strengthening the partnership: access to data processing, management service, education, joint purchasing advantages, and so on. Hospitals too can profit by the contributions increased medical staff involvement will bring.

While many think of Kaiser Permanente as simply a health maintenance organization, on a regional level the Kaiser system is an example of a successful HCVAP. Kaiser consists of three components: an "insurance" company, physicians, and hospitals. Each of the constituent parts understands that if it fails to temper self-interest and weakens one of the other partners, the entire enterprise will suffer. Accordingly, while San Francisco Bay Area hospitals were passing their inefficiencies along to Blue Cross and Blue Shield and other insurers, Kaiser was steadily gaining market share. If the Bay Area providers (and providers in areas Kaiser has targeted) cannot form effective and efficient integrated relationships (like HCVAPs), Kaiser will continue to gain market share. In many markets, the first health care group to form an effective integrated HCVAP that combines risk limitation (insurance), physician care, and acute care (not just preferred provider organization discounting arrangements) will be able to obtain significant competitive advantages.

Integrated Health Systems

Thus, on a broader level, those health care providers that are able to become part of an integrated approach to health care can enjoy a superior competitive position. It is for this reason that system approaches to health care have been advanced (McManis 1987; Davis 1988; Senge and Asay 1988). Heretofore, the largest problem with health care integration has not been the system concept, but its implementation. Providers have generally attempted to implement integrated systems using unified ownership and control. This approach encountered the usual difficulties experienced by integrated companies: misplaced incentives, internal competition for resources, lack of responsiveness, and loss of specific management expertise.

Those providers who have not joined integration efforts resisted, by and large, because they feared loss of identity and self-determination. Those who have joined have met with frustration as a result of the difficulties that attach to operation of a unified, wholly owned system.

The HCVAP may provide a way for health care providers to form effective integrated systems. Thus, an HCVAP might consist of one or more hospitals, long-term care facilities, medical groups, home health agencies, primary care facilities, ambulatory surgeries, diagnostic imaging centers, and other specialty health care providers, even an insurance function. Each of the partners would retain its own identity, ownership, and control, as shown in Figure 4. Partnership activities might include contracting on a group basis with payers, joint purchasing, joint educational activities, joint planning and marketing, or sharing of overhead to the extent that it results in economies of scale and more effective patient referrals. The partnership may find that it has much greater leverage in terms of access to capital and input into the legislative process.

The HCVAP can obtain fiscal success by obtaining economies of scale and joint marketing power for its members. The HCVAP takes the form of a partnership or even a looser coalition or association of parties with consistent interests. Each member will retain the incentive to maintain its expertise and to operate in an efficient manner. This too should translate into added profitability as it has with McKesson and Kaiser.

Putting the HCVAP into Operation

The Impetus for Forming HCVAPs

The most challenging aspect of the HCVAP is not its conceptualization. Cooperation, even in the face of a hostile environment, has intuitive as well as

Figure 4
A Health Care Value-Adding Partnership

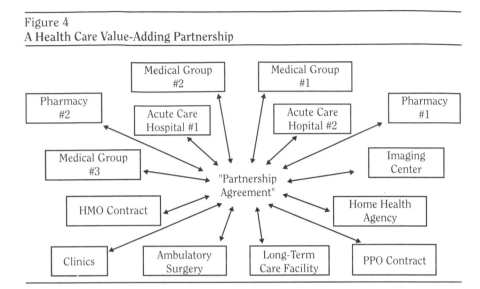

intellectual appeal. Rather, the challenge of the HCVAP is its implementation, particularly because the form that any particular HCVAP can take is infinite.

Given such diversity, what, if anything, can be said about implementing HCVAPs? Is the HCVAP just another idea that sounds good but is impossible to implement? We think not. The HCVAP becomes viable at that point in time when two or more entities recognize that cooperation will provide them with definite and distinct advantages (whether in terms of control of costs, enhanced marketing, contracting power, access to information, and so on). An HCVAP becomes the mechanism or model of choice when the providers who recognize the advantages of cooperation conclude that unified ownership and control is either not possible (politically or economically) or will produce demonstrable disadvantages. Some groups can and will accomplish successful formation of HCVAPs. The first successful HCVAPs will have significant advantages not only over independent providers but also over other HCVAPs that form later. The advantages of becoming the first HCVAP in the market with the best service and the most compatible partners adds some sense of urgency to the idea of forming an HCVAP.[5]

Faced with the vagaries of the health care industry, we cannot predict when or how HCVAPs will be implemented. We do believe that the stress of the current environment, coupled with the potential power of the HCVAP makes successful formation of some HCVAPs inevitable (Axelrod 1984). While we cannot predict the specific form these HCVAPs will take, or even the process by which they might be formed, we can consider some mechanisms that may enhance the change for successful formation.

The Formation Process

Successful formation of an HCVAP will require one or more persons who have sufficient vision to recognize the advantages that can be obtained from the HCVAP and who have sufficient communication and persuasion skills to convince others of the power of the vision. The vision might encompass some preliminary idea of the ways that the HCVAP can provide competitive advantages, the service that might be offered by the HCVAP, the geographic area that might be served, and some idea regarding who might be good potential partners. In essence, the HCVAP will need one or more "advocates." Any number of persons might fill the advocacy role. Through training and experience a hospital CEO might be the best candidate, although board members, physicians, planners, educators, and even insurance company executives can play a crucial role.

Group dynamics will be important. The visionaries must persuade potential partners to discuss the HCVAP in greater detail. Group interaction will determine whether or not the HCVAP can be formed and once formed, how effective it will be. As with any dynamic processes, intangibles like leadership, the history of past dealings between and among the parties, the character of the parties (e.g., their willingness to take risks, to undertake commitments, to consider change, and so on) will enter into the equation. Again, each case will be unique. By and large, however, the more sophisticated the parties are in the process of group dynamics the greater the likelihood of success.

A history of competition and mistrust among the partners need not be debilitating. The HCVAP concept recognizes and emphasizes the importance of self-interest. Partners do not need to like one another and even do not need to trust one another in order to cooperate. They need only to respect the contribution that the potential partners can bring to the partnership and to have assurance that all partners understand the need to follow the HCVAP's rules.[6] In essence, they only need to understand the "prisoner's dilemma" nature of their situation.

At the heart of any successful HCVAP is its operating rules. The rules must be "fair," as simple as possible (to minimize disputes), and above all, enforceable. If the rules are not enforceable, the partnership will have to be maintained solely on trust. At key junctures the incentive to defect many be too tempting. If the rules are enforceable, the likelihood that they will have to be enforced becomes remote, particularly if there are advantages to HCVAP membership and a breach would risk loss of membership. Needless to say, mere adoption of rules is not enough; the partners must enforce them.

Leadership

The HCVAP members will have to address the leadership issue head on, which may prove to be the single most difficult hurdle. The HCVAP will not be successful without strong leadership. At a facile level, anyone who has a vision cannot be bashful about trying to convince others. However, strong leaders may not be trusted. The presence of two or more strong leaders can lead to a power struggle that will undermine the HCVAP. Also, if weaker HCVAP members insist on disproportionate leadership and control, stronger members may not commit enough energy and resources to the HCVAP. Disproportionate benefits for stronger members can diminish the strength of the weaker members, weakening the HCVAP. There are strategies that can be used to deal with the leadership situation. However, the most important realization is simple and overriding: the partners are involved in a prisoner's dilemma. Tempering self-interest is an essential part of cooperation for joint gains (Schelling 1978).[7] At some point, any benefit demanded by one of the partners will weaken another partner and thereby weaken the HCVAP. If the partners understand and internalize this concept, the opportunity for success will be enhanced.

Conclusion

Value-adding partnerships offer a way for health care providers to cooperate in the midst of a competitive environment. Those providers who can cooperate will have a distinct advantage over those who do not enter into such alliances. The HCVAPs themselves can offer substantial benefits in comparison with enterprises that rely on unitary ownership and control. Those who can cooperate and work together in a hostile world will have a much better opportunity to survive and to prosper; HCVAPs may be the key.

Notes

1. We make no value judgments herein regarding either conflict/competition or cooperation. Each concept has its uses and "abuses." For example, cooperation allows persons or enterprises to accomplish as a group what no single group member could. Competition spurs competitors to become efficient and to innovate. However, competition can destroy those less able and can drive out cooperation. Excessive cooperation can lead to waste, inefficiency, and lack of innovation. It would seem that the optimum situation would call for some sort of creative balance or tension.

2. See chapters 4 and 5 of R. Duncan Luce and Howard Raiffa's *Games and Decisions* (New York: John Wiley & Sons, 1957).

3. In actuality, the entire industry suffers, including the payers, if payment to providers is driven so low that the quality of care provided to patients suffers, if there is insufficient capital for new technology and for new plant and equipment, and if there is no incentive for the "best" to seek careers in health care. The payers may gain in the short run but will lose in the long run.

4. The need for "responsiveness" is why the concept of "employed" physicians has substantial drawbacks. We should want each and every physician to treat each patient as if his or her reputation and continued income stream depends on the best possible care.

5. Some care must be exercised that antitrust laws are not violated. Sound legal advice in this area is readily available and events of the last several years tend to diminish the antitrust law's role in joint health care activity. The main concern of the HCVAP's participants should rest on business matters.

6. It will help if the parties recognize the "prisoner's dilemma" nature of the situation. Theoretically, it might be to the advantage of one or more parties to continue to compete if the rest cooperate. However, if this happens, none of the parties will cooperate and all will lose. Accordingly, if cooperation can begin, it will be to the distinct and continuing advantage of each of the participants to continue to cooperate, even though the advantages derived thereby might not be as great for each individual partner as they might be if the partner could continue to act selfishly while the rest cooperated.

7. Chapter 3 of Schnelling 1978 presents an eloquent analysis of situations in which "rational self interested" individual behavior leads to less-than-optimum results for all and must be tempered.

References

Axelrod, Robert. *The Evolution of Cooperation.* New York: Basic Books, Inc., 1984.

Cowan, Dale H. *Preferred Provider Organizations.* Rockville, MD: Aspen Systems Corp., 1984.

Davis, L. J. "The M.D. Who Would Be a Tycoon." *New York Times Magazine* (25 September 1988): 28.

Deutsch, Morton. *The Resolution of Conflict.* New Haven, CT: Yale University Press, 1973.

Fuchs, Victor R. *The Health Economy.* Cambridge, MA: Harvard University Press, 1986.

Goldsmith, Jeff Charles. *Can Hospitals Survive?* Homewood, IL: Dow-Jones-Irwin, 1981.

Johnston, Russell, and Paul R. Lawrence. "Beyond Vertical Integration: The Rise of the Value Adding Partnership." *Harvard Business Review* 66 (July–August 1988): 94, 98–99.

Kriesberg, Louis. *Social Conflicts,* 2d ed. Englewood Cliffs, NJ: Prentice-Hall, 1982.

McManis, Gerald L. "Evolving Health Care Systems of the 1990s." *Clinical Management Review* (January–February 1987): 17, 20–21.

Porter, Michael E. *Competitive Advantage.* New York: Macmillan, Inc., 1985.

Schelling, Thomas C. *Micromotives and Macrobehavior.* New York: W. W. Norton & Co., 1978.

Senge, Peter, and Diane Asay. "Rethinking a Health Care System." *Healthcare Forum Journal* 31 (May–June 1988): 32.

Starr, Paul. *The Social Transformation of American Medicine.* New York: Basic Books, Inc., 1982.

Sugden, Robert. *The Economics of Rights, Cooperation and Welfare.* London: Basil Blackwell, 1986.

Part II

Management

Hospital managers who began their careers in the halcyon 1950s and 1960s confronted environments that were remarkably free of turmoil and conflict. Financial pressures were largely unknown; strategic and business plans were virtually absent from the executives' lexicon and were usually translated into decisions to expand facilities, programs, and services. It was assumed that cost-plus reimbursement would take care of equity and access. Quality management was not in vogue at that time, nor was it well understood.

Since then, shifts in institutional power have enabled CEOs to abandon "facilitative" roles for more powerful line positions. Simultaneously, emphasis on the business of health care has engendered different management styles, concerns, and methods that more closely resemble those of the corporate sector.

John R. Griffith (Chapter 6) recognizes the exceptionally complex structure of today's hospital and prescribes five factors that differentiate the well-managed community hospital: (1) Success is measured by market share at a satisfactory financial margin and an acceptable level of quality; (2) The business of a hospital is medical care, which means that doctors must be its allies; (3) Planning and budgeting decisions are the arena where trustees, executives, clinical professionals, and managers have their most frequent and meaningful collaboration; (4) Facts, and therefore information systems, are the key to successful planning and budgeting decisions; and (5) Rewards are routine and generous to members of the hospital team who contribute to overall success.

Howard S. Zuckerman (Chapter 7) examines the role of the CEO cast in terms of three metaphors: the *Perimeter Player*, who ensures that the organization is adaptive and responds to the external environment; the *Interior Designer*, who is concerned primarily with operations management issues; and the *Leader of the Band* to whom the basic values of the organization are entrusted.

Chapter 8 focuses on the role of physician leaders in hospital strategic decision making. Anthony R. Kovner and Martin J. Chin present a contingency model that is heavily dependent on physician leadership characteristics.

The role and function of middle management is a neglected aspect of organizational design and development. Arnold D. Kaluzny (Chapter 9) suggests various guidelines for executives and middle managers that will serve to enhance decision-making activities.

George C. Burke III and Michael O. Bice (Chapter 10) ask health executives to consider personal renewal and change in their own lives, which will enable them to breathe life into their institutions. They point out that numerous barriers interfere with executive renewal, including time pressures, fatigue, cultural factors, and trustee attitudes. The essay suggests various approaches that health care executives should consider.

Chapter 6

Principles of the Well-Managed Community Hospital

John R. Griffith

John R. Griffith is Andrew Pattullo Collegiate Professor, Department of Health Services Management and Policy, School of Public Health, The University of Michigan, Ann Arbor. He is a Fellow of the College.

This article was published in *Hospital & Health Services Administration* 34, no. 4 (Winter 1989).

Today's environment for operating community hospitals (American Hospital Association 1987a) is the most demanding in 50 years. Financial constraints are severe, medical staff relations are demanding, there is a nursing shortage, and quality and utilization standards are rising. Many hospitals and hospital executives are in trouble. Yet some hospitals are doing very well. Their debt ratios are low; their market share is rising; their surplus funds are growing; doctors, nurses, and patients seek them out; and their executives are well paid and happy.

The difference between the successful and the unsuccessful hospital may be luck as well as management, but in some cases management is obviously different. The right decisions get made, on time, without rancor. The management recognizes individual needs and deals with them effectively. The various services are responsive to one another, and requests are met promptly and accurately. As a result, work environment is more attractive to doctors and nurses, quality of work is superior, patients are more satisfied, demand is higher, and costs are lower. The position of the institution relative to its competition improves. Underlying this ability to make the right decisions and to respond effectively is an organization design—a framework of information, communication, procedures, and traditions that stimulates a more effective decision-making process. Behind the successful design is a body of guiding principles influencing the organization's performance in the same sense that the genetic code influences the biological organism.

Five Principles

The principles of the well-managed community hospital must relate an exceptionally complicated organization to an environment that is unusually dynamic and demanding. For the hospital to be successful, these principles must be valid in the context of people who can support or threaten the hospital's continued existence (Blair 1988). It goes almost without saying that principles coordinating the perspectives of large numbers of people must be consistent over time. Perhaps less obvious is that they must also be integrated; excellence on one or two of the principles is not effective if others are ignored. They must also be understood and therefore they must be simple; large numbers of trustees, managers, and doctors must know the principles well enough for them to guide daily decisions. Principles used in this way must be valid at a level more abstract than *what* a hospital does (expands, merges, divests, relocates, etc.), focusing instead on *how* to change (identifying and evaluating variation; selecting, retaining, and diffusing successful models) (Aldrich 1987).

As the principles are applied to different parts of the hospital, they are expanded with examples and specific applications. Each solution to a recurring problem, such as a budget process to control costs or a planning process to support recruitment, takes on its own life and becomes rich with detail. The result expands to a book, or even a library. The principles themselves become only the common core or essence of the management philosophy. I believe the following five premises comprise the essence that distinguishes today's well-managed community hospitals.

- Success is measured by market share at a satisfactory financial margin and an acceptable level of quality.
- The business of a hospital is medical care, and doctors must be its allies.
- Planning and budgeting decisions are the arena where trustees, executives, clinical professionals, and managers have their most frequent and meaningful collaboration.
- Facts, and therefore information systems, are the key to successful planning and budgeting decisions.
- Rewards are routine and generous to members of the hospital team who contribute to overall success.

1. Success is measured by market share at a satisfactory financial margin and an acceptable level of quality.

Success is defined by the achievement of goals, and it is important to understand what these goals are and how achievement is measured. Success occurs because the institution emphasizes responsiveness to change. A declining or senescent hospital is one that has lost that innovative ability. Life cycles and declines of organizations occur, in part, because the organization outgrows its ability to change (McKelvey and Aldrich 1983).

One important aspect of avoiding senescence is finding an easily understood central measure of how well the organization is maintaining the overall dynamic equilibrium. The choices are market share, profit, and quality, and the answer depends on the corporate structure. In for-profit enterprises, profit is the central measure. It is the recurring concern that influences all management decisions because, despite its limitations, it summarizes the interest of the owners. Much of the debate and thought surrounding for-profit decision making is actually about the limitations of the central measure, such as the risks associated with forecasts, the conflicts between short- and long-run profitability, and the trade-offs between owners' goals, workers' goals, and social goals such as quality. The use of profit as a central measure does not eliminate or simplify these important issues. Rather it provides a focusing objective that identifies and illuminates them.

The central measure for not-for-profit community hospitals should be market share. The hospital's owners are the community, and the success of the hospital is properly measured by the community's willingness to use it in preference to competing alternatives. Adoption of the market-share measure as central focuses the efforts of the governing board and management on the owners' interests and creates a criterion for appropriately subordinating other important goals. The more patient care needs a hospital fills, the more patients it attracts, and the more successful it is. The more patients a hospital attracts, the more doctors and other clinical professionals it will need. The better the hospital fills the needs of clinical professionals, the more of their effort or resources it will attract, and the more patients it will be able to serve.

Profit, although essential to long-term success and frequently proposed as the central measure for not-for-profit hospitals, should become an important but subordinated consideration. Profit is not what the owners are seeking. (If they were, presumably they would reorganize in a for-profit structure.) The minimum profit necessary to sustain and expand market share must be earned, but beyond that, emphasis on profit can lead to the discontinuance of unprofitable services, inconvenience to some community members, and a reduced market share (Griffith 1987).

Quality of care is an essential but subordinated consideration in both for-profit and not-for-profit structures. Minimum acceptable quality—that which would be acceptable to the participants for themselves or their loved ones—is always required, but the maximization of quality should be subordinate to the maximization of market share. Practically, quality is such a vast and confusing subject (Donabedian 1980) that it cannot be measured well enough to be the central measure. Philosophically, one should not maximize quality beyond the point where it causes a loss of market share. The question is: Whose quality standard is to prevail in cases of dispute? the technocrat's or the patient's? By setting market share as the central measure, we endorse the latter.

It is useful to understand some of the implications of the market-share measure. It is a practical admission that subjects the hospital to the discipline of the marketplace. It is not inconsistent with older notions of "need" or "community benefit," if one assumes that the customers are the best people to define their needs and benefits. By defining the mission, it can be adjusted to specific markets. A hospital with a charitable mission, for example, might define the market for charity (poor people), and measure its share of that market. The process for a children's hospital is analogous. Similarly, one might aggregate several specific missions and markets. The principle suggests that selected missions should be judged for practicality—whether profit and quality constraints can both be met—and also by comparison with the market-share possibilities of other missions.

Several other important but subordinate measures fit easily into a scheme of maximizing market share, subject to necessary profit and acceptable quality. Measures of productivity and customer satisfaction become important means to the end. Cost, in particular, assumes new conceptual clarity. A service should be added or expanded if it can be produced and sold at a price the community wishes to pay, (that is, a competitive price) because that price will increase market share.

Having a central measure does not automate the decision process, but it clarifies the debate, and focuses attention on the proper decisions. It also clarifies the job of the executive. The executive has to keep the idea of market share as the measure of success in front of everybody from the trustees to the porters. Then he or she must devise procedures that produce a steady flow of market-share-increasing proposals.

2. The business of a hospital is medical care, which means that doctors must be its allies.

The buyers and users of hospital services are increasingly articulate about what they want. They want high-quality care at the lowest possible price, and they will increase the market share of any hospital they believe provides it. Obviously, doctors and nurses are essential to building market share, but the premise is more complex than it seems. It actually has three parts.

a. Medical care—any hands-on patient care, not just traditional hospital services—is the appropriate business of hospitals. People do not come to hospitals because they want a bed; they come because they want medical care. Communities operate hospitals because they want to recruit doctors and have access to medical care at both outpatient and inpatient levels. Therefore, the adequacy of medical care in every aspect is the appropriate concern of the hospital governing board and raises the question of how to develop relationships with doctors and other professionals so that the community gets what it wants.

b. Medical care is the unique business of hospitals. Businesses or missions outside the broad definition of medical care are extraneous. Hospitals need to be quite careful about the risks of entering businesses outside medical care. Prudent trustees and executives immedi-

95

ately question their ability to run businesses other than their own unique business.

c. One cannot run any organization where the mission is at odds with the people who control the core technology. Therefore, doctors and nurses have to be the allies of hospitals. These professionals obviously have certain rights. Among these are the rights to a reasonable income and lifestyle, and the right to use, within established limits, their professional skills. They also have rights to professional recognition and to participation in decision making. Alliance begins with the mutual recognition of rights (Wegmiller 1988).

With physicians, the two points that seem to cause the greatest confusion are the hospital's right to recruit and reward physicians meeting community needs and the doctor's right to a competitive income and a practice comparable to his or her peers. Doctors obviously also have a unique business of medical care. It is necessary to define the contributions of both doctor and hospital so that they become complementary, rather than conflicting. This can be done if the hospital accepts an obligation in its recruitment commitments to help the doctor achieve his or her monetary and professional goals, so long as these are consistent with the marketplace and prevailing standards of practice. The doctor accepting privileges at a well-managed hospital can assume that obligation will be honored, but he or she must also assume that the hospital will resist efforts to earn excessive compensation by exploiting patients or to endanger the quality of care. The alliance is formed on just these agreements.

Nursing presents many parallels. Well-managed hospitals do not have permanent nursing shortages (American Hospital Association 1987b). When shortages threaten, they examine work conditions, professional opportunities, and compensation and make successful adjustments so that they can recruit. They form an alliance with their nurses toward their mutual goal of improving patient care. The well-managed hospital must form alliances not with just any doctor or nurse, but with the most suitable and best qualified available. Thus the hospital is usually the suitor, even in cases where the profession is in oversupply. One key to the hospital's suit is the existence of a medical staff plan and a nurse staffing plan that guarantees each doctor and nurse adequate work and sufficient income. A second key is the operation of a high-quality overall program and the opportunity to associate with like-minded peers. The third is the opportunity to participate meaningfully in decisions affecting the mutual future (Griffith 1987). Meaningful participation implies that all professional opinions can be freely expressed and objectively received. That is, it implies that the interprofessional bigotry and sexism that plagues us has no place and will be systematically discouraged.

If these keys are well implemented, there need be no theoretical or inherent conflict between the hospital and its professional staffs. Although disagreements will certainly arise, they can be resolved by applying the market share maximization goal as a mutual benefit criterion. The goals of good professionals and the hospital goal of increased market share must be made synergistic, rather than competing. The principle recognizes that qualified professionals attract market share, and if the organization is carefully structured and managed, high market share increases each professional's rewards.

The role of the executive who successfully fulfills this premise is to recruit wisely, keep operations effective, and integrate doctors and nurses into all the hospital's decisions. Most of the rewards that affect the hospital's marginal ability to recruit are nonmonetary. The first reward that distinguishes one hospital from another is often the effectiveness of its clinical and plant services. At bottom, then, this premise implies sound general management. The second most important reward may be assurance of participation in the organization's decisions. Broad participation in decisions becomes possible when the central measure is clear. It becomes mandatory with a commitment to a decision-making criterion of mutual benefit.

Executives who cannot form the alliance, or cannot implement it as well as the competition, face serious problems. Often the steps necessary to provide income, respect, and participation to clinical professionals lie outside the clinical activities themselves, in finance, budgeting procedures, recruitment and training policies, medical staff organization, information systems, or the corporate culture.

3. Planning and budgeting decisions are the arena where trustees, executives, clinical professionals, and managers have their most frequent and meaningful collaboration.

The first two principles imply an organization that is broadly participative in form and is coordinated by widespread understanding of the central measure. They suggest a cooperative or a social club with little or no specialization of function or role—models too simple for the modern hospital. In reality, there are several kinds of decisions involved in running a complex organization, and there is role specialization for the participants. It is possible conceptually to classify decisions by level of abstraction from the day-to-day work, or conversely, by their centrality to the owners' needs.

1. The most abstract from the workplace and most central to the owners is the setting of the mission and the definition of its measure.
2. Decisions about process, accountability structures, communications channels, and information systems come next. These identify who will translate goals to actions.
3. Resource allocation decisions are in the third group, beginning with the translation of the mission to the long-range plan and then to a capital budget and an operating budget.
4. Procedural decisions for specific tasks and recurring decisions of operations, including the professional decisions regarding individual patients are the most concrete and the most removed from the direct surveillance of the owners.

There are relatively few decisions in the first two groups, many more in group three, and very large numbers in group four. The traditional focus of the professions is on group four, where they often have specific legal mandates. Group one is the traditional focus of the governing board, and group two of the executive. The resource allocation decisions in group three are frequently the source of disagreement. In a sound theory, no level of decision should be considered the exclusive domain of one group of people. However, the practicalities of time constraints and limited interests make careful selectivity of participation essential.

The resource allocation decisions in group three offer important practical opportunities to broaden participation. Quality, cost, marketing, and potential tangible rewards are bound up in these decisions. Everyone's interest is visibly at stake, and to the extent feasible, everyone should participate. Using well-designed planning and budgeting procedures and extensive information bases, these decisions can be debated by many members of the organization. Doing so has multiple advantages. It allows realistic participation, provides an intrinsic reward to clinical professionals, encourages innovation, and improves the fact base. It also can be used to build consensus and train leaders. Participation in planning and budgeting decisions offers a concrete introduction to the complexities of management, illustrates the importance of group four decisions, and encourages sensitivity to the more abstract group one and two decisions. With modern information technology and a well-designed process, it is not difficult to allow at least 50 doctors, nurses, trustees, and executives to be involved in the annual environmental assessment, plan revision, and budget guideline setting that begins the budget cycle. The entire management group and most key professionals outside management should be involved by the conclusion of the budget cycle.

The implication of this approach to resource allocation decisions is that executives must pay very close attention to the process, structure, and information decisions in group two. It is environmental reality that determines good resource allocation decisions. Knowledge of this reality is as important as the skills of the individuals who make the decisions. To get successful results, the executive must pay more attention to the process of planning and budgeting and the quality of the information available to support the decisions than to the decisions themselves.

That is to say the executive's job is to get the right facts to the table with the right players at it. The players, not the executive, will make the resource allocation decisions, and their collective judgment will be superior to any individual's. While this formulation of decision making may seem radical, it is actually consistent with established thought on management and the executive role. Mintzberg (1973), for example, identified ten interlocking roles, which he groups as "interpersonal," "informational," and "decisional." "Resource allocator" was only one of four decisional roles. While Mintzberg's manager is not voiceless in resource allocation decisions, particularly at the most fundamental or strategic level, it is clear that he or she must do more structuring, listening, fact finding, answering, and negotiating than ordering or deciding (Mintzberg 1973). More recent work remains consistent with this view (Zuckerman 1989).

The executive must avoid the danger of being manipulative. As leaders mature in the clinical group, their skills will be required in group two decisions, and their interests will broaden. The truly skillful executive will encourage their participation in group two decisions, and they will find little to criticize as they review the history of these decisions.

4. Facts, and therefore information systems, are the key to successful planning and budgeting decisions.

Objective information builds consensus and drives good decisions. The more of it the decision makers use, the better their decisions will get. The process for resource allocation decisions must meet three almost equally critical goals. It must ensure that overall control of the organization remains in the hands of the trustees. It must incorporate environmental realities, including realistic limitations on individual and group performance. Finally, it must be open to near-universal participation among management and interested physicians yet protected from both selfishness and well-intentioned naiveté (Austin 1988). This balance is achieved by using an explicit system of control and review that relies heavily on the distribution of facts. The facts required are many and varied, and they must be presented so that they are communicated quickly and reliably. A well-designed computerized information system is now essential to do the job in all but the smallest organizations (Griffith 1987).

The first job of the control system is to coordinate the planning activities in a coherent whole. This is most easily done by having the governing board set explicit goals on the basic measures of success at the outset of the budget cycle. These goals, usually called the budget guidelines, specify limits on next year's costs, profits, and capital expenditures. Ideally, each guideline should be set in the light of measures directly linked to future market-share considerations. They may also highlight general concerns or priorities, such as deficiencies in quality or service that must be addressed. (Specific concerns will be added at appropriate organization levels as the decision requirements are transmitted (Berman, Weeks, and Kukla 1986).)

Setting the guidelines is the board's biggest opportunity to carry out its trust to the community. Directly or indirectly, the board determines the scope of services, quality, amenities, cost, profitability, debt ratio, and risk exposure of the institution. The budget guidelines must also be fact-driven. They require clear presentation and analysis of three major sources of information: (1) surveillance of the external environment, (2) summary of the actual performance from last year drawn from the previous budget and financial reports, and (3) integration of past decisions not yet implemented but recorded in the long-range plan. Each source now requires a multipart data base. Quality, market trends, patient satisfaction, employee and doctor satisfaction, and price are as important as cost data. The computer capabilities are used for rapid access, thorough analysis, and effective display.

The better the data base, the less acrimonious the debate. The risks of selfishness and naiveté are overcome by using objective facts and by competitive review within the organization. Since costs, profit, and capital expenditures are set in the guidelines, all budget requests are subject to scrutiny at higher levels as the totals are compiled and compared to the guides. In a well-established system, the governing board's role in approving the final budget is pro forma; the guidelines have been met and the arguments have been resolved by collegial review.

Modern information systems are essential to meet the information needs of a large number of decision makers without losing the central focus on market share. The automation of many professional and managerial activities and the development of extensive marketing data bases have expanded the kinds of information that now can be made routinely available. Data base management systems can now organize, retrieve, and analyze the information quickly and economically. The technology to do this is evolving rapidly, and the ability of management to use the information naturally lags its availability. For some years to come, the best hospitals will be investing and improving in their information systems. The executive's role is to see that these investments and improvements occur in a timely and competitive manner.

5. Rewards are routine and generous to members of the hospital team who contribute to overall success.

The final premise rests on a fundamental truth about the behavior of people in organizations. Rewards and incentives are essential to excellence. Sanctions, coercion, and threats can, at the very best, achieve mediocrity; they will probably do worse. This suggests that hospitals must offer deliberate and identifiable rewards for loyalty, for participation, and for contribution to increased market share. The basic employment or privileges contract and the corporate culture must be modified to include these rewards and to establish them as incentives.

It is not difficult to do this once one recognizes that money is not the only important compensation (Strasser and Bateman 1983). Other factors, such as professional opportunity and satisfaction, answers to work-related questions, participation in key decisions, and a congenial workplace, are always important when clinical professionals select a hospital. Given that competition will tend to erase any difference in monetary compensation, these other factors become a critical weapon. They offer the opportunity to maintain the margin that allows selection of the best and most empathetic people. The hospital attracts workers who believe in the first four principles and apply them in daily actions. The principles are soon embedded in the corporate culture. People who disagree with them tend to go somewhere else. A program that identifies the opportunities for reward and uses them to reinforce behavior that leads to increased market share is the next step.

Installing both intangible rewards and monetary rewards in a hospital is a matter of further use of the group two decisions. Training programs for leaders should reinforce the key ideas of the system. It may not matter that most of these are on-the-job. The critical factor may be that the promising beginner is recognized and moved through assignments with increasing responsibility and reward. Formal training may be necessary where large numbers of people are concerned. It should emphasize both operational process—correct group four decisions—and management processes—supervisory skills, human relations, and the correct use of information. The measures of performance, once understood, are their own reward. Recognition and promotion based on these measures quickly imbeds them in the corporate culture.

Hospitals that achieve a program of incentives and rewards will have a major advantage; they will have their pick of the best physicians, nurses, and employees generally. The health care world has become one of sanctions, punishments, and negative feedback. The litany of malpractice charges, utilization review queries, professional review organization denials, and publication of mortality statistics in today's world has created a climate that is inherently negative and discouraging. The organization must be used as a shelter and an example of a better concept: a place where good is done and work is enjoyed. The most powerful reward we have is the satisfaction from giving good medical care as a loving act.

The executive must build a system that allows everyone to do good work and by doing so, win both emotional and monetary rewards. A program that also makes sophisticated use of monetary reward is the next step. There is as yet no publicized answer or model.

Implementation

A pragmatic approach might be to try these five principles and see if they can be made to produce the desired results, that is, increase the hospital's market share, subject to constraints on profit and quality. Begin at the group two decisions (those dealing with process, accountability structures, communications channels, and information systems), in particular by disseminating the market-share and profit measures. Facts on cost, quality, and satisfaction should follow as soon as possible. Educate people by feeding them facts, and build on that by deliberately improving the decision processes and accountability structure to use the information.

There is an inescapable boot-strapping quality to the initial efforts. The immediate goal is to produce an improved process leading to a long-range plan, including a preliminary medical staff plan and a prudent financial plan. The information necessary to produce this plan will be incomplete. The act of planning itself will produce extensive demand for improvement of information leading to a component of the long-range plan directed at information systems improvement. The overall plan, with its several components, must be understood as living documents, subject to annual revision and extension, but serving in the meantime as a device to coordinate efforts to improve market share. In other words, start by implementing a fact-based, market-driven planning system, and let the market and the facts direct the decisions that an increasing number of people participate in. The success of the theory is measured by market-share increases.

In some situations, substantial preliminary work may be necessary. The chief executive must be both committed and professionally capable. The governing board must be committed to the principles and the demonstration. The board's bylaws, and those of the medical staff, may need review. Legal counsel is required to avoid the antitrust implications of a poorly developed medical staff plan. A small cadre of medical staff leaders and upper-level managers must be educated in the principles. In some cases, reeducation or replacement of key leaders may be required.

In many hospitals, consultants and outside management development programs will be necessary. In the most complex cases, merger or contract management may be needed to gain the skills required. The contribution of a larger, more experienced organization may be the only way to reeducate the people involved, or to avoid an impractically long learning period. The record of multihospital systems is not encouraging however. Few have demonstrated the growth of subsidiaries or affiliates, and some have encountered serious difficulties at both unit and corporate levels (Shortell 1988). Certainly a hospital shopping for a partner would be well advised to ask for evidence of real and steady improvement in performance of the system and its units, as measured by market share, profit, and quality.

References

Aldrich, H. "New Paradigms for Old: The Population Perspective's Contribution to Health Services Research." *Medical Care Review* 44 (Fall 1987): 257–77.

American Hospital Association. *Hospital Statistics.* Chicago: The Association, 1987a. p. ix. The definition includes virtually all nonfederal short-term inpatient institutions except mental.

———. *Nursing Demand.* Chicago: The Association, 1987b.

Austin, C. J. *Information Services for Health Services Administration,* 3d ed. Ann Arbor, MI: Health Administration Press, 1988.

Berman, H., L. Weeks, and S. Kukla. *The Financial Management of Hospitals,* 6th ed. Ann Arbor, MI: Health Administration Press, 1986.

Blair, J. D. "Too Many on the Seesaw: Shareholder Diagnosis and Management for Hospitals." *Hospital & Health Services Administration* 33 (Summer 1988): 152–66.

Donabedian, A. *Explorations in Quality Assessment and Monitoring. Vol. 1, The Definition of Quality and Approaches to Its Assessment.* Ann Arbor, MI: Health Administration Press, 1980.

Griffith, J. R. *The Well-Managed Community Hospital.* Ann Arbor, MI: Health Administration Press, 1987.

McKelvey, B., and H. Aldrich. "Populations, Natural Selection, and Applied Organizational Science." *Administrative Science Quarterly* 28 (March 1983): 101–28.

Mintzberg, H. *The Nature of Managerial Work.* Englewood Cliffs, NJ: Prentice-Hall, 1973.

Shortell, S. M. "The Evolution of Hospital Systems: Unfulfilled Promises and Self-Fulfilling Prophecies." *Medical Care Review* 45 (Fall 1988): 177–214.

Strasser, S., and T. Bateman. "Perception and Motivation in Health Care Management." In *Health Care Management, A Text in Organization Theory and Behavior*, edited by S. Shortell and A. Kaluzny. New York: John Wiley & Sons, 1983.

Wegmiller, D. "Boards Must Address Regional Issues." *Health Management Quarterly* 10 (Fall 1988): 3–5.

Zuckerman, H. S. "Redefining the Role of the CEO: Challenges and Conflicts." *Hospital & Health Services Administration* 34 (Spring 1989): 25–38.

Chapter 7

Redefining the Role of the CEO: Challenges and Conflicts

Howard S. Zuckerman

Howard S. Zuckerman is Professor, School of Health Administration and Policy, College of Business, Arizona State University. He is a Faculty Associate of the College.

This article was published in *Hospital & Health Services Administration* 34, no. 1 (Spring 1989).

Continuing and often dramatic changes in the external environment and within health services organizations have altered the context for strategic decision making. Pressure to contain the rate of increase of health care costs; the need to respond to both competition and regulation; and significant changes in the payment system, which have altered the incentives for organizational and managerial behavior, serve to create a turbulent environment. Major demographic and epidemiological changes, a threatening political climate, and a reemergence of social issues add to external uncertainty. Further, economic and ethical issues associated with technology and growing demands for organizational and professional accountability confound the environment surrounding health care.

At the same time, health care organizations have become larger and more complex, calling for increased coordination, information, and communication. Tensions among occupational groups, multiple and sometimes conflicting relationships among key organizational actors, and redistribution of power also represent substantial changes within health care organizations.

These changes in the external environment, as well as those internal to the organization, suggest the growing centrality of the role of the chief executive officer. The CEO sits at the intersection of the organization and its environment and, simultaneously, at that of the managerial level of the organization with the technical core where the work gets done (Parsons 1960). The CEO may be seen at the "strategic apex" of the organization (Mintzberg 1979), serving as the focal point for strategic decisions that will enable the organization to adapt to its environment and to manage itself internally. Likewise, the CEO bears major responsibility for integrating the elements of the organization in pursuit of its mission and goals, consistent with the organization's underlying values and needs of key stakeholders.

The evolving roles of the CEO may be cast in terms of three categories. First, there is a set of activities involving adaptation of the organization to its external environment. Such activities include assessment of the environment, recognition that the environment-organization linkage is a two-way interaction, and development of adaptive strategies. This role of the CEO is entitled *Perimeter Player*. Second, the CEO must tend to the internal operations of the organization. Involved herein are such activities as designing the structure of the organization; assuring attention to key tasks such as management of costs and quality; maintaining requisite communication, coordination, and information flow; managing conflict; allocating resources; and managing human resources. This role of the CEO is entitled *Interior Designer*. Finally, the CEO is seen as *Leader of the Band*. In this role, the CEO provides the strategic vision and direction for the organization. Further, the CEO serves as keeper of the corporate values, assuring that the organization remains true to its mission and responsive to its key influential constituencies.

This article outlines and highlights the key elements of three emerging roles, particularly in the context of hospitals and hospital-based systems. It is not intended to be an exhaustive treatment, but rather serves as an outline of the CEO as the increasingly central figure in health care organizations facing dynamic external and internal environments. Finally, the article addresses both the challenges and the conflicts as the CEO plays out these multiple roles.

The Perimeter Player—
Adapting to a Changing Environment

Scanning the Environment

The CEO must assure a continuing outward look to identify and assess developments in the environment that may affect the organization. The nature of the environment makes this function more important than ever. The CEO must, through his/her own networks as well as through resources of other organization stakeholders, monitor relevant signs and signals from the external environment.

It has become quite clear that health care is part of the economic, social, and political fabric of society and is directly affected by environmental change. For example, when the U.S. auto industry lost ground in its ability to compete in world markets, there were plant closings and attendant loss of jobs. Over time, many auto workers lost their health insurance but not their need for medical care. The loss of benefits led to the deferral of needed care. When care was finally sought, these workers often required more intensive services, yet did not have the ability to pay. Health care organizations then were faced with sicker patients without insurance. It is for reasons such as this that scanning and understanding environmental changes and interrelationships will be of fundamental importance in the years ahead.

Influencing the Environment

The linkage between environment and organization should be viewed as a two-way interaction. That is, the adaptive manager not only will react to the environment but will seek to influence it as well. In essence, the CEO has a role as an advocate for the organization, for the constituencies that it represents, and for the populations that it serves. CEOs should and do seek to influence the formulation and implementation of public policy. Health care organizations are fundamentally community service organizations, designed to serve the public interest (Vladeck 1986). Thus, CEOs have a legitimate responsibility to seek to affect policy decisions that, in turn, affect the public interest. The call for political, social, and economic response to such issues as

107

care of the indigent, financing services for the elderly, and the uninsured population highlight this aspect of the role.

Lessons from Other Industries

Health and hospital care may be characterized as having many unique attributes. The system of financing, relations with federal and state government, governance structures, arrangements with physicians and medical staffs, and, in many cases, linkages with the church are among these special characteristics. However, it is also true that health and hospital care has attributes similar to those of other industries. There are, in fact, other industries that bear striking similarity with regard to structure, strategy, and focus on service. Other industries have gone through or are going through comparable evolutions and transformations, often for the same reasons. Such other industries have moved along a similar continuum from regulation toward competition and deregulation. There are valuable lessons to be learned, both positive and negative, from the experiences of other industries.

This suggests that we need an expansion of the field of vision to put health care in a larger context. Specifically, it could be argued that there is merit in comparing industry structure in fields such as airlines, banking, and communication, both prior to and following deregulation, and comparing changes to those being developed and implemented in health care. For example, removal of barriers to entry and exit, new entrants, mergers and consolidations, introduction of price competition, and elimination of guaranteed revenue streams characterize some of the structural shifts common to health care and other industries. Likewise, it is instructive to observe shifts in the strategies of these industries as they sought to respond to many of the same kinds of environmental forces and pressures. Such strategic shifts include greater attention to costs and cost structures, more emphasis on marketing and distribution, use of strategic alliances and networking, diversification, new pricing mechanisms, and increased reliance on information technology. Further, changes in the performance of these industries is also of interest. The effects of changing strategy and structure on financial performance, market share, productivity, resource utilization, quality/safety, and customer satisfaction within these other industries could provide indicators that might be useful in forecasting the effects of such changes within health and hospital care.

Broadening the Boundaries of the Field

As yet another element of this adaptive role, the CEO must lead the organization toward redefining the boundaries of the field. It continues to be important to identify other existing organizations that are now or may become collaborators or competitors to evaluate the relative strengths and weaknesses of such organizations and to assess the implications of their strategies. It is equally important, however, that the CEO assess the strengths and weaknesses of his/her organization as well and identify those competencies and capabilities that are distinctive.

Beyond this, it is also important to identify and assess new or potential entrants to the field as well as those organizations offering substitute services and products (Porter 1980). These new players often fill market niches at the expense of existing organizations. In broadening the boundaries, careful consideration should be given to changing roles among suppliers and buyers. Suppliers, for example, are becoming increasingly concentrated, which may serve to increase their relative bargaining power. Further, there is some evidence of a threat of forward integration by suppliers into delivery of service. It is quite clear that there has already been a significant shift of power from the provider sector to the buyers of health care. In addition, there is some indication of backward integration by buyers into the delivery arena. The emergence of new participants and changing roles of existing participants would seem to call for a broadening of the boundaries of the field and ongoing, systematic assessment of the roles of these various players.

Adaptive Strategies

Among the leading strategies for adaptation to a changing environment are horizontal integration, vertical integration, and diversification. Horizontal integration, involving organizations at the same stage of the production process (e.g., hospital linkages) will undoubtedly continue. The intent of such integration is to achieve economies of scale, improve utilization of resources, enhance access to capital, increase political power, and extend the scope of the market. It is such horizontal integration that, until very recently, has characterized the thrust of the development and growth of multiple hospital systems. Much attention is now being devoted to vertical integration, linking organizations at related stages of the production process. Such integration aims to ensure source of supply and/or markets for services or products (Conrad et al. 1988). Vertical integration would thus move beyond inpatient acute care toward multiple levels of care and a more comprehensive range of services. A third strategy involves diversified activities that may or may not be related to health care. Diversification may involve new products or services, new production technologies, and/or entry into new markets (Clement 1988). Diversification has been viewed as a means to generate new sources of revenue and to provide opportunities for growth and expansion.

It is anticipated that a good deal of the horizontal and vertical integration will be operationalized along regional lines. Regions, which may be defined as metropolitan, local, or state, will be organized around common market areas. Emerging regional networks or clusters are aimed at protecting and dominating markets, a strategy similar to the "hub and spoke" approach used by the airlines. Such models appear consistent with how care is delivered and where service populations, hospitals, and physicians are located. It is also presumed that these regional networks will be organized in the context of some form of managed care, calling for the linkage of delivery and financing. The evidence to date suggests that our ability to link financing and delivery is not very well developed. Nevertheless, the adaptive CEO will likely see such linkage as essential and will not deal with the question of whether, but rather how, such linkage is to be accomplished.

The challenges and opportunities of horizontal and vertical integration as well as diversification are not without conflict, however. For example, as regional networks evolve and seek increases in market penetration and market share, it is necessary that, given environmental conditions, such increases for one organization will likely come at the expense of another. Some organizations will be hurt in this process. For many, this will be a new and often painful experience. Even more important will be the effects of such efforts on the communities and populations served and the purchasers who share in the financing.

As efforts continue to link financing with delivery, the issue of conflicting incentives emerges as organizations attempt to be both providers and insurers (Tresnowski 1986). That is, as providers, the motivation is to increase volume and utilize services; as insurers, the motivation is quite the opposite, thus the incentives are contradictory. It may be that vertically integrated systems, with multiple levels of care and the opportunity to move patients within the production process to the most appropriate placement, enable convergence of the incentives for delivery and financing. While the financing/delivery linkage appears to be pivotal, difficult and expensive lessons are being learned about product development, marketing, and the time and expense of introducing insurance products.

Diversification represents a particular source of concern and potential conflict. It has been argued that organizations should do what they do best and not get into businesses they do not know how to manage (Drucker 1980). Further, organizations have been cautioned not to be distracted from their core business and that diversification should be consistent both with purpose and capability. At least some diversification efforts may hurt rather than help the core business. For example, diversified activities that require subsidies may prove to be a drain on the very business they were supposed to assist. In addition, there is a question as to the public perception of the appropriateness of some areas of diversification, particularly nonhealth-related endeavors. To the extent that health care organizations compete with local tax paying businesses, diversification may fuel arguments for elimination of tax-exempt status. Entry into diversified businesses requires very careful evaluation of what makes a difference between success and failure, what constitutes competitive advantage, what distinctive competencies are required, and whether the benefits will exceed the costs.

Finally, adaptation to a changing environment requires a shift from a product orientation to a market orientation. A market orientation requires that a delivery organization understands who its customers are, how they may be characterized, and how their needs and demands can be identified. It is essential to segment the components of the market, specify what factors will influence target populations, and then, and only then, develop and market products and services. This orientation will undoubtedly place greater emphasis on the market research function.

In sum, as *Perimeter Player,* the CEO, through personal activities and through encouragement of others, is thus engaged in a variety of actions and approaches designed to enable the organization to adapt to a changing and uncertain environment.

The Interior Designer— Organizing the Organization

Managing Costs and Utilization

The management of cost will continue to be one of the major concerns for the CEO and for the organization. The cost issue will remain problematic as long as the cost of health care rises as a proportion of the gross national product, the medical care price index increases faster than inflation, personal health expenditures grow, and corporate health benefits costs climb. With the governmental component of health expenditures exceeding 40 percent, federal, state, and local concern undoubtedly will continue. Business and industry, seeing health insurance premiums affect the prices of products and services and thus impede their ability to compete in world markets, will likewise continue to press for control of costs. The management of cost will be a central issue regardless of how the financing system evolves. That is, managing costs is fundamental to pricing in a competitive market, to being able to benefit from a regulated price structure, or to succeed under a capitated system.

Health care organizations will continue to be pushed to increase productivity, reduce excess capacity, and improve utilization of human, financial, and physical resources. Wide variation in utilization of services and facilities, observed virtually at every level of analysis (Griffith et al. 1981; Wennberg and

111

Gittelsohn 1973) remains a crucial concern. Admission rates, surgical inci-
dence rates, and per capita costs have been shown to vary widely within states,
regions, and across the country, thus far defying explanation. Importantly,
these variations have not been shown to be related to differences in health
status.

Managing Quality

Quality is reemerging as a major issue and will require substantial organizational attention. There is renewed focus on defining quality not only in the
inpatient setting but in alternative settings as well. It appears that quality no
longer will be defined only by physicians and hospitals, nor will it be defined
only in professional and technical terms. Purchasers, payers, and patients will
insist on participation in new definitions of quality. Further, such definitions
will include customer perception of and satisfaction with the quality of care
received.

Health care organizations will be obliged not merely to proclaim quality but
to demonstrate it through the use of objective measures. These measures
increasingly will focus on outcomes. Indeed, the development of outcome
indicators is the essence of the "Agenda for Change" of the Joint Commission
on Accreditation of Healthcare Organizations (Robinson 1988). In addition,
organizations will seek to make quality an integral part of the production and
distribution process along lines similar to those that Deming (1986) taught
the Japanese. Finally, organizations will see quality as a means to differentiate
themselves and also as a vehicle for competitive advantage.

Managing Human Resources

In many ways, success in managing cost and quality will be a function of an
organization's ability to manage its human resources. It will be increasingly
important to motivate employees, to exact commitment to the organization,
and to provide incentives to enhance productivity and performance. Organizations will need to encourage continuing educational and developmental programs, seeking to enable individuals to maximize their potential.

Health care organizations are called upon to reassess their responsibility to
employees. In *Service America!*, Albrecht and Zemke (1985) argue that employees should be seen as the "front line" in serving patients. In large part,
customer satisfaction is determined by how they are treated by employees. In
turn, how employees treat patients is influenced by how management treats
employees. This work, and others, would suggest that investment in human
resources is an important mechanism if an organization is to control its costs
effectively and enhance its quality.

The management of cost, quality, and human resources is not without conflict. For example, as efforts to control costs continue, what will be the impact on quality? Some of the recent evidence can be seen as unsettling (Shortell and Hughes 1988). As organizations seek to control costs, it is not uncommon to find cutbacks in programs and services, along with employee layoffs, among the tactics being used. How do such tactics relate to the values of health care organizations? How will organizations manage conflict between cost-control demands, on one hand, and the common role of the hospital as a major employer in the community on the other? How are the growing ethical, as well as economic, issues related to resource allocation, rationing of services, and caring for the indigent to be addressed? As decisions to merge or close facilities are made, how will such community issues as access to care and availability of services be reconciled?

It is not yet clear how physicians and hospital managers will react to the likely participation of buyers, insurers, employers, and other customers in the definition and assessment of quality. In addition, as the focus shifts toward outcome measures of quality, it will be important not to lose sight of the need to relate structure and process to such outcome measures. If, in fact, there is to be understanding of why outcomes are as they are, and if the requisite changes to improve outcomes are to be made, the relationship among all three factors must be taken into account.

Information Systems

The development of timely, accurate, and useful information systems is essential to both management of the internal organization and adaptation to the environment. Integrated clinical and financial information systems are pivotal to the effective management of costs and quality. Likewise, such systems are important for comparative analysis of performance within the organization and between organizations. In addition, to monitor the environment, assess competitors and collaborators, undertake industry analysis, and perform market research, a sound information system is crucial. It is the role of the manager to define information needs. Control cannot be abdicated to technicians who may or may not design systems consistent with the needs of management. If, in fact, systems to provide information, and not simply data, are to be designed, needs must be defined by the key users, namely, managers.

Structuring the Organization

In designing the organization for the future, the CEO must assure that the structure be flexible and adaptable. The demands of the environment and the interests of the internal organization require that there be both integration and differentiation (Lawrence and Lorsch 1967). Integration should facilitate achievement of overall organizational goals, enable coordination across the organization, and take advantage of synergies so that the whole is greater than the sum of its parts. At the same time, organizations need to be sufficiently differentiated so as to encourage innovation, creativity, and rapid response to environmental changes (Moore 1987). This point is of particular interest with regard to multiple hospital systems and other multicorporate organizations.

Spanning almost two decades, the research literature on systems consistently suggests that the promise of systems exceeds their performance (Zuckerman 1979; Ermann and Gabel 1984; Shortell 1988). It may well be that, at least in part, this results from such organizations being structured as systems, but not functioning as such. That is, they are not sufficiently integrated to take advantage of synergies, of economies of scale, and of opportunities for exchange of services and expertise across the organization. Such integration will continue to be important as pressure for economic and production efficiency grows. At the same time, the press toward regionalization, along with the need for rapid and flexible responses to market conditions, will require an appropriate balance of differentiation.

Involving Key Constituencies

Governance

In many ways, changes in the role of governance parallels the changing role of the CEO. That is, the role has become more demanding and challenging. As the environment has become turbulent, trustees often must deal with conflicting pressures concerning social imperatives, public expectations, community need, cost control, financing, quality assurance, and technological development, among others. As health care organizations have, in turn, become more complex, new relationships, authorities, and responsibilities are established, not always with great clarity. For example, in the context of multiunit organizations, one might well find governance structures for the local hospital, subsidiary corporation, regional office, and corporate system entity. How well integrated are those multiple levels of governance, and how are policy-formulation and decision-making functions divided? What levels of governance are best suited to address the key strategic issues facing the organization? Given the rapid and often dramatic changes in the environment and within organizations, to what extent are governance structures and processes keeping pace?

The CEO, as the key resource person for the board of trustees/directors, will be central to successful evolution and strengthening of the governance. It will be necessary to assure that focus in trustee selection is on performance and not merely representation. Trustee education will have to provide the requisite knowledge about the changing environmental and market conditions and the skill to deal with the inevitable conflicts involved in allocation of resources, policy formulation, and strategic decision making.

Physicians

A major challenge for CEOs will be the integration of physician and organizational interests. This will require new models for physician involvement in the governance and management of hospitals and hospital systems. The imperatives of managing costs and quality, of improving productivity and resource utilization, and of adaptive strategies such as vertical integration and managed care, cannot be achieved without such physician involvement. Physicians must play a significant role in policy formulation, decision making, resource allocation, and the formulation, implementation, and evaluation of organizational strategy. The underlying assumption is that the destinies of hospitals, hospital systems, and physicians are inextricably intertwined. These new relationships, while they will undoubtedly assume various forms and evolve in various ways over time, call for the development of mutual trust and commitment.

It will be necessary to specify the expectations and the anticipated benefits and costs of physician involvement, particularly in management. Clarity as to responsibilities, accountabilities, authorities, and relationships will be needed. The factors that facilitate or serve as barriers to physician involvement must be identified. A variety of models for physician roles in management are beginning to evolve. The characteristics and relative merits of these alternatives should be assessed, as should the conditions under which different models appear most appropriate. It will also be important to identify the skills and knowledge needed and for organizations to commit resources to the education and development of physicians assuming these emerging roles. A key issue lies in the incentives that will prove sufficiently powerful to attract physicians to such new roles.

As these arrangements evolve, it will be necessary to assure that a new dual structure is not created within our organizations, leading to duplication and conflict. While collaborative arrangements are desirable, it is likely that there will be competitive relationships in some areas. What is at issue is the management of these multiple relationships and the avoidance of "unnecessary" competition.

The Leader of the Band— Direction for the Future

It has been suggested that the CEO must lead the organization in adapting to the external environment and in managing the internal organization. The CEO also plays an overarching role, however, in providing strategic direction and vision to the organization, serving as keeper of the corporate values, and assuring that the organization achieves its mission.

The strategic vision for the organization requires that the CEO maintain a long-term view. Despite the many external and internal pressures that have been discussed, it is the CEO who must cling to the broad picture of the future. This means that the CEO cannot manage only with an eye toward the bottom line of the next quarter (Work et al. 1988). It means that the CEO must be prepared to make short-term sacrifices to secure long-term gains. It means that the CEO will stick with ideas likely to add value to the organization over time (Prokesch 1987).

The CEO plays the key role in ensuring that members of the organization know, understand, and accept the values of the organization. As keeper of the corporate values, the CEO must live the values of the organization, show their relevance in decision making, and integrate them into the evaluation and reward system of the organization (Rossy 1987). If such values are to have meaning, the behavior of the organization must be consistent with these values. Phrases such as "the customer comes first" has meaning only if customers are treated with respect and dignity. "We are a people-oriented company" has no meaning if people are treated as expendable. "We are a risk-taking, innovative company" has no meaning if the organization does not reward risk taking and innovation. Saying so does not make it so. In the long run, the extent to which managerial decision making reflects the basic values of the organization will be of fundamental importance (Bice 1986).

The CEO must assure that the organization is true to its values and aspirations, takes advantage of environmental and market opportunities, builds on competencies and resources, and meets its obligations to society (Andrews 1980). Health care organizations are first and foremost public service organizations, accountable to society in general and the communities they serve in particular. This does not underestimate the importance of economic responsibilities, but rather reminds us that no organization can sacrifice its basic values and remain viable over time (Kaluzny and Shortell 1987). The challenge to the CEO, then, is to lead the organization toward an appropriate balance to assure that it is true to its fundamental social mission while remaining sensitive and responsive to its economic burden.

Conclusion

We have viewed the evolving role of the CEO in terms of three metaphors: *Perimeter Player*, *Interior Designer*, and *Leader of the Band*. Each of the metaphors holds both challenges and conflicts. In light of a turbulent and often hostile environment, the *Perimeter Player* must ensure that the organization remains adaptive and responsive to changing external conditions. At the same time, the *Interior Designer* must manage and integrate the internal operations of the enterprise so as to achieve effectiveness and efficiency. In the face of environmental uncertainty and organizational complexity, the *Leader of the Band* is entrusted to maintain the basic values of the organization and to reflect such values in managerial decision making. It is the necessity to strike a balance among these multiple and often conflicting demands that perhaps represents the greatest challenge. Successfully meeting this challenge may well serve to reinforce the centrality of the CEO to health care organizations facing dynamic external and internal environments.

References

Albrecht, Karl, and Ron Zemke. *Service America!*, Homewood, IL: Dow Jones-Irwin, 1985.

Andrews, Kenneth R. *The Concept of Corporate Strategy* (revised edition). Homewood IL: Dow Jones-Irwin, 1980.

Bice, Michael O. "Corporate Cultures and Business Strategy: A Health Management Company Perspective." *Hospital & Health Services Administration* 31 (September–October 1984): 7–15.

Clement, Jan P. "Vertical Integration and Diversification of Acute Care Hospitals: Conceptual Definitions." *Hospital & Health Services Administration* 33 (Spring 1988): 99–110.

Conrad, Douglas A., Stephen S. Mick, Carolyn Watts Madden, and Geoffrey Hoare. "Vertical Structures and Control in Health Care Markets: A Conceptual Framework and Empirical Review." *Medical Care Review* 45 (Spring 1988): 49–100.

Deming, W. Edwards, *Out of the Crisis*. Cambridge, MA: MIT Press, 1986.

Drucker, Peter F. *Managing in Turbulent Times*. New York: Harper & Row, 1980.

Ermann, Dan, and Jon Gabel. "Multi-Hospital Systems: Issues and Empirical Findings." *Health Affairs* 3 (Spring 1984): 50–64.

Griffith, John R., Joseph D. Restuccia, Philip J. Tedeschi, Peter A. Wilson, and Howard S. Zuckerman. "Measuring Community Hospital Services in Michigan." *Health Services Research* 16 (Summer 1981): 135–60.

Kaluzny, Arnold D., and Stephen M. Shortell. "Creating and Managing Our Ethical Future." *Healthcare Executive* 2 (September–October 1987): 29–32.

Lawrence, Paul R., and Jay W. Lorsch. *Organization and Environment*. Homewood, IL: Dow Jones-Irwin, 1967.

Mintzberg, Henry. *The Structuring of Organizations.* Englewood Cliffs, NJ: Prentice-Hall, 1979.

Moore, Thomas. "Goodbye, Corporate Staff." *Fortune,* 21 December 1987.

Parsons, Talcott. *Structure and Process in Modern Societies.* Glencoe, IL: Free Press, 1960.

Porter, Michael. *Competitive Strategy.* New York: The Free Press, 1980.

Prokesch, Steven. "Remaking the American CEO." *New York Times,* 25 January 1987.

Robinson, Michele L. "Sneak Preview: JCAHO's Quality Indicators." *Hospitals* 62 (5 July 1988): 38–43.

Rossy, Gerard L. "The Executive's Role in Ethics: The View from Business and Industry." *Healthcare Executive* 2 (September–October 1987): 17–21.

Shortell, Stephen M. "The Evolution of Hospital Systems: Unfulfilled Promises and Self-Fulfilling Prophesies." *Medical Care Review* 45 (Fall 1988): 177–214.

Shortell, Stephen M., and Edward F. X. Hughes. "The Effects of Regulation, Competition, and Ownership on Mortality Rates Among Hospital Inpatients." *New England Journal of Medicine* (18 April 1988): 1100–07.

Tresnowski, Bernard R. "The New Health Care Problems, Solutions, Values." Hospital Administration Alumni Association Distinguished Lecture, The University of Michigan, Ann Arbor, Michigan, 7 April 1986.

Vladeck, Bruce C. "Health Care Executives, and Their Communities: The Gintzig Memorial Lecture." *Hospital & Health Services Administration* 31 (September–October 1986): 7–15.

Wennberg, John, and Alan Gittelsohn. "Small Area Variations in Health Care Delivery." *Science* 182 (December 1973): 1102.

Work, Clements P., Beth Brophy, Andrea Gabor, Robert F. Black, Mike Tharp, and Alice Z. Cuneo. "The 21st Century Executive." *U.S. News and World Report,* 7 March 1988.

Zuckerman, Howard S. "Multi-Institutional Systems: Promise and Performance." *Inquiry* 16 (Winter 1979): 291–314.

Chapter 8

Physician Leadership in Hospital Strategic Decision Making

Anthony R. Kovner
Martin J. Chin

Anthony R. Kovner is a professor in the Health Policy and Management Program, Robert F. Wagner Graduate School of Public Service, New York University. He is a Faculty Associate of the College. Martin J. Chin is senior vice president for corporate affairs, Mercy Health Corporation of Southeastern Pennsylvania, Bala Cynwyd, Pennsylvania. He is a Nominee of the College.

This article was published in *Hospital & Health Services Administration* 30, no. 6 (November/December 1985).

Hospitals are facing greater competition, and their freedom to make changes in the scope of clinical services is becoming more restricted by financial and regulatory constraints. These environmental pressures are recognized by hospital officials, but there has been little attention paid to the role of physician leaders in strategic decision making.

The changing relationship between hospitals and their physicians requires study by both parties as resources become more scarce and as competition increases. This article identifies key variables that influence hospital strategic decision making and presents three models of physician participation in hospital strategic decision making and the findings from a study of eight acute general hospitals.

Definitions

Physician leaders are those physicians who occupy formal positions of authority in the hospital organizational structure. Such positions include chiefs of clinical services, officers of the medical board, and occupants of formal administrative posts such as medical director, director of medical education, or chief of the medical staff.

The emphasis of this article is on formal leaders who control many of the channels relating to strategic planning, channels available for interaction between managers and the medical staff. Managers ultimately must communicate with and seek out the formal physician leadership even if the informal physician leadership is very influential. Formal leaders are often informal leaders as well.

One special group excluded from the group of physician leaders includes those physicians who serve as chief executive officers (CEOs) of hospitals. In these cases, physician CEOs are considered to be managers because they are held accountable for their managerial performance, not their performance as physicians.

Strategic decisions are choices made by hospital officials to initiate, expand, diminish, or close clinical programs and services. These decisions involve changes in hospital scope of service, usually referred to as changes in product mix.

Strategic decisions involve major changes in the commitment of resources in terms of financing, personnel, equipment, facilities, and organization. Examples of strategic decisions are discontinuance of inpatient pediatric or obstetric service due to low volume, expansion of cardiac diagnostic capabilities, establishment of a hospital-sponsored health maintenance organization (HMO), acquisition of a nursing home, participation in a multi-institutional system, and creation of a clinical or research institute.

The Literature

There has been limited research on the subject of physician participation in hospital strategic decision making. Most research has focused on how physicians affect hospital operational outputs such as costs and utilization. These articles reflect the prevalent method of study of hospital-physician relations, which is to examine structural characteristics of physicians and hospitals (e.g., how many doctors, what size of hospital) and relate these to hospital cost and utilization performance.

While this research addresses the role of physicians in hospital operational, rather than strategic, decision making, there are findings from this research that apply to both forms.

Shortell and his colleagues have produced the major body of research on the characteristics of physicians and their impact on hospitals. In a paper on physician involvement in hospital decision making, Shortell (1983) argues that environmental changes are causing both for-profit and not-for-profit hospitals to move from dual and separate authority structure (where physicians and managers control different types of decisions) to shared authority in hospital decision making.

Shortell and Evashwick (1982) studied characteristics of the medical staffs of 4,212 acute general hospitals. They found that medical staffs could be differentiated according to the extent to which all physicians had a contractual orientation toward their hospitals and according to the level of participation of physicians on governing boards. They found that for-profit hospitals tended to have higher proportions of physicians in a formal contractual relationship than not-for-profit hospitals. Larger hospitals also tended to have greater proportions of contracted physicians. Medical staff participation on governing boards also was greater in for-profit hospitals, but there was less medical staff participation on governing boards in larger hospitals (less than 500 beds) than in medium-sized hospitals (300–499 beds).

Pauly (1978) suggested that coordination and control of hospital output (where output is defined by units of service, such as an inpatient day) becomes more difficult as this output is dispersed among a larger number of physicians. Harris (1977) critiqued the decision-making structures of hospitals by depicting the hospital as made up of feudal territories. These fiefdoms were controlled by competing chiefs of services who dominated the resource allocation process. He called for changes in the regulation and organization of hospitals in order to deal with the lack of coordinated resource allocation.

Sloan (1980) echoed this notion by noting that, "very few hospitals can afford to be managed by a loose coalition of attending physicians." Sloan found that the vast majority of hospitals do not place limits on the ability of its physicians to have close relations with other hospitals, although this differs substantially between hospital-based physicians (such as pathologists and radiologists) and non hospital-based physicians.

All of these authors allude to the increasing complexity of hospital operations and the concurrent need for more formal structures for decision making.

Sloan and Becker (1982) conclude that a more decentralized medical staff structure (more control at the departmental level) results in higher hospital costs. Thus, if chiefs of clinical services have more delegated powers, they must also have strong accountabilities, otherwise the hospital will experience poorer cost and utilization performance. This study suggests that having physicians paid by hospitals is not alone sufficient, but that there must exist other structures that integrate physicians into the hospital management structures such as having more formal control systems, regular reporting relationships, and performance appraisal systems. Once again, formal structures for control and communication are cited as necessary for improved hospital performance.

In one of the few studies of the process of decision making, Heyssel (1984) concludes that contractual relationships for physician leaders must be supported by other organizational control devices. Costs were found to be lower where there were salaried chiefs who were accountable for their performance as managers and supported by managerial staff at the departmental as well as at the hospital level. This suggests that greater integration of management staff with physician leaders improves operating performance.

A Normative, Conceptual Scheme

This article offers a normative, conceptual scheme for selecting an appropriate model of physician participation in hospital strategic decision making. The model is normative in that performance on each of the independent variables determines which model of decision making is most appropriate. The model is applied to acute general hospitals.

The dependent variable, strategic decision making, is operational in terms of three models: fractionated, dual domain, and integrated. The four independent variables consist of: the competitiveness of the hospital's environment, the complexity of the strategic decisions facing the hospital, the strategic orientation of physicians in leadership positions, and the contractual relationships of these physician leaders to the hospital.

The following five sections in this article deal with independent and dependent variables. Findings from an empirical study of eight hospitals are also presented.

122

Independent Variables

Competitiveness of the Environment

Health delivery organizations compete for patients, physicians, capital funds, and for the right to offer new services through the certificate-of-need process. Competitors include other hospitals, private physician groups, or alternative delivery organizations such as HMOs and freestanding ambulatory care centers. A more competitive environment is characterized by a greater number of competitors over a wide scope of services.

The competitiveness of the environment is an important independent variable for selecting a decision making model because it determines how many and how quickly decisions must be made. If the environment is highly competitive, this suggests that a hospital must confront a greater number of strategic decisions, which may necessitate a more sophisticated model.

Complexity of Strategic Decisions

Hospitals vary in the scale or impact of these decisions on their organizations. Complexity of decisions refers to the scale of decisions that a hospital must consider, relative to its size and sophistication. The complexity of decisions is particularly great if a hospital considers a major change from the existing mission.

Decisions are more complex if they: represent a major change in the hospital mission, entail greater risk and uncertainty, consume a larger proportion of hospital resources, affect several departments or services, or require major organizational restructuring.

Strategic Orientation of Physician Leaders

Physician leaders assume their positions for different reasons, and there is substantial variation in the willingness of physicians to participate in strategic decision making. Some physician leaders have more advanced management skills, greater knowledge, and an eagerness to participate; others are either unwilling or unable.

In many hospitals, there are physicians in key leadership positions who choose to be informed and who are active participants in the assessment of strategic choices and in the making of decisions about services that do not directly relate to their own personal clinical domains. In the same institutions, other physician leaders may choose to focus on the delivery of clinical care, teaching, or research and will leave the overall strategic decisions to be made by managers. They will only interact on strategic issues that directly relate to the services they control.

The strategic orientation of physician leaders is high if there are physicians in formal leadership positions who have the following characteristics:

- Knowledge of a hospital's competitive position and willingness to communicate this to other decision makers.
- Interest in working on administrative committees, task forces, and work groups.
- Ability to distinguish between personal, departmental, and hospital-wide objectives and acknowledgement of these distinctions.

Contractual Relationship of Physician Leaders

The literature suggests that the formal relationship of physican leaders to the hospital may be an important determinant of the ability of hospitals to effectively make decisions. Given the loose coupling of physicians to most hospitals, contracted physician leaders may serve a vital function in improving the contribution of physicians to hospital strategic decision making.

Contracted physician leaders have loyalties and biases that are favorable to medical staff–hospital relations. The contractual relationship of physician leaders is measured on a hospitalwide basis by the number of physician leaders who have a formal, specified financial arrangement with the hospital and the number and extent of formal reporting and accountability responsibilities that physician leaders must fulfill.

Dependent Variable: Three Models

Fractionated Model of Decision Making

The fractionated model of decision making is characterized by the absence of formal systems for strategic decision making. These decisions are made with few data or analyses concerning the hospital's market conditions, competitive position, or financial plans. Long-range planning is not considered to be valuable or feasible, thus the issues that are considered have a short (one-year) time frame.

Under the fractionated model, one to three key decision makers assume all responsibility for assessing the environment and evaluating alternatives. There is little awareness and no influence over the strategic choices on the part of anyone in the hospital's management or medical staff other than the one to three key decision makers.

Figure 1
Normative Conceptual Scheme for Selecting the Most Appropriate Model of Strategic
Decision Making

Independent Variables	Recommended Model of Strategic Decision Making		
	Fractionated	Dual Domain	Integrated
Competitiveness of the environment	Low	High	High
Complexity of decisions faced by the hospital	Low	Low	High
Strategic orientation of the M.D. leaders	Low	Low	High
Contractual relationship of the M.D. leaders to the hospital	Low	Low	High
Total	Low	Medium	High

Hospitals able to make strategic decisions effectively under this model face environments that are noncompetitive and slowly changing. Such hospitals are geographically isolated from competing provider organizations, are in areas of short supply of inpatient facilities relative to the population needs, and serve well-insured patient populations.

Decision making tends to be of low complexity because relatively few decisions are made; these decisions involve limited choices and are made as responses to short-term crises. The longer-term, strategic problems are seen primarily in terms of short-term threats or opportunities. Thus, there is little need for a formalized system of gathering data, setting priorities, and selecting actions.

Fractionated decision making is appropriate for hospitals that face little environmental change, where physicians lack a strategic planning orientation, and where physicians do not have contractual accountability to the hospital for managerial responsibilities. This occurs in geographically isolated hospitals, hospitals that serve more affluent populations, and smaller hospitals that have defined their market niche as being that of a low-cost, low-technology institution. Fractionated decision making is also appropriate where management is nonspecialized or lacking in financial and personnel resources to conduct a formal strategic-planning program.

However, there are examples of hospitals that attempt to retain fractionated decision making even when the environment changes.

Dual Domain Model of Decision Making

The dual domain model is characterized by a division of responsibility and authority to make strategic decisions. Under this model, managers engage in formal strategic planning, but the scope of services that can be affected by this planning process is limited to the domain not closely guarded by physician leaders.

Hospitals that operate under the dual domain model face environments they see as becoming more competitive. Managers set the planning agenda, collect the data, and then work with selected board members and physicians to select the courses of action. Managers may seek physician input but discourage proactive participation of physician leaders because they may not want physicians to alter the managerially determined agenda. They may not completely trust the physicians, or they may not want too many parties participating in the decision making process. In the dual domain model, physicians are informed and are asked to react to strategic initiatives posed by managers.

Physician leaders in hospitals that typify the dual domain model see their primary roles as clinicians and not as managers of their departments. Most of them are elected by their peers rather than appointed or hired by the CEO.

While the strategic planning process is largely influenced by managers and trustees in dual domain hospitals, changes in scope of service and product mix do occur (as they do under the fractionated model), largely as a result of changes in the day-to-day physician practice patterns, not from any centrally planned policy.

Service changes occur as a result of new admitting practices, referral patterns or treatment preferences of individual physicians and not as the result of a strategic redirection of resources. The consequence is a divided course of action; some decisions derive directly from the formal strategic planning process, while others derive from uncoordinated physician behaviors.

Dual domain hospitals are characterized by a reluctance or inability on the part of the formal strategic planning bodies to make decisions regarding acute care services. In dual domain hospitals, rarely are decisions made that involve major changes in the mission of the hospital.

When managers and trustees attempt to make decisions in these areas, physicians often resist because they are unwilling to allow nonphysician intervention in clinical services. The motivation for the resistance may be economical or philosophical.

Because of this resistance, many managerially controlled strategic planning efforts focus on services that fall outside of the main interests of most physicians. Many managers and trustees find it is easier to strategically plan for long-term care services, hospices, and alcoholism services because these do not directly touch on acute inpatient care.

Thus, if there is a low level of complexity of decisions, the dual domain model is recommended because decisions do not require extensive interaction between physician leaders who dominate the traditional major clinical services and managers who dominate other services.

Today, the dual domain model may be the most common form of strategic decision making used in hospitals. Many hospital managers have become comfortable only recently with the tools and techniques of strategic planning, particularly as applied to the major clinical departments. Many hospitals lack information about which services comprise separate markets, and they lack data to evaluate the hospital's market niches. However, they have pursued formal strategic planning in the hopes of improving the sophistication and influence of the process for a later use.

The dual domain model is inappropriate when the skills of the managers do not allow them to carry out a formal strategic decision making process or when the environment is so competitive that individual physician leaders cannot make decisions that serve both the interests of key physicians in their departments and the interests of the hospital as a whole.

Some hospitals may inappropriately rely on the dual domain model because managers fail to recognize that physician participation is crucial when the environment is most competitive or because managers have not yet sufficiently developed their own staff's skills in strategic planning.

Integrated Model of Strategic Decision Making

Under the integrated model, regular communication occurs among managers, board members, and the physician leadership. There is a regular formalized process for soliciting physician input in decisions regarding changes in service mix. Physician leaders assist in specifying which data should be gathered to study strategic options.

There is a formal process by which key physicians, board members, and managers jointly determine the courses of action. Hospitals that operate under the integrated model assume that formal strategic planning is a necessary and routine activity. They also assume that active physician leader participation is essential for the process to be effective.

Hospitals that operate under the integrated model also have the ability to consider a broader range of decisions, but they have difficulty prioritizing the choices. The process also tends to be slow and prone to miscommunication due to the larger number of people analyzing issues and contributing to the process.

The integration of physicians into strategic planning may take different forms. Physician leaders may be held directly accountable for their managerial performance by board members, other physicians, or managers. Chiefs of services may be required to take on full- or part-time managerial duties and an associated salary. New physician leader positions entitled "vice president for medical affairs" or "medical director" may be created to serve as a liaison between managers and physicians.

Empirical Findings from Eight Case Study Hospitals

We conducted structured interviews with 120 physicians in formal leadership positions, 20 trustee board members, and 40 administrators in eight, not-for-profit, nongovernmental, acute general hospitals (greater than 200 beds) in the Northeast. The interviews consisted of a set of open-ended questions related to the four variables described above. Questions were asked regarding:

- *Competitiveness of the environment.* How many competitors and how intense was the competition? In what service areas was competition most keen?

- *Complexity of decisions.* What were the major strategic issues considered by the hospital during the period 1980–1982? What difficulties were encountered in the process of decision making?

- *Strategic orientation of physician leaders.* How were physicians involved in strategic decision making? What types of information did they receive, and what input did they provide to the process?

- *Contractual relationship of physician leaders.* To what extent were physician leaders contractually obligated to the hospital? What formal accountability was required of physician leaders to hospital officials?

The interviews were conducted by a team of six researchers who worked in pairs. Interviewers were randomly assigned. Notes from each interview were transcribed and used by the interviewers to assist them in rating each hospital's performance on four independent variables.

A four-point measurement scheme was used for each of the four variables. The six researchers rated each hospital on each of the four variables. Raters relied on the interview notes and their personal experiences in the interviewing process. The highest and the lowest scores from the six raters were dropped for each variable. The mean of the remaining four scores was calculated, and this provided the final score for each variable. The scores on the four variables were added to create a total score for each hospital.

A test of agreement was conducted to investigate whether there was consistency among the ratings provided by the six researchers. Using the agreement rule of five out of six raters scoring within one point, we found agreement in 75 percent of the 32 scoring trials. Based purely on chance, this kind of agreement would occur only 22 percent of the time. Thus, there was strong evidence that the raters had agreement that was not due to chance.

Once total scores for each hospital were obtained, these were used to classify each institution in one of the three models. The categories for these total scores were: fractionated model—4.0–6.99; dual domain model—7.0–12.99; and integrated model—13.0–16.00.

The categories were constructed so that a hospital would have to score low (1 or 2) on most variables to be classified in the fractionated model. To be classified as an integrated model, a hospital would have to score high on most variables.

By design, this classification scheme has a wider range of scores for the dual domain model. Having a larger central category was preferable to uniform assignment of scores for categories to ensure that the fractionated model was truly differentiated from the integrated model.

Findings

Our interviews in eight hospitals suggest there may be different levels of strategic orientation and contractual relationship of physician leaders for different types of hospitals. Figure 2 shows how the scores on the four variables placed each of the case study hospitals in one of the three models of strategic decision making.

Discussion and Implications

Physician leaders serve an important function by bridging the gap between attending physicians and the hospital trustees and managers. Their role in strategic decision making may be minimal as under the fractionated model; it may be limited to specific areas as under the dual domain model; or it may be highly proactive as under the integrated model. As changing financial, regulatory, and competitive pressures are brought to bear on physicians and hospitals, the role of the physician leader becomes increasingly complex and difficult.

The results indicated that the strategic orientation of physician leaders was low in many hospitals. Chiefs of services often had large private practices and did not identify with the strategic concerns of hospital officials. Physician leaders in these hospitals were primarily concerned with their private practices and tended to see the interests of the hospital from the viewpoint of independent practitioners rather than as hospital clinical managers. Managers and board members may have discouraged these physician leaders from attaining a higher strategic orientation because they did not trust physicians' judgment or loyalty to the hospital.

Figure 2
Scores for Eight Case Study Hospitals on the Independent Variables

	Competitive-ness of the Environment	Complexity of Decisions Faced by the Hospital	Strategic Orientation of the Physician Leaders	Extent of Contractual Relationship of M.D. Leaders	Total Score	Model
Affiliated Hospital	3.25	3.25	3.5	3.75	13.75	Integrated
Catholic Hospital	3.75	3.75	1.5	3.75	12.75	Dual
TATCH	3.5	2.5	2.25	4.0	12.0	Dual
Hope Medical Center	3.5	3.5	1.75	2.25	11.0	Dual
Borough Hospital	3.0	3.25	1.5	2.5	10.25	Dual
Inner City Hospital	1.25	2.25	2.0	3.25	8.75	Dual
Community Hospital	2.5	1.75	1.0	1.0	6.25	Fractionated
Union Hospital	2.25	1.75	1.25	1.0	6.25	Fractionated
	$\bar{x} = 2.875$	$\bar{x} = 2.75$	$\bar{x} = 1.844$	$\bar{x} = 2.689$		

The physician leader must balance the often conflicting responsibilities of representing colleagues versus protecting the larger interests of the hospital. He or she runs the risk of either being perceived by attending physicians as selling out to managerial pressures or being seen by managers and board members as guarding the parochial interests of physicians. This balancing of interests must be considered by physician leaders, although the role of the physician leaders varies under each different model of strategic decision making.

Seven out of the eight hospitals in our study were freestanding community general hospitals. These freestanding hospitals were 300–700 beds and were not part of an academic medical center. Freestanding community hospitals and their physician leaders may be in the most precarious strategic position. They are faced with many complex decisions regarding their mission and scope of services.

Figure 3
Expected Physician Leader Characteristics and Hospital Setting

		Contractual Relationship of Physician Leadership with the Hospital	
		High	Low
Strategic Orientation of the Physician Leadership	High	Multihospital system	Smaller, geographically isolated hospital
	Low	Academic health center	Freestanding community hospital

The hospital may lack some specialized market and planning staff that larger entities may possess. They may face more competition than smaller, more isolated, and locally dominant hospitals. They may be unable to muster the resources needed to sustain a complete research and teaching program that is found in academic medical centers.

Figure 3 illustrates how the strategic orientation and contractual relationship of physician leaders may vary by type of hospital. For freestanding community hospitals to make strategic decisions that are timely and sufficient, they may be forced to move toward one of the other cells depicted in Fugure 3. Since the constraints to becoming an academic health center are increasingly formidable, most freestanding community hospitals may be forced to move, either to become part of a multi-institutional system or to become a hospital that is more limited in terms of its market served and the services offered.

There is nothing in the literature to indicate that multi-institutional systems score higher on strategic orientation or contractual relationship of physician leaders. Such multihospital systems do tend to have sophisticated planning and marketing capabilities to support physician leader integration.

Strengths and Limitations

There are several strengths to this conceptualization of strategic decision making in hospitals. First, the emphasis of these models is on the role of the physician leader. Previous studies focused on the medical staff as a whole and ignored the dominant role of medical officials. By focusing on the chiefs of services and appointed medical officials, a model for exchange among managers, board members, and specifically identified physicians can be developed.

A second strength of this conceptual scheme is its reliance on a recommended model of decision making that is contingent on a hospital's performance on selected environmental and physician leader variables. The recommendations for change are conservative. Hospitals and physician leaders should not engage in sophisticated forms of strategic planning unless the conditions are largely satisfied.

A third strength of this conceptual scheme is the ability to make recommendations for different types of hospitals. The role of physician leaders can be substantially different in small community hospitals than in academic medical centers; these in turn may differ greatly for physician leaders in multiunit hospital systems. The variables used to select strategic decision making models are flexible enough to apply to different types of hospitals.

There are several limitations to the concepts and models proposed in this article. First, the models assume that there is homogeneity of requirements among physician leaders; that is, all chiefs of services will require similar levels of strategic orientation or similar contractual relationships. Clearly this is an oversimplification, since in any hospital there is likely to be wide variation by service as to competitive situation and complexity of decisions.

There are differences in the power of physician leaders as well. In some hospitals, only one or two physicians may be strategically oriented, yet this may be sufficient to move the hospital toward an integrated model. In other hospitals, the vast majority of physicians may be strategically oriented, but a few key physician leaders may be resistant. This could prevent the adoption of an integrated model. Interphysician variation can be important and should be considered in analyzing strategic decision making in any hospital.

The ability to assess the informal power relationships among physician leaders, board members, and managers is another limitation. The variables used for these models relate to formal and visible characteristics of managers and physician leaders. This article avoids questions of informal influence, historical relationships, and personality traits—important determinants of organizational behavior in the hospital settlng. If the board members and physician leaders have strong informal or social ties to each other, this can drastically alter the selection of the most effective model of strategic decision making.

A third limitation concerns the identification of clear boundaries among the three different types of strategic decision making. This is an inherent problem for any organizational model. The determination of which model a hospital fits into can be muddied by scoring on the independent variables. As a result, we sometimes are faced with hospitals on the border of different categories. Further work on operationalizing the independent variables and separating out their effects is required to refine the classification rules.

A fourth limitation is the sample of hospitals on which observations were based and generalizations grounded. These were eight medium- to large-sized, not-for-profit hospitals in the Northeast. Our models are biased to the extent that these hospitals are not representative of hospitals in other parts of the country.

We suggest further research to see if the models in specified hospitals are associated with changes in the scope of clinical services, a result of strategic decisions.

References

Harris, J. E. "The Internal Organization of Hospitals: Some Economic Implications." *Bell Journal of Economics* 8 (1977): 467–82.

Heyssel, R. M., et al. "Decentralized Management in a Teaching Hospital: Ten Years at Johns Hopkins." *New England Journal of Medicine* 310 (1984): 1477–80.

"Decentralized Management in a Teaching Hospital: Ten Years at Johns Hopkins." *New England Journal of Medicine* 310 (1984): 1477–80.

Pauly, M. V., "Medical Staff Characteristics and Hospital Costs." *Journal of Human Resources* 13 (Supplement 1978): 77–111.

Shortell, Stephen M., "Physician Involvement in Decision-Making." In *The New Health Care For Profit: Doctors and Hospitals in a Competitve Environment,* edited by B. H. Gray. Washington, DC: Institute of Medicine, National Academy Press, 1983.

Shortell, Stephen M., and Connie Evashwick. "The Structural Configuration of U.S. Hospital Medical Staffs." *Medical Care* 19 (1982): 419–30.

Sloan, F. A. "The Internal Organization of Hospitals: A Descriptive Study." *Health Services Research* 15 (1980): 203–30.

Sloan, F. A., and E. R. Becker. "Internal Organization of Hospitals and Hospital Costs." *Inquiry* 18 (1982): 224–39.

Chapter 9

Revitalizing Decision Making at the Middle Management Level

Arnold D. Kaluzny

Arnold D. Kaluzny is Professor, Department of Health Policy and Administration, School of Public Health, and Senior Associate, Cecil G. Sheps Center for Health Services Research at the University of North Carolina at Chapel Hill. He is a Faculty Associate of the College.

This article was published in *Hospital & Health Services Administration* 34, no. 1 (Spring 1989).

D espite efforts of top management, the health care industry continues to be plagued with costs that are rising faster than gains in productivity. Good programs and strategies often are not implemented or are not implemented well, and high rates of absenteeism and turnover abound among personnel who once took pride in their work and their organizations. When we think about possible causes of these problems, a likely explanation is simply that we have focused too much attention on enhancing the abilities of top executives to manage strategic change and too little attention on preparing middle managers to run the day-to-day operations of health care organizations. These middle managers include department heads, clinical managers, unit supervisors, charge nurses, and numerous other people who have some managerial responsibilities within their organizations.

Nature of the Problem

Health care organizations and hospitals in particular are under siege, and the industry is responding with a host of new strategies such as downsizing, cost reduction, vigorous marketing efforts, and vertical integration. A central theme in all these strategies is the idea of control. Moreover, each strategy is characterized by a great deal of attention to job definition, assigned accountability, measurable standards, and status differentials. As described by Walton (1985), "At the heart of this traditional model is the wish to establish order, exercise control and achieve efficiency in the application of the work force."

The control model translates into a set of norms that describes how many middle managers feel they should act (Bradford and Cohen 1984).

- The good manager knows at all times what is going on in the department.
- The good manager should have more technical expertise than any subordinate.
- The good manager should be able to solve any problems that come up (or at least solve the problem before the subordinate).
- The good manager should be the primary (if not the only) person responsible for how the department is functioning.

These norms implicitly or explicitly guide managerial decision making throughout health care organizations. While the "control" approach has always had difficulty, its limitations are becoming increasingly apparent given a number of developments within the health care field.

- *Technology*. Health care organizations are characterized by an ever-expanding technology that contributes to increasing cost. The development of new organizational roles and forms to assure the delivery of this technology presents difficult organizational problems partly because of the emergent nature of the technologies and structures but also because the processes and interrelationships are quite incompatible with the requirements of the control paradigm. For example, through the development of the National Cancer Institute–funded community clinical oncology programs, community oncologists are able to provide patients with the latest in treatment and cancer control technologies heretofore only available in large metropolitan teaching centers. Participation, however, involves interorganizational collaboration of medical oncologists, surgeons, primary care physicians, and appropriate support personnel—coordination efforts that depart from the traditional control model.

- *Environmental uncertainty*. Unprecedented changes in sociodemographic, competitive, and regulatory environments are a major concern for upper echelon managerial personnel and are equally important at the middle and lower levels of management. At all levels these changes are being met with increased reliance on a variety of planning methodologies that emphasize clarity of job definition, accountability standards, and other "traditional" control approaches. The level of uncertainty, however, may be beyond the capacity of the control paradigm and in fact may be dysfunctional. As described by McKelvey and Aldrich (1983):

What may be radically wrong with many clients' strategic processes is that they are too organized. By the time they have defined what they mean by mission, goal, strategy, objective, plan, business unit, and the like, they may have so narrowly defined the boundaries as to proscribe experimentation.

- *Work force changes*. Changes in the work force itself are likely to stress further the utility of the control model. As increasing numbers of women move into medicine and health care management positions, the traditional gender-based division of women holding lesser positions in the health care hierarchy is likely to be challenged.[1] Moreover, there is mounting evidence that workers are less willing simply to follow orders on the basis of positional authority. Research suggests that younger managers are less inclined to defer to authority and that

137

they have few needs for dominance (Lawler 1987). An equally important finding is that employees would like to have significantly more influence on a range of issues including how they do their work, scheduling of work, pay raises, promotions, hiring, and making organizational policy (Lawler, Renwick, and Bullock 1981).

Effective Decision Making at the Middle Management Level

To meet the challenges of the 1990s requires a major paradigm shift similar to what has occurred at the apex of health care organizations with respect to management and the environment. Middle level managers must redefine their role, and managers at the executive level must also redefine their roles vis-à-vis the middle management level. A model of involvement and commitment (I/C)—not control—and a new way of thinking about superior-subordinate and professional-nonprofessional relationships must pervade each health care organization.

While not particularly new, the idea of building employee commitment to the organization through substantive involvement in decision making has gained increased recognition among industrial organizations in the face of global competition and deregulation (Walton 1987). This approach changes the way management and personnel think about their organization and the manner in which individuals function within it. A premium is given to adaptability, and middle and lower level managers are given much broader responsibility with greater involvement of all personnel in the decision-making process.

Under the involvement/commitment model, information and decision making do not simply flow from the top with the expectation of only trivial modifications. Instead, the model places a great deal of emphasis on individual initiative to upgrade constantly the system. Since variety of skills and perspectives are necessary to adequately perform the tasks, interdisciplinary teams become the basic accountability units. Information is shared widely, with full assurance that candid and thoughtful participation will not result in loss of jobs or stature within the organization.

Equally critical to this approach is the movement away from the control model's emphasis on surveillance, inspection, and discipline to a cycle of continuous improvement (Deming 1986). This approach builds on the involvement of all personnel in decision making and restructures the role of management in the decision-making process.

The Middle Management Role

What is the role of middle management in the new model of involvement and commitment? First, as Drucker (1988) suggests, there may be fewer middle managers in the future simply because organizations will be composed largely of "specialists" who direct and discipline their own performance through feedback from colleagues, customers, and headquarters. Moreover, the middle managers themselves will be technical experts and what Lorsch and Mathais (1987) term "producing managers"—i.e., individuals who are both formally responsible for managing activities and actively engaged in the provision of client services.

Secondly, what specific skills and activities are required? The general management literature and studies of health services have tended to focus on the role of top management vis-à-vis the total organization. Studies of middle managers have emphasized training within a control paradigm rather than an involvement/commitment model. However, recent developments within the industrial and health care literature give new attention to middle management skills and the kinds of activities that are required of "producing managers" in health service organizations.

Redefinition of Quality as an Integral
Part of the Total Production Process

Historically within health services, we have relied on physicians and "quality assurance coordinators" to define and monitor quality. The movement toward an involvement/commitment paradigm requires that individuals within the organization be involved and committed to something of substance—and there is no better candidate than the idea of "quality." Middle managers can take a leadership role in developing an organizationwide quality consciousness and designing delivery systems for quality.

This approach to quality, as conceptualized by Deming (1986) for industrial organizations, has been adopted by the Hospital Corporation of America (HCA) as the foundation for its quality improvement process. Using principles of operations research to differentiate "special causes" from "common causes" of variation, HCA uses this knowledge to improve the patient care process. Special causes of variation are deviations from intended process specifications that are due to controllable, attributable, and nonrandom events. Such variations can be controlled through direct interventions without fundamental changes in the ongoing patient care process. Common causes, on the other hand, are random variations that are derived from the patient care system itself even though it may be running strictly in accordance with its design. For example, within nursing, the assignment of general duty nurses to units according to some nurse/patient ratio may result in a variety of performance problems when some of these assignments require a particular level or type of expertise. Although the system is clearly working according to plan—that is, the ratios are being maintained—individual nurses or their supervisors are being held accountable for the resultant problem—that is, common cause variations. This is even more frustrating when these problems are defined as "special causes" within the unit—in other words, they are viewed as being controllable. Clearly, this is a situation in which management needs to redesign the assignment system to reduce variation from common causes.

The role of middle level management is to distinguish between common and special causes and understand the pattern of variation that may provide clues to initiate corrective action. This action should be based on basic statistical tools developed within the discipline of operations research and middle level managers will increasingly be required to know these quantitative methodologies. As described by Berwick and Batalden (1988) in their application of the cycle of continuous improvement to the provision of medical care:

> Health care quality assurance to date has rarely, if ever, made the theoretically fundamental distinction between special causes and common causes of variation. In general, those who assess health care quality tend to assume implicitly that all causes of undesired deviation from specifications are likely to be special and identification of such deviation therefore is tantamount to corrective action. This assumption ignores a common observation that 85% or more of variation in systems is from random causes—workers in a production process who are held accountable for common cause variation can easily become demoralized, angry and disconnected from their work; holding someone accountable for random events can drive them crazy. It is the job of leaders (mid-level managers) to redesign the system to reduce variation from common causes.

The approach clearly focuses on the use of knowledge to improve decision making at the level of middle management. Improvement occurs through the design and redesign of patient care systems—not by inspecting final "products" of health care or by blaming individual workers within the health care organization. Efficient use of information coupled with the techniques of group process, group decision making, and organizational development is the basic tenet for changing the system to better assure quality and productivity.

The pervasive focus on quality throughout the organization and the critical role of middle management is a central theme of the emerging Joint Commission on the Accreditation of Healthcare Organization's "Agenda for Change." While the specifics of this program are currently in the process of development, discussion is centered on the role of quality as a function of *all* personnel within the organization and the linking of both incentives and structure to the further assurance and continued improvement of quality.

Building an Involved and Committed Team

Given the clear mandate for quality throughout the patient care process, the inclusion of a range of disciplines relative to that process requires a high level of interdependency. As described by Bradford and Cohen (1987):

> The problems of bringing together all the necessary information and producing all the coordination are growing each year at increasing speed . . . .The solution is not to work harder and run faster, but instead to build a team that shares in the responsibility of managing a department.

The advantage of a team approach to departmental or unit management is that each individual is able to participate in complex decisions and to add relevant expertise. This level of involvement not only facilitates the performance of the group/unit but also enhances the overall level of commitment within the organization.

A variety of planning processes are available that can be systematically applied to build an involved and committed team. These processes tend to focus on defining mission, identifying critical success factors, identifying what has to be done to meet these success factors, and then targeting those factors that will have the biggest impact on achieving the designated mission. Critical to the success of the entire effort, however, is involving all the key players in the planning process, achieving unanimity, and assuring follow through. All members of the team must be involved from the onset. As described by some proponents (Hardaker and Ward 1986):

> . . . if even one member of the team cannot attend—wait. [The process] requires a buy in from everyone not only to identify what is needed but also to commit to the process.

Involvement will not be achieved without a certain amount of conflict. Bright, dedicated people interacting on substantive issues are likely to disagree on fundamental points—particularly given the level of uncertainty facing health service organizations. Thus, middle management requires special skills in negotiation and conflict management. The issue is not how to avoid the problem but how to structure the group and interpersonal processes to assure successful negotiations.

Development of Individual Skills

A team is composed of individuals and individuals who must have certain skills if the group is to function effectively. Since the involvement/commitment paradigm requires that individuals have both technical and behavioral skills, the role of middle management is to develop these skills among subordinates to improve team decision making. Special attention must be given to the development of interpersonal skills since these skills are least developed and most critical to consensual decision making and mutual influence characterizing the involvement/commitment model.

How can this be accomplished? A range of options is available including continuing education programs, career counseling, etc. However, in reality, the development of technical and behavioral skills is probably best served by an inhouse developmental process (Bradford and Cohen 1984). Under this approach, tasks are assigned to broaden subordinates' knowledge and skills with appropriate coaching and feedback by middle managers.[2] The approach provides an opportunity to constructively convert behavioral problems into learning opportunities and can be quite motivating to both mid-level managers and their subordinates. Obviously not all individuals have the appropriate levels of interest, motivation, and ability; yet, the role of management is to assure that all individuals have the opportunity to realize their full potential.

Determining and Building a Common Departmental Vision

Middle level managers need to infuse their respective groups with a vision of the unit vis-à-vis the larger organization. Given the focus on cost, it is all too easy to forget about the basic mission of the organization—particularly at the level of middle management. Thus, the focus on quality as the overarching goal of the organization and its restatement within various departments and roles provides a critical base for building a common departmental/organizational vision. The approach fulfills several functions (Bradford and Cohen 1984); unites and inspires members thus justifying extra effort; establishes criteria on which to make decisions; makes clear the direction toward which the unit should be striving; and defines the future.

New Directions

The workers are handicapped by the system and the system belongs to management. (Deming 1986)

Traditional efforts to deal with middle management training have focused primarily on programmatic solutions that, in isolation, fail. The assumption that the implementation of a quality circles program (McKinney 1984), a financial system for middle managers (Shyavitz, Rosenbloom, and Conover 1985), or a performance/productivity evaluation system (Dailey 1988; Kotch et al. 1986), as discrete activities, will resolve major organizational problems is overly simplistic. The challenge centers on the transformation to a new organizational paradigm to fit the needs of middle managers. These alterations have nontrivial implications for how the human and material resources of health care organizations are deployed and managed.

The transformation will not be easy and is particularly risky for middle managers who are no longer in charge of simply maintaining the system but now are charged with the responsibility of improving the system. Moreover, health service organizations suffer from a combination of "genetic" and "iatrogenic" disorders that inhibits the transformation. Genetically, these organizations have high levels of inertia because of their structural characteristics and because of the characteristics of certain key actors. Structurally, health care organizations in general and hospitals in particular are "loosely coupled." Their organizational units are not coordinated in any systematic manner and while they may share a common mission, there are few integrating mechanisms to sustain coordinated activities over time. With uncoordinated units, it is different to initiate and to sustain change since each unit has the option to sabotage, veto, or simply ignore the process.

Health service organizations are composed of individuals who by background and technical training have commitments and orientations independent of their organizations. In contrast to many industrial organizations where the main line of advancement is into general management positions, health professionals have limited interest in or expectations of becoming managers. In fact, many have considerable contempt for the entire management process.

An iatrogenic disorder that cannot be ignored is a level of cynicism among health care personnel. For the past ten years, health care organizations have been in constant transition, and there is a pervasive attitude among personnel that "we have seen it all." Hospital personnel have been subjected to DRGs, MBO, performance evaluation systems, and quality of work life programs—all with high expectations for solving major organizational problems. Since each program has fallen far short of expectations, any new attempts to transform health care organizations along the lines that we have suggested will have to overcome employee skepticism.

What steps can be taken to facilitate the paradigm shift? It begins with top management and requires courage, knowledge, and sustained support. Only the executive level can articulate a vision of how the new paradigm will operate and specify the role of mid-level managers within the paradigm. Moreover, only the executive level has the resources necessary to sustain the process over time. While there are no simple algorithms to follow, a number of guidelines are helpful.

- Develop a basic and realistic understanding of the change process. Any change involves a series of stages beginning with the recognition of a problem and then proceeding to the identification of a solution vis-à-vis that problem, implementation, and finally institutionalization of the change within the organization. Because organizations and units within these organizations will be at different stages in the change process, an accurate identification of stage is critical. Failure to stage accurately the organization/unit will greatly limit our ability to facilitate the paradigm shift. For example, efforts to build involved and committed teams or "continual improvement programs" are likely to encounter resistance if the problems that the solutions address are not recognized. Equally critical is the recognition that different units and components of the organization may be at different stages, and where discrepancies exist, management must be capable of recognizing these differences and acting accordingly.

- Develop some level of dissatisfaction with the existing state. Several approaches are possible. First, managers might provide opportunities to compare the organization with similar organizations. Comparative data have historically been used to highlight performance gaps, thereby initiating a search for viable solutions. While this approach may be worthy of further exploration, one major limitation is the fact that it tends to foster denial and defensive behavior on the part of critical actors within the organization and thus reinforces the control model. An alternative approach is for the organization to compare itself over time. Research reveals that when results fall short of what individuals desire, motivation for change increases (Lawler 1988). This strategy is far less threatening and provides an opportunity for a great deal of learning on the part of organizational decision makers.

144

- Lead the process to define what the organization means by the term "quality" and learn new ways to use clinical and financial information, as part of that definitional process. As part of that process top management must define and recognize new constituent groups and ways to implement change (Berwick and Batalden 1988). For example, the development of a "quality improvement program" is a substantive step to implementing change—yet in hospitals under labor contract, failure to recognize and involve organized labor in the design and development of the program limits the transformation at its onset.

- Appeal to the social as well as economic motives of health care personnel. While involvement is never a substitute for adequate remuneration, failure to recognize or to underestimate the importance of social motives will limit the ability of management to operate within the new paradigm. Protecting and advocating for their patients is an equal, if not stronger, motivational force than purely economic rewards for most health care personnel. The challenge is to channel this energy in a constructive direction given financial, logistical, and cultural constraints (Shea 1988).

- Finally, capitalize on the basic value compatibility between the health care organization and the involvement/commitment paradigm. In contrast to many industrial organizations undergoing similar transformations (Walton 1987), health services organizations emphasize individual worth and justice—values that are central themes of the involvement/commitment paradigm. Emphasizing this compatibility rather than apologizing for the apparent structural anomalies of health care organizations will facilitate the transformation and in so doing, revitalize the important role of middle management within health care organizations.

Obviously these guidelines are not the panacea for a complex and understudied area of health services management. Moreover, each of these points is not new in absolute terms. Yet, these guidelines highlight the key points so often ignored as senior managers struggle with the very survival of the organization. The ability to instill a realistic understanding of the change process, to provide a foundation for change through a shared recognition of the organization's potential, to lead in the process of defining "quality," to appeal to the social as well as the economic motives of health care personnel, and to capitalize on the basic value compatibility between health care organizations and the involvement/commitment paradigm are critical to the revitalization of decision making at the middle management level.

Acknowledgments

Thanks are given to the following for their helpful comments and suggestions: Martha McKinney, Jenifer Ehreth, Geoff Hoare, Steve Shortell, Howard Zuckerman, and Paul Batalden. Thanks are also given to Susan Baldwin and her colleagues for their logistical and typing support at the Department of Health Services, School of Public Health and Community Medicine at the University of Washington, Seattle.

Notes

1. An alternative and less charitable interpretation is that the influx of women into medicine and middle management will simply reinforce the control paradigm since women may be willing to accept a subordinate role within the larger corporate structure at reduced pay.

2. Middle managers themselves will require mentoring and support over time as they engage in these activities. In the implementation of the Hospital Corporation of America's continuing improvement program, each manager has a designated mentor to provide counseling and support.

References

Berwick, D. M., and P. Batalden. "An Alternative Theory of Health Services Quality: The Cycle for Continuous Improvement." Hospital Corporation of America unpublished manuscript. Personal communication with P. Batalden, 1988.

Bradford, D. L., and A. R. Cohen. *Managing for Excellence.* New York: John Wiley & Sons, Inc., 1984.

Dailey, R. C. "Productivity Monitoring Systems in Hospitals: A Work Group Focus." *Hospital & Health Services Administration* 33 (Spring 1988): 75–88.

Deming, W. E. *Out of the Crisis.* Cambridge, MA: MIT Press, 1986.

Drucker, P. "The Coming of the New Organization." *Harvard Business Review* 66 (January–February 1988): 45–53.

Hardaker, M., and B. K. Ward. "Getting Things Done." *Harvard Business Review* 65 (November–December 1986): 112–15, 118–20.

Kotch, J. B., C. Burr, W. Brown, A. Abrantes, and A. D. Kaluzny. "A Performance Based Management System to Reduce Prematurity and Low Birth Weight." *Journal of Medical Systems* 10, no. 4 (1986): 375–94.

Lawler, E. E., III. "Transformation from Control to Involvement." In *Corporate Transformation*, edited by R. H. Kilmann and T. J. Covin. San Francisco: Jossey Bass, 1988.

―――. *High Involvement Management.* San Francisco: Jossey Bass, 1987.

Lawler, E., P. A. Renwick, and R. J. Bullock. "Employee Influence on Decisions: An Analysis." *Journal of Occupational Behavior* 2 (1981): 115–123.

Lorsch, J. W., and P. F. Mathais. "When Professionals Have to Manage." *Harvard Business Review* 87, no. 4 (July–August 1987): 78–83.

McKelvey, B., and H. Aldrich. "Applied Population Science." *Administrative Science Quarterly* 28 (March 1983): 101–28.

McKinney, M. M. "The Newest Miracle Drug: Quality Circles in Hospitals." *Hospital & Health Services Administration* 29 (September–October 1984): 74–87.

Shyavitz, L., D. Rosenbloom, and L. Conover. "Financial Incentives for Middle Managers: Pilot Program in an Inner City, Municipal Teaching Hospital." *Health Care Management Review* 10, no. 3 (1985): 37–44.

Shea, G. "The View from the Union." Paper presented for the 24th Annual Forum on Hospital and Health Affairs, Duke University, May 1988.

Walton, R. E. *Innovating to Compete.* San Francisco: Jossey Bass, 1987.

———. "From Control to Commitment in the Work Place." *Harvard Business Review* 85, no. 2 (March–April 1985): 76–84.

Chapter 10

Renewal and Change for Health Care Executives

George C. Burke III
Michael O. Bice

George C. Burke III is Associate Professor and Coordinator, Graduate Program in Health Care Administration, Southwest Texas State University, San Marcos. He is a Fellow of the College. Michael O. Bice is President and CEO, Allegany Health System, St. Petersburg, Florida. He is a Member of the College.

This article was published in *Hospital & Health Services Administration* 36, no. 1 (Spring 1991).

One cannot step twice in the same river, for fresh waters are forever flowing around us.

—Heraclitus

Much attention has been given to the subject of change in today's health care organizations, but less to the subject of change in the life of the individual executive. As change agents, health care executives must be capable of managing change in their own lives if they are to implement major change in their organizations. Executives who succumb to arteriosclerosis during their career can hardly serve as role models for the organization. Health care executives must consider renewal within their own personal careers if they seek to breathe life into their own institutions. The appointment and support of the chief executive officer (CEO) is, according to Griffith (1988), one of the nondelegable duties of the trustees of voluntary hospitals. Health care executives have a corresponding fiduciary responsibility to maintain their own edge and vitality. We are, in a sense, trustees of our own careers.

The literature is rich with information about change in the organization. Experts tell us that CEOs and their senior managers are at the apex of change. Not all change is good, of course, but the issue is the direction and effectiveness of the change. Dyer (1984) states that "changes in human conditions, be they societal or organizational, are going to occur. Nothing is static. . . .For those in positions of management or leadership the issue is, how can we plan change with reasonable assurance that the desired consequence can be achieved?" Gardner (1963) says that "renewal is not just innovation and change. It is also the process of bringing the results of change into line with our purposes." Bice (1984) discusses the role of health care leaders in shaping changes through an understanding of corporate culture. Silverzweig and Allen (1976) point out common pitfalls in the cultural change process when there is only lip-service commitment from the CEO. No sustained change will occur unless the leaders model the desired behavior each day. People react to deeds, rather than words, and are quite adept at reading mixed signals. For example, CEOs who encourage their staff to "stay close to the customer," yet themselves remain locked into a daily office routine have only themselves to blame if the organization is not market sensitive. On the other hand, if they get out and talk to patients and families, there will be a profound impact on a staff who observes this activity.

Schein (1986) refers to leaders who "embed and transmit culture." They do this in a number of ways, such as what they pay attention to in meetings and through deliberate role modeling, teaching, and coaching. According to

Schein, leadership for managed change requires perception and insight, motivation and skill, emotional strength, ability to change the cultural assumptions, and depth of vision. These are qualities that must be continually cultivated, lest they become eroded as the strength of the marathon runner is sapped by the sheer distance of the race. The challenge is to find a second wind—again and again.

Barriers to Individual Change and Renewal

While we may acknowledge the need for positive change and renewal, barriers to change are real and powerful and require a continuous effort on the part of the CEOs to overcome. In fact, we may not recognize the barriers because they are so embedded in our culture that we accept them as the modus operandi. Among the barriers to change are

- *Time pressures.* As Quick et al. (1985) point out, time pressure is a "source of stress for most hospital administrators and is related to the 24-hour duties and activities in which the administrator engages." Pressure to accomplish much in a short time often leads us to neglect the long-run considerations such as professional development.

- *Fatigue.* Health care executives put in long hours, typically 55 to 70 hours per week, in nonstop activities requiring them to shift gears rapidly. While many executives thrive on the action (positive stress), there are often negative aspects of stress that may take their toll. I reported role overload to be a common perception among hospital executives in a particular study (Burke 1989). Quick et al. (1985) point out that burnout is a distressful consequence of work overload. The executive who feels burned out does not look beyond the horizon for creative ideas but instead tries to merely survive the day.

- *The Protestant work ethic.* Embedded in our society's culture is the notion that hard, unstinting effort will carry the day, and that doing well has its own rewards. While these values are important for health care executives, amidst the unstinting effort there must be space for renewal. Some may see renewal as "soft" and not for the strong of heart. Workaholics of both sexes assume that busyness equals productivity, and they cannot be bothered with what appears to be a non-productive activity.

- *On-the-job retirement.* When successful, we may assume that change is not necessary. We may see the myriad changes taking place and

151

decide to play it safe to avoid risks. The result is that some executives seem to retire while still on the job. Because the field is changing, so must we. On-the-job retirement is not an affliction reserved for those approaching formal retirement (though such may occur), but it can be a problem for any executive whose professional attitude is to continually play it safe and be reactive rather than proactive.

- *Corporate culture.* It's hard to go against a corporate culture that may say "if it ain't broke, don't fix it." A number of organizations seem to have this as their credo, but it is clearly anathema to any marketer. Bice (1984) points out that some hospitals have conservative, nonrisk-taking corporate cultures and that it is difficult for an individual executive to turn around corporate cultures. CEOs, as keepers of the culture, set the tone for renewal. If they do not encourage and reward renewal, it will not happen. Health care executives who embrace positive change encourage the development of subordinates. To respond to a key manager's suggestion with "we tried that before" or "it'll never work" is demoralizing to the subordinate who is ready and willing to make a contribution to the organization. Yet executives who are tired, inflexible, and threatened by new ideas and change, are apt to make such a reply.

- *Trustee indifference.* Some CEOs who embark on renewal may have to start without trustee support. It is not advisable to do so, yet the dilemma could arise. Trustees often represent conservative views or focus on the bottom line to the exclusion of the personal needs of the CEO. Lloyd (1987) suggests that the annual CEO objectives include a "career/personal development" category and become part of the annual review process. This would open a dialogue with the trustees on the matter.

OK, Ponce, Where's This Fountain of Youth?

Just as Ponce de Leon never found the fountain of youth, there's no magic formula for renewal and change among health care executives. Here are, however, some suggestions.

- *Self-assessment and goal setting for professional and personal goals.* This assumes that executives have some systematic way to evaluate their professional knowledge and career advancement. The American

College of Healthcare Executives, with its self-assessment seminars, serves as a major resource in this area, and executives should plan for such an assessment at least every five years. Another suggestion is to use the services of a professional outplacement firm. An array of tests are utilized to develop a personal profile. Executives receive an unbiased (and confidential) view of their strengths and weaknesses. Many executives have benefited from such services, which can be completed in one day.

- *Career or job change.* Reassessment generally leads to recommitment to the present job, but it can also lead one to conclude that it's time to move on. Drucker (1977) suggests that managers look at their jobs from two perspectives: (1) What can I contribute to it? and (2) What can it contribute to me? He suggests that when the executive is no longer growing in the job (and if the individual is still younger than late middle age) that it is time to move on. It is the content of the job, rather than the perquisites, that bring satisfaction over the long haul, and executives may find that they need a new challenge in order to grow professionally. A job change may be a path for renewal, providing deeper soil when we are root-bound in the present job. Even an involuntary job change can be liberating and a renewal experience, provided that the individual is able to work through the grief process, learn lessons, and get on with new adventures.

- *Process vs. outcome.* There is a tremendous emphasis on the bottom line, and certainly institutions cannot live on red ink. Yet managing processes—such as team building, market research, strategic planning, and cultural change—also produce valuable (though less quantifiable) results. If our tenure as CEO is marked by a high profit margin but loss of team spirit and corporate values, have we really made a contribution to our social institution? Oliver Wendell Holmes, Jr., once said, "Life is a painting, not doing a sum." Perhaps he meant that as we go about our daily work, we will have a richer day when we think of ourselves as painting a picture instead of merely keeping score.

- *Solitude.* Oglesby (1985) says that health care leaders have learned the art of introspection. Introspection and self-assessment require the solitude that some health care executives seem to avoid. If executives entered health care administration because of its nonstop action, they may be uncomfortable with quiet space. Yet each of us needs some amount of unstructured time to recharge our batteries and to reaffirm our own activities. Solitude is often difficult to find and must be scheduled on the calendar. (You routinely schedule an hour per week for the medical director; is not your career as important?) Others find solitude in an early morning jog or walk, with additional benefits gained from exercise. Periodically we all benefit from a half-day or day off for the sole purpose of reflecting on the past and future.

- *Networking.* Participating in a network of health care executives is stimulating and yields various rewards. For hospital executives, participating in a network with insurance executives, consultants, and health maintenance organization (HMO) executives can be beneficial. Networks are important support structures during difficult times and serve as reliable sources of job opportunities and references. Oglesby (1985) refers to successful health care executives as professional networkers who seek counsel and advice from those they consider to be successful. They develop networking relationships that allow them to tap into their environments and test their ideas. Stolp-Smith (1986) points out the benefits of local health care executive groups, including educational programs, camaraderie, opportunities for leadership roles for young executives, informal support from the American College of Healthcare Executives, and social interaction. As with any relationship, maintaining communication within networks takes time and effort. Caver (1989) encourages executives to engage in networking both in and outside their organizations, pointing out that it is a two-way street. He encourages executives to volunteer for projects that will enable them to interact with people outside of their own areas.

- *Lifelong learning.* Oglesby (1985) encourages health care executives to establish a set of activities that allow them the ability to continually develop or stretch. He refers to "a life-long process of learning for which there are no shortcuts. . . ." Likewise, high-performing health care organizations exhibit an ability to stretch themselves and maximize learning (Shortell 1985). For the individual executive, lifelong learning could include additional formal education, but what is more likely among health care executives is that they will be in attendance at seminars. Attending those seminars related not only to aspects of your own present job but also those related to changes in the health care industry in general is important. The goal should be to be prepared to move to any health care organization and "hit the ground running." Indeed many health care executives are challenged today to do just that. While becoming specialized may be an attribute, it can become a liability if executives allow themselves to become obsolete in the process. The American College of Healthcare Executives has taken the lead in assisting its affiliates in remaining current in all areas of health care management through the self-assessment process and sponsorship of seminars.

- *Surrounding oneself with change agents.* We will never be able to single-handedly keep up with all the changes in the field. Our best strategy is to surround ourselves with a staff of executives willing and able to accept and implement positive change. It is then the role of the CEO to set the direction so that subordinates make changes in line with organizational objectives. Pointer (1985) suggests that CEOs identify individuals or groups of individuals who can play the role of ideator (one who is the source of new ideas); the champion (one who is willing to promote the idea); the benefactor (one who is willing to grant initial support and funding); and the orchestrator (one who assumes primary responsibility for managing the innovation phase). It is then incumbent upon the CEO to support a climate or corporate culture in which change can occur. The attitude of the CEO toward change is an important factor in whether subordinates will be risk-takers or will instead play it safe.

- *Business travel.* Gardner (1963) discusses the value of travel in breaking us out of our present perspectives and gaining new insights. Yet many executives jet in and out of new places without seeing the community, fashioning their travel in the style of the "Accidental Tourist," a movie in which a writer advises executives on how to travel without feeling that they've ever left home. The unfortunate reality is that funds appear to be waning these days for such executive travel, a concession for short-term savings at the expense of long-term development. Business travel for development can and should be included in the health care executives' annual objectives that are reviewed and approved by the trustees. Enlightened boards will expect their key management teams to keep current by attending conferences.

- *Sabbaticals.* Rountree (1979) suggests that a sabbatical may be effective in renewal of health care executives. While sabbaticals are more common in the university and research settings, they may be appropriate for certain health care executives who seek to benefit from the learning curves of other industries. Health care corporations could also benefit by using executives on loan from (or exchanges with) other industries such as banking, information systems, marketing, consulting, etc. It is suggested that in such instances salary be held at existing levels and return to the initial organization guaranteed.

- *Outside interests.* Drucker's (1977) statement that "nobody can live to age 50, especially in a big organization, without major frustrations and setbacks" may be particularly applicable to health care executives. He suggests that to survive, executives need an outside interest to gain a proper perspective—to help the executive realize that the world is bigger than just the company. An avocation or hobby can do just that for an avocation is not just a hobby but another identity. Whether gardening, sports, community volunteer work, music, or art, it allows us to see that our identities are more than our work. We should try to find an activity that we are as passionately committed to as our work. Interestingly, one study of graduates of a health care administration program reported that high levels of compensation were associated with relatively low undergraduate grade point averages and high levels of participation in undergraduate extracurricular activities (Porter and Galfano 1987). This finding could point to the importance of being a well-rounded individual. Reading outside the health care field can also be of benefit in this regard. Since few of us have the time or inclination to read all of the trade journals in the field of health care, we can probably benefit from reading one or two high-quality health care publications and a variety of other materials, including fiction, history, and biographies. Charles Ewell (1989) suggests that CEOs read what their board members do, including the *Wall Street Journal* and *Fortune.*

- *Mentors.* It is all too easy to be caught up in the job pressures and to lose an objective picture of self, strengths, weaknesses, and career path. Renewal can be enhanced by a mentor who can serve as an unbiased observer. Ross (1984) points out that mentoring benefits not only the protègè but also the mentor. For the protègè it results in a sharing of values, experiences, and professional contacts. For the mentor, it provides a different perspective and allows a sharpening of the mentor's ability to understand various viewpoints. Levey, in the Association of University Programs in Health Administration's *Survey of Early Career Opportunities* (1987), discusses the importance of mentoring and encourages educational programs to consider this aspect in establishing linkages with various health care institutions. The executive who can periodically turn to a mentor for a realistic perspective or can serve as a mentor is fortunate and has an additional resource for continuous growth and renewal.

- *Learning from mistakes/failures.* We need to put our failures in perspective—not dwell on them inordinately, nor shy away from the lessons to be learned. We need a retrospective review of what went wrong, why, and what we can do differently next time—all done in a spirit of "no fault." There are few outright failures; there are lessons to be learned. Thomas Edison once said he "failed his way to success."

- *A sense of humor and perspective.* The job itself is deadly serious, and yet we must maintain a sense of humor and a sense of perspective. Essayist Norman Cousins claimed that humor extended his life; perhaps it may also extend ours. It's essential to take the job seriously, but sometimes we take ourselves too seriously. Management, like sword-fighting and golfing, is sometimes most effectively performed by maintaining a relaxed, yet effective, grip.

- *Faith/spiritual reflection.* Religious faith is an anchor in troubled times and a source of personal renewal. As our personal and professional lives overlap, recommitment to our religious/spiritual values can lead to increased commitment to our professional careers in this helping profession. Early hospitals were founded to serve the poor and destitute, and our forebears had few resources other than their faith as they provided care under adverse conditions. Health care executives today have incredible technical resources at their disposal, but money and equipment are not enough. Periodically we need to tap our religious and spiritual roots. We recommend reading Kubler-Ross' *On Death and Dying* (1970) for deeper insight into the grief and change process and Henri Nouwen's *The Wounded Healer* (1979) for his discussion of the spiritual aspects of healing.

- *Family and friends.* Last but certainly not least is the importance of close personal relationships. Family and friends are a source of stability during life's storms. A child is the embodiment of new life and can teach adults much about creativity. Balancing the personal and professional goals in this demanding environment is perhaps the penultimate challenge health care executives face today.

Conclusions and Implications

With the health care industry undergoing tremendous structural changes, individual health care executives face substantial barriers to their professional renewal. The rapid and seemingly accelerating rate of change may easily induce what Toffler (1970) calls "future shock." In this state, individuals have lost the ability to cope with the rate of change and have begun to exhibit dysfunctional behavior. A high-stress environment demands a frequent self-assessment as a proactive response to this danger. In a rapidly changing situation, success at personal balance and the achievement of renewal takes work. We cannot look elsewhere—to the board, peers, or boss—for our own development.

It is the individual health care executive who must take responsibility for growth and renewal. The American College of Healthcare Executives serves as a marvelous resource for professional development, but it cannot promote growth without individual commitment. Self-assessment and analysis must occur regularly, and effective time managers will make room in their schedule for this important activity.

Obviously, renewal does not happen as a result of a program or seminar. Like weight control, it will take sustained effort over time to achieve. Renewal is a way of life, a lifelong process characterized by continuous learning. Oglesby (1985) hypothesizes that successful executives are those who stretch more, who commit themselves to lifelong learning, goal setting, and professional self-renewal. If this prescription is true, it tells us something about the role of a manager.

As managers and professionals, our obligations exceed self-interest. We must lead and inspire, not just direct. Thus, our own efforts at renewal will serve as a model to the organization. The CEO and senior management have the responsibility to make renewal important within the organization's value system—organizations catch the values of their leaders. High-performing organizations tend to stretch themselves and to exhibit a commitment to maximization of learning (Shortell 1985). John Gardner (1963) advocates "a system or framework within which continuous innovation, renewal, and rebirth can occur." As individual executives, we would do well to incorporate such a framework into our careers and organizations. While renewal starts with and is the responsibility of the individual, the organizational culture nurtured by senior management can do much to encourage and foster the process.

References

Bice, M. O. "Corporate Cultures and Business Strategy: A Health Management Company Perspective." *Hospital & Health Services Administration* 29, no. 4 (1984): 64–79.

Burke, G. C. "Understanding the Dynamic Role of the Hospital Executive: The View Is Better from the Top." *Hospital & Health Services Administration* 34, no. 1 (1989): 99–112.

Caver, M. D. "Career Planning: Your Competitive Edge." *Healthcare Executive* 4, no. 6 (1989): 24–25.

Drucker, P. *The "How To" Drucker.* New York: AMACOM, 1977.

Dyer, W. G. *Strategies for Managing Change*. Reading, MA: Addison-Wesley Publishing Co., 1984.

Ewell C. M. "Strengthening Board/Physician/Management Relationships and Effectiveness." Presentation at the Congress on Administration of the American College of Healthcare Executives, Chicago, 15 February 1989.

Gardner, J. W. *Self-Renewal*. New York: Harper & Row Publishers, 1963.

Griffith, J. "Voluntary Hospitals: Are Trustees the Solutions?" *Hospital & Health Services Administration* 33, no 3 (1988): 295–310.

Levey, S. Interview. *Health Administration Employment: A Survey of Early Career Opportunities*. Arlington, VA: Association of University Programs in Health Administration and Korn Ferry International, 1987.

Lloyd, J. "Where Did I Go Wrong?" *Healthcare Executive* 2, no. 3 (1987): 18–21.

Oglesby, D. K. "The Executive Stretch: Professional Self Renewal." Unpublished manuscript. Presentation at the Texas Hospital Association, Dallas, 3 June 1985.

Pointer, D. D. "Responding to the Challenges of the New Healthcare Marketplace: Organizing for Creativity and Innovation." *Hospital & Health Services Administration* 30, no. 6 (1985): 10–25.

Porter, J., and V. J. Galfano. "MHA Admission Criteria and Program Performance: Do They Predict Career Performance?" *Journal of Health Administration Education* 5, no. 4 (1987): 549–69.

Quick, J. C., J. E. Dalton, D. L. Nelson, and J. D. Quick. "Health Administration Can Be Stressful...But Not Necessarily Distressful." *Hospital & Health Services Administration* 30, no. 5 (1985): 101–11.

Rountree, G. D. "Renew Your Career—Take A Sabbatical." *Hospital & Health Services Administration* 24, no. 4 (1979): 67–80.

Ross, A. "The Mentor's Role in Developing New Leaders." *Hospital & Health Services Administration* 29, no. 5 (1984): 21–29.

Schein, E. H. *Organizational Culture and Leadership*. San Francisco, CA: Jossey-Bass Publishers, 1986.

Shortell, S. M. "High-Performing Healthcare Organizations: Guidelines for the Pursuit of Excellence." *Hospital & Health Services Administration* 30, no. 4 (1985): 7–35.

Silverzweig, and R. F. Allen. "Changing the Corporate Culture." *Sloan Management Review* 17 (Spring 1976): 47–48.

Stolp-Smith, S. C. "Local Healthcare Executive Groups: Tapping Networking Opportunities." *Hospital & Health Services Administration* 31, no. 6 (1986): 103–13.

Toffler, A. *Future Shock*. New York: Random House, 1970.

Part III

Financial Strategies

In their attempts to increase patient revenues, hospitals have undertaken a spectrum of strategic adaptation initiatives such as horizontal and vertical integration, reorganization, and diversification. Hospital operating margins have dipped in recent years, and various forecasters have stated that 20 to 30 percent of facilities are in precarious financial straits. Indications are that the gap in fiscal health between the most profitable and least profitable institutions is widening.

Stephen M. Shortell, Ellen Morrison, and Susan Hughes (Chapter 11) write that hospitals have engaged in a variety of diversification activities over the past several years, many of which have not met expectations. From a nationwide study of 570 hospitals belonging to eight leading hospital systems, four factors are identified that differentiate winners from losers. These include strategies for working effectively with physicians, learning to combine centralized and decentralized strategic planning approaches, understanding partially related diversification, and effectively applying the experience curve.

William O. Cleverley and Roger K. Harvey (Chapter 12) emphasize that executives who fail to recognize competitive factors in their strategy formulation and implementation expose their organization to risk of financial losses and even failure. The central theme of the article is that hospital executives should create and maintain a competitive advantage for their hospital by formulating strategies linked to performance. Through the study of experiences of successful and unsuccessful hospitals, strategic "principles" are presented that will help hospitals enhance performance and reduce the risk of failure.

Thomas R. Prince (Chapter 13) reports on a three-year study of financial outcomes for 1,297 community hospitals. The hospitals are classified into five categories: (1) 121 hospitals in a crisis status, (2) 203 hospitals in a warning status, (3) 511 hospitals with average results, (4) 312 hospitals with excellent performance, and (5) 150 hospitals with outstanding performance.

Cleverley's second article (Chapter 14) provides an analysis of key differences between a small sample of high-performing and low-performing hospitals where performance is defined as return on equity. Significant findings are: (1) High-performing hospitals achieve their superior performance through cost control rather than higher prices; (2) High-performing hospitals minimize their investment in plant assets and accounts receivable; they are also likely to have a newer plant than low-performing hospitals; (3) High-performing hospitals are not afraid to use debt in their capital structure, but they use significantly less debt than low-performing hospitals; (4) High-performing hospitals have set aside greater reserves for future plant replacement, which helps them to keep their level of debt reasonable and generates significant amounts of investment income; and (5) High-performing hospitals have greater market share than low-performing hospitals.

Chapter 11

The Keys to Successful Diversification: Lessons from Leading Hospital Systems

Stephen M. Shortell
Ellen Morrison
Susan Hughes

Stephen M. Shortell is the A. C. Buehler Distinguished Professor of Health Services Management and Professor of Organization Behavior at the J. L. Kellogg Graduate School of Management and Director of the Program on Organization Behavior in Health Care at the Center for Health Services and Policy Research at Northwestern University, Evanston, Illinois. He is a Fellow of the College. Ellen Morrison is Associate Director of the Health Care Program at the Institute for the Future, a non-profit research and forecasting organization in Menlo Park, California. Susan Hughes is Associate Professor in the Department of Community Health at Northwestern University Medical School and Director of the Program in Gerontological Health at the Center for Health Services and Policy Research and Senior Health Scientist in the Center for Cooperative Studies in Health Services at Hines VA Hospital. She is a Member of the College.

This article was published in *Hospital & Health Services Administration* 34, no. 4 (Winter 1989).

"The hope was that diversification would not only help feed the base hospital business but be profitable in its own right as well. So far, we've achieved neither," says a hospital system executive.

This statement reflects most hospitals' experience with diversification over the past several years. Like other service industries that have diversified (e.g., financial services, airlines), health care has experienced a fundamental change in its environment that has been marked by prospective payment for services based on fixed rates, increased competition, new technological developments emphasizing outpatient care, and growing employer and consumer demands for more cost-effective care. The net result is a fundamental change in the strategies, structures, and underlying power relationships of the industry. Strategies have changed from an internal operations focus to an external, market-driven focus. Structures have changed from functionally oriented service lines to services organized along divisional or product lines within multicorporate organizations. Power has shifted from the providers of care to the purchasers and consumers of care.

Faced with these and related challenges, hospitals have responded by diversifying into new services and new markets (Coddington, Palmquist, and Trollinger 1985; University of Chicago 1987). Examples include ambulatory surgery centers, outpatient diagnostic centers, rehabilitation centers, home health care, durable medical equipment, sports medicine, occupational health, health promotion, and behavioral medicine programs among others. The objectives have been to (1) develop additional revenue streams, (2) preempt competitors, (3) feed the core business (i.e., acute inpatient care) through referrals, (4) facilitate earlier hospital discharge, and (5) develop an integrated package of services that can help contain cost, promote continuity of care, and be marketable to local employers.

Many of these objectives have not been achieved. A recent Booz Allen study of 30 large regional health care systems indicated that only one-third received more than 5 percent of their revenues from nonhospital activities (Fox 1988). Few of the initiatives have preempted competitors because of the inability to erect barriers to entry. As one hospital planner commented: "We attract competitors like flies. It doesn't seem to matter what we do." Referrals for inpatient care have frequently been far less than expected. Early discharge to post-hospital facilities have been hampered by a lack of coordination and poor discharge planning, as well as related problems of managing vertical integration (Mick and Conrad 1988). The ability to develop an integrated package of services has been impeded by the lack of systemwide planning and lack of a common set of incentives.

What are the reasons for these negative experiences? Is it because diversification is so new to health care? Is it because health care is so different from other industries? What distinguishes the more successful from the less successful diversifications?

Based on a three-year study of 570 hospitals belonging to eight leading hospital systems (Shortell, Morrison, and Friedman 1990) and conversations with industry leaders, four sets of "best practices" that appear to distinguish the winners from the losers in the health care diversification game have been identified. They are

- Working effectively with physicians
- Combining centralization and decentralization of strategic planning
- Understanding partially related diversification
- Effectively applying the experience curve.

Methods

The eight hospital systems studied ranged in size from four hospitals to over 200 and, together, owned or managed 570 general acute care hospitals in 45 states. Three of the systems are investor-owned, two are not-for-profit religious, and three are not-for-profit secular. All were founded in the late 1960s or early 1970s.

The investor-owned system hospitals are somewhat larger, have somewhat higher occupancy rates, and are more likely to have some degree of teaching involvement than other investor-owned system hospitals at large. The not-for-profit system hospitals are smaller, have somewhat lower occupancy rates, and are less likely to have teaching involvement than other not-for-profit system hospitals. The participating not-for-profit system hospitals are somewhat smaller, have somewhat lower occupancy rates, and are somewhat less likely to have teaching involvement than all U.S. freestanding not-for-profit hospitals. Thus, while the results cannot be statistically generalized to the U.S. population of hospitals at large, the findings and lessons to be discussed hold substantive significance for nearly all hospitals in the country, with one exception. The exception is that freestanding hospitals do not have access to corporate office resources or assistance in undertaking diversification initiatives. Thus, if anything, the challenges and lessons derived from examining diversification among system hospitals may have additional significance for freestanding hospitals. This is particularly true for issues pertaining to physician involvement, understanding partially related diversification, and effectively applying the experience curve. Issues involving the centralization and decentralization of strategic planning primarily pertain to hospitals that are system members.

The findings presented are based on a combination of 127 in-depth semi-structured interviews conducted in 1985 and an additional 37 phone interviews conducted in 1987 with top corporate executives including the president, chief operating officer, vice president for strategic planning, vice president for marketing, and vice president for finance among others; two waves of questionnaires requesting detailed information on approximately 40 diversified services at the individual hospital level; and a survey of each chief executive officer's (CEO) assessment of market share, growth potential, and profitability for 15 specific service lines.[1] Completed response rates were 96 percent for the first wave diversified services questionnaire, 90 percent for the second wave, and 87 percent for the CEO assessment questionnaires. The focus of analysis was primarily on diversification at the individual hospital level.

Descriptive Findings

Table 1 shows the differences in type and extent of diversification by ownership. As indicated, not-for-profit hospitals are more diversified at the *hospital level* than are investor-owned system hospitals. This in part reflects the more diverse constituents served by not-for-profit community hospitals as well as the investor-owned systems' traditional emphasis on acute hospital care. The major exception, National Medical Enterprises, is a broadly diversified health care company overall (e.g., nursing homes, psychiatric hospitals, and rehabilitation hospitals) but not at the individual-hospital level.

Table 1 also indicates that not-for-profit system hospitals are significantly more involved in health maintenance organization (HMO) ownership or sponsorship and somewhat more involved in economic joint-venture relationships

Table 1
Diversification and Managed Care Activities

Item	Investor-Owned System Hospitals (N = 451)	Not-For-Profit System Hospitals (N = 74)
Average number of diversified services offered (bed-size adjusted)	8.83	12.67*
Percent with HMO ownership or sponsorship	3.3%	32.4%*
Preferred provider organization involvement	22.1%	23.0%
Economic joint-venture involvement	23.3%	32.4%**
Percent services reported as profitable	35.0%	37.4%

*$p \leq .001$.
**$p \leq .05$.

with their physicians than investor-owned system hospitals. Interview data indicated that investor-owned hospitals were more interested in cutting losses as quickly as possible once they realized that they did not really know the HMO business. In contrast, not-for-profit system hospitals saw their HMO activity as a central part of their local strategy to develop a continuum of care for retaining and enhancing market share. As such, they were more likely to stay with the HMO strategy even in the face of operating losses. The somewhat greater tendency of not-for-profit hospitals to engage in economic joint-venture activities with their physicians than investor-owned system hospitals is due in part to the historical reluctance of many investor-owned hospitals to undertake any activity that might be viewed as interfering in the practice of medicine. As a result, they have been somewhat slower than their not-for-profit counterparts in developing such initiatives.

Interview data also indicated that the corporate office usually set the overall thrust and direction for the diversification activities. Each hospital, however, was generally free to choose its own set of activities that appeared to fit its own local market needs and circumstances best. Among the most frequently offered services were ambulatory surgery, chemo/radiation therapy, outpatient diagnostic services, outpatient and in-home rehabilitation programs, health screening, and wellness programs. Most of the efforts were in operation for at least two years, and some are best described as second- and even third-generation diversification activities. An example of the latter was a freestanding ambulatory surgery center that subsequently added a birthing center and most recently has evolved into an integrated medical campus offering a wide range of ambulatory health care services (Goldsmith 1989). Overall, 75 percent of the services were provided independently by the hospitals themselves, 14 percent were offered jointly with an outside party, and 11 percent were joint-ventured internally within the corporate system.

The criteria for successful diversification included both the financial viability of the venture itself as well as the extent to which it contributed to the hospital's overall financial viability and achievement of its strategic objectives. For example, a satellite clinic might not have been profitable on its own, but it was considered successful if it channeled patients to other physicians within the system and generally preempted the market from other competitors. Considering both direct and indirect operating costs, Table 2 presents a summary of the most frequently reported profitable and unprofitable services. Overall, approximately one-third of the diversified services were reported as profitable but approximately 50 to 60 percent of the efforts might be considered successful if one takes into account the role that the service played as a loss leader or feeder of patients to other physicians or to the hospital itself, or otherwise helped the hospital to meet its strategic objectives.

Table 2
Most Frequently Reported Profitable and Unprofitable Services*

Profitable	Unprofitable
Ambulatory surgery	Crisis intervention
Chemotherapy/Radiation therapy	Outpatient psychiatric/mental health services
Rehabilitation program	Urgent care/immediate care centers
Cardiac rehabilitation/conditioning	Geriatric assessment/consultation/case
Outpatient respiratory therapy	management
Durable medical equipment	Geriatric day care
In-home infusion therapy	Home-delivered meals to seniors
In-home physical therapy	Health screening services
In-home respiratory care	Immunization services
In-home extended therapy services (not	Occupational health services
physical therapy)	School health exams
Outpatient radiology	Wellness programs
Outpatient CT scan	Disease/condition-specific counseling and
Outpatient nuclear magnetic resonance or	education
magnetic resonance imaging	Community health lectures, classes, and
Outpatient ultrasound	health fairs
Outpatient hematology/biochemistry lab	Family planning and preparation: parenting
Outpatient neurological diagnostic services	and sibling education
Outpatient cardiovascular diagnostic	Hospice
services	Intermediate care/skilled nursing facility
Outpatient nuclear medicine	Hospital-sponsored primary care group
	practice

*Profitability = operating revenues minus operating costs (direct and indirect).

The Four Keys

The Physician Factor

What most distinguishes health care from other industries is the role played by physicians. Most physicians are not hospital employees, and many belong on the staffs of competing institutions. What physicians do or do not do and what they say or do not say can affect all hospital decisions—including the decision to diversify into new services and new markets. Imagine IBM trying to develop the personal computer while working with a group of "voluntary" engineers and scientists who at the same time also work with Apple or Zenith.

Almost every participating executive mentioned the importance of developing effective working relationships with physicians. Physicians generally opposed hospital diversification efforts for three reasons: encroachment on physician turf, such as when a hospital sponsors a primary care center that competes with staff physicians for patients; philosophical opposition to what physicians perceive as the "corporate practice of medicine"; and lack of involvement in the planning and decision-making process. In other cases, the hospital serves as a symbolic target of criticism reflecting physician frustrations with the many social and economic changes affecting physician income and the way in which medicine is practiced. The problem is also compounded when specific diversification efforts pit one group of physicians against another. For example, one hospital faced a fiasco when its desire to open an ambulatory surgery center was seen by key physicians as favoring one group of surgeons over another.

To deal effectively with these challenges requires both across-the-board and targeted strategies. Successful hospitals learned that a key across-the-board strategy was to get meaningful physician involvement into the governance and management of the institution. This includes involving physicians as voting members of the hospital board, as key participants in the strategic planning process of the institution, and as members of the hospital's top management team. At one Midwest hospital this was reflected in physician involvement throughout the organization. Among 15 voting board members, three were physicians from the hospital and a fourth was a respected outside physician from a neighboring community. Three physicians serve on the hospital's strategic planning committee. There is also a full-time executive vice president for medical affairs (a physician) whose job is to oversee all of the hospital's quality assurance activities and to ensure integration between the hospital's strategic plan and physicians' interests. The hospital feels that these mechanisms help to assure that physician ideas, interests, and concerns receive regular attention. They also serve as a forum through which the hospital educates physicians regarding challenges facing the institution and the need to consider new opportunities.

This grass roots involvement at the individual hospital level needs to be extended to the regional and corporate levels of hospital systems. At least five of the eight systems studied created physician executive positions at corporate and regional offices. These positions were usually charged with the responsibility for overseeing systemwide quality assurance efforts, assessing future trends in medical practice, and helping to assure that the system's plans were sensitive to, informed by, and consistent with physician interests at local hospitals throughout the system. In a few cases, physicians were responsible for overseeing the system's diversification plans, such as in the area of HMOs and managed care.

The across-the-board involvement approach provides a climate or culture supportive of diversification efforts, but it is not enough. Also needed are specifically focused strategies that speak to physicians' economic and professional interests. This involves the need to identify those physicians who are

169

most interested in specific diversification initiatives, those who are likely to be neutral, and those who may be opposed. Some strategies for promoting the former while neutralizing the latter are discussed here.

An East Coast hospital began formulating its diversification strategy by surveying medical staff members regarding their assessment of the hospital's strengths and weaknesses, the need for new programs, and their own practice plans. From this survey, the hospital identified three areas for possible cooperative activity: an outpatient magnetic resonance imaging (MRI) center, an outpatient cardiac rehabilitation program, and a home health care agency. Each initiative, however, also had detractors. A joint hospital-physician committee was appointed to explore the pros and cons of each activity. After much study and discussion, the committee decided to proceed with the MRI as a 50/50 economic joint venture between the hospital and physicians, allowing all physicians on the staff to invest in the venture if they desired rather than limiting it to those who would directly benefit from the relationship. Cardiac rehabilitation plans were temporarily put on hold pending recruitment of an additional cardiologist. An agreement for joint ownership of a home health care agency with a neighboring hospital was approved by physicians with the understanding that they were not required to refer their patients to the agency. Referrals would depend on the quality of services provided by the agency. Two physicians were appointed by the hospital to the home health agency board.

Faced with pressure from HMOs and other managed care entities, a West Coast hospital and its physicians decided to first form a joint corporation *before* considering any specific diversification opportunities. They decided that it was important for both parties to be at economic risk or reward, to have equal involvement in governance and management, and to develop criteria for evaluating specific activities that would be consistent with the new corporation's mission and purpose. Among these criteria were the extent to which specialists would benefit (through increased referrals) from programs designed to increase primary care physician practices, and the extent to which primary care physicians would benefit (through increased institutional prestige) from programs desired to enhance specialists' capabilities. These considerations led to the formation of a ten-person board (five hospital representatives and five physicians), the appointment of a physician executive, and development of a committee to screen proposals. After four years the corporation has developed a successful preferred provider organization (PPO), several successful outpatient diagnostic centers, one ambulatory surgery center, and a very successful physician practice management program.

Among the specific lessons to be gleaned from the above experiences are the following:

There is the need for a clear statement of mission and purpose not only for the organizational entity charged with diversification but also for each specific *diversification activity.* As stated by one hospital's home health care activity:

> The goal of our home health care program is to keep patients within our health care system by providing a coordinated array of medical, social, and support services in an accessible, affordable and convenient manner. We will evaluate our success through patient, family, and physician satisfaction surveys; by attempting to achieve at least one-third market share within the first two years; by breaking even financially after the first two years; and by tracing the number of patients who use other services within our system.

The selection of physicians who understand and are willing to take some financial risks is important. As one executive commented: "Some physicians' idea of a joint venture is when they get all the *adventure* and stick us with the *joint.*"

A clear specification at the outset of each others' roles and responsibilities must be made. Physicians often operate on short time frames and, thus, expect financial rewards sooner than can be realistically achieved. Executives must carefully explain the short-run and long-run risks and communicate realistic financial scenarios. Services that are well reimbursed and less subject to cost-containment pressures such as ambulatory surgery and outpatient diagnostic testing are more likely to be immediately profitable than less well-reimbursed services such as hospice care and geriatric services. Criteria should also be developed by which each party may dissolve its interest in the joint venture.

A detailed business plan should be developed for each specific program. The plans should include target market characteristics, market size, projected market share by segment, projected revenues and expenses (broken out by fixed and variable), and delineation of backup or contingency plans.

There should be shared (hospital and physician) governance in management of the joint activity consistent with the nature of the risk/reward relationship. Fifty/fifty financial arrangements should be matched with approximately 50/50 decision making authority and influence. In cases where one or the other party bears more of the risk/reward relationship (for example, 75/25), governance and managerial decision making should be matched accordingly.

Appropriate forums need to be established for managing conflict. In smaller undertakings, this can be done successfully through close, almost daily interaction between the CEO and key physician leaders. Important unresolved disagreements can be handled by the board. In larger organizations, task forces may be created to oversee troublesome areas. It is particularly important that interested individuals with the appropriate expertise and knowledge be involved in these deliberations. The process must be seen as fair by all involved.

Sufficient autonomy must be given to the diversification or joint venture unit. Ambulatory surgery, home health care, health promotion, and sports medicine are very different from providing acute inpatient care. Attempts to impose the hospital's culture, rules, and decision-making paradigms on these new kinds of activities failed time and time again. A diversification unit must be free to experiment and to learn what best serves its needs.

Finally, it is important that information systems be developed to match the needs of the diversification activity so that corrective action may be taken in a timely fashion. A number of HMO and PPO activities failed in part because of lack of sufficient or accurate data on projected enrollment and utilization by market segment.

Combining across-the-board physician involvement in the management and governance of the institution with specifically focused joint-venture strategies were the hallmark of the "best practices" of the more successful diversifiers. The degree of specific physician involvement required generally depends on the extent to which the new activity directly threatens physicians' economic and professional interests. As shown in Figure 1, this will be very high for such programs as ambulatory surgery and outpatient diagnostic centers and less so for such undertakings as health promotion and health education.

To Centralize or Not: Achieving Strategic Integration

It is widely recognized that health care is delivered locally and is therefore subject to local traditions, preferences, and physician practice styles. This makes it difficult for national and even regional hospital systems to develop

---

Figure 1
Degree of Physician Involvement Required

Higher   Lower

$\longleftarrow$ ————————————————————————————————— $\longrightarrow$

Ambulatory surgery	Industrial medicine	Home health	Health promotion
Outpatient diagnostic center	Sports medicine		Health education
Outpatient cardiac rehabilitation unit			

172

new products and services to meet the needs of different local markets. If one tailors such services specifically to each market, one loses some of the economies of scale of being a system. On the other hand, failure to do such targeting may result in rejection by the local market. Thus, it is difficult at the corporate level to develop a diversification strategy that is strategically integrated with the system's acute care strategy. One hospital planner highlighted the dilemma as follows: "Our inpatient care strategies differ somewhat from market to market but compared to our other activities they're a piece of cake. Everyone needs basic medical, surgical, and obstetrics care. But deciding to put dollars on behavioral medicine versus retirement homes versus fitness centers is chancy. Many of our communities are very different from each other."

To diversify usually requires some degree of innovation. This, in turn, usually requires some degree of autonomy that often runs counter to the needs of multidivisional organizations such as hospital systems for some degree of centralized control (Gupta 1987; Hill and Hoskisson 1987). Centralization appears to facilitate certain "induced" processes such as formal environmental assessment and competitor analysis while decentralization favors various "autonomous" processes that are spontaneously generated by individuals in the course of dealing with everyday challenges (Burgelman 1983b; Mintzberg 1978). In the present study, the more successful diversified hospitals met this challenge through a combined centralized-decentralized approach to strategic planning rather than an either/or approach. In these systems, the overall direction and some market analysis were conducted centrally, but each hospital was left free to determine the mix and amount of services to meet local market needs. Once the broad guidelines were set, serving the local market well became the basis for strategic integration. A hospital located in a young growing community emphasized women and children services, health promotion and health education, sports medicine and fitness centers. A hospital located in a community with a growing elderly population emphasized long-term care services including nursing home care, adult day health care, hospice care, and continuing care retirement centers.

The following cases illustrate a centralized-decentralized approach.

- A moderately sized investor-owned hospital system experimented in the early 1980s with centralizing its planning process. Standardized reporting forms were used, the results were analyzed by corporate planning staff, and the decisions were largely made by corporate executives. Central themes or product lines were identified such as urgent care centers and occupational medicine clinics. Directives encouraging all hospitals to initiate such activities were issued. Local hospital executives struggled to "fit" these programs to their own environment, with some successes but more failures. In many communities

173

these programs simply did not meet local needs or take into sufficient account local competition despite their appeal from the vantage point of corporate strategic analysis. Recognizing their mistake, the system reorganized its planning process. Market analysis is now done locally but with assistance from the regional and corporate office. Based on such analysis, local hospitals' strategic plans are developed and forwarded up the corporate chain for review and comment. Local hospital executives now participate in regional and corporate planning task forces. Corporate and regional planning, marketing, and financial staff are called on by local CEOs as needed. The implementation process is directed by the local hospital. Test markets are developed for targeted programs such as lower back pain clinics. If successful, they are then made available to other interested hospitals—typically hospitals operating in a similar market and with similar competitive circumstances as the test site. The net result for the system has been the development of a process of transfer learning.

- A hospital system operating in the West recognized that its attempts to diversify into ambulatory care centers, pharmacy management, and dietary services, while marginally profitable, were diverting resources that might better be employed elsewhere. The CEO commented, "We can't be all things to all people." Most of these strategies have been developed centrally. The problems of implementation occurred locally and were largely due to physician opposition. The system recognized the need for local physician input into the process, as previously stated. They have now decentralized the planning process with particular emphasis on assessing local physician needs and interests. Through this process they have identified several "cluster markets" of hospitals and associated physicians where they believe synergies can be achieved through programs of selective diversification that will support both hospital and physician interests. Examples include diagnostic testing centers and industrial health exams.

- A third case illustrates the need for some degree of centralization and control. Philosophically committed to decentralization and local hospital autonomy, several diversified programs have been developed by local hospitals, particularly in regard to HMOs and care for the elderly. These programs face strong competition and are less profitable than expected. Part of the problem was the reluctance of local hospitals to "pull the plug" on activities in which they had a heavy emotional investment. The system recognized the need for a more formal and somewhat more centralized planning process that would provide greater discipline and accountability. A "top down-botton up" process was initiated in which the corporate office provides overall guidelines and strategic directions. Hospitals then develop their own plans within these guidelines, which are then submitted for corporate office review, comment, and approval. The plan is monitored throughout the year by both individual hospital and corporate office staff. A staff planner commented, "A certain amount of direction and control is necessary to achieve consistency with our mission, but there is only so much we can do at corporate. A lot of the action remains local and that's probably where it should be."

The health care corporations studied are continuing to experiment with their planning systems. There is greater recognition that strategic planning is as much a line management function as it is a staff function and of the consequent need for greater preparation of line managers in strategic thinking (Gray 1986). In general the larger and more geographically diversified the system, the greater the decentralization of the planning process. Aside from the assessment of national trends and competitive factors, most functions are being done by regional offices or local hospitals. Corporate office plays primarily an advisory and integrative role.

The smaller the system and the more geographically concentrated and homogeneous the markets, the easier it is for more centralized planning to be effective. Even here, however, there is greater involvement of local hospital executives and physician leaders than was true in the past.

Partially Related Diversification

What went wrong in the following situations?

- A midwestern hospital decided to diversify by starting a primary care group practice. A popular staff physician agreed to head the group, and the practice was successful in recruiting several new primary care physicians. The practice was established as a subunit of the hospital's ambulatory care division. Many of the hospital's personnel policies, budgeting, purchasing, billing, reporting, and information systems were established for the group. After six months, two of the three physicians resigned from the group citing frustrations with the "hospital's bureaucratic approach to the practice."

- A hospital in the Rocky Mountain area identified a market need for a health promotion or wellness program. The nurses charged with development of the program felt it would be natural to organize it as part of the hospital's nursing department. After several months in which hospital rules, policies, and practices threatened program growth, it was reorganized as a separate unit with its own leadership and charged with responsibility of developing its own policies and practices.

- Several hospital systems in the 1980s became involved in HMO ownership. After sustaining considerable losses, several withdrew, citing price cutting on the part of established health care insurance carriers, lack of actuarial underwriting skills, and alienated physicians as the reasons for their withdrawal.

The common thread throughout these scenarios is that the parties involved *misjudged the relatedness* of these activities with the hospital's mainstream acute care business. This was a pervasive problem for almost all hospitals and systems studied. Delivering primary care, developing a health promotion program, and running an HMO are quite different activities than delivering acute inpatient care. What hospital executives thought of as related diversification under the general rubric of health care services was, at best, only partially related. Hospital efforts to manage these activities as they did the acute care business spelled failure.

More successful diversification efforts were marked by greater attention paid to assessing the *clinical* and *managerial* relatedness of the services undertaken. Clinical relatedness dimensions include

- Compatibility with existing technology
- Consistency with existing technical skills and knowledge
- Ability to build synergies with existing clinical services, such as outpatient cardiac rehabilitation, complementing a strong inpatient cardiology program
- Compatibility with the interests of clinical staff.

Managerial relatedness criteria include

- Consistency with the hospital's mission and philosophy
- Consistency with existing managerial skills, knowledge, and resources
- Compatibility with existing management systems
- Ability to serve relevant hospital markets.

176

Findings from other industries generally suggest that related diversification, because of the ability to leverage human and technological resources, is more successful financially than unrelated diversification (Rumelt 1976; Montgomery 1982). Our findings, contrary to previous studies of health care diversification (Clement 1987) also support this notion. Services that were clinically and managerially more related to the provision of acute inpatient care such as ambulatory surgery, outpatient chemotherapy and radiation therapy, CT scans, nuclear medicine, ultrasound, and cardiovascular/pulmonary diagnostic services were more profitable than less-related services such as fitness centers, adult day health programs, and health promotion programs (see Table 2). However, our evidence also suggests that such partially related services as home health care, geriatric care, primary care, sports medicine, and occupational health can be successful if it is recognized that the technological, managerial, and cultural requirements for success are *different* from those involved in providing acute inpatient care. As previously mentioned, this means giving those involved with such activities sufficient autonomy to manage them. As one executive noted, "You cannot manage this kind of activity [a primary care center] as you do the hospital's radiology department. They won't stand for it. The needs are different—different markets, different kinds of staff, different technologies. We found that they didn't even want to use our purchasing system because they [the primary care center] felt they could build good will by purchasing from a local vendor. We learned quickly."

The extent to which diversification efforts are clinically and managerially related to the acute care business also influences the way in which hospitals choose to develop new services and new markets. In general, the more related the diversification and the more familiar the hospital is with the new services and new markets, the more appropriate is internal development by the hospital itself. Internal development, such as for an ambulatory surgery center, results in a higher degree of control over the service. In contrast, the more unrelated the proposed service, the more likely it is that joint ventures and alliances become more appropriate entry strategies (Roberts and Berry 1985). These strategies enable hospitals to share the cost and risk and to maximize learning opportunities, although they result in some loss of control and the need to manage the transaction costs among the joint venture or alliance partners. Intermediate entry strategies include internal corporate ventures (Burgelman 1983a) such as for a cardiology rehabilitation center and internal corporate joint ventures (Shortell and Zajac 1988), particularly for partially related diversification activities such as hospital-sponsored primary care centers where external joint-venture possibilities may not exist. These intermediate strategies have the advantage of promoting innovation while enabling the hospital to maintain some degree of control. Major challenges, however, involve balancing the autonomy needs of the venture unit with the control needs of the hospital.

In the hospitals studied, there was emerging evidence that entry strategies were being matched more appropriately to diversification opportunities. For example, the initial entry strategy of many systems into the HMO business was through internal development or acquisition. These systems quickly learned that they lacked the necessary knowledge and expertise to make such an entry strategy viable. Many switched to a joint venture strategy such as Hospital Corporation of America's joint venture with Equitable Insurance (Equicorp) and the Voluntary Hospitals of America's (VHA) joint venture with Aetna.

Entry strategies can of course be sequenced and used in combination. For example, a joint-venture strategy might be used to gain greater knowledge of a new business in a new market and then brought in house for greater control for purposes of long-run expansion.

Timing, the Experience Curve, and the First Mover Advantage

The experience curve suggests that those who are "first movers" into a market with a new product or service can build volume quickly and translate the learning involved into continued process improvements that can result in creating a barrier to entry for would-be competitors (Ghemawat 1985). Whether or not organizations that are first movers can sustain the initial advantage depends on their ability to keep the learning or experience curve advantages proprietary (i.e., within the firm) and, in general, keep their overall strategy from being imitated by others (Lieberman and Montgomery 1988; Barney 1988). Where this cannot be accomplished great demands are placed on the need to continually differentiate the product or service (Porter 1985) to sustain competitive advantage. The hospitals that were more successful at diversification understood better than the less successful the circumstances and conditions under which the experience-curve effects could be realized. The following examples illustrate the point.

- Hospital X faced a market in which two HMOs had already enrolled over 100,000 subscribers. The hospital, having lost the first mover advantage, nonetheless decided to develop its own HMO to protect its existing patient base from further erosion. As the vice president for strategic planning commented, "We were late into the HMO market. Our enrollment is less than one-third of our major competitor. We lost $1 million our first year. But 90% of employers in the area offer the HMO option. So we feel we have to be involved to prevent further erosion and to be a full-service provider." The hospital is essentially involved in a rear guard defensive strategy. An alternative developed by a hospital in another community was a joint venture with an established HMO and, thereby, an opportunity to share in the learning gained by the more established organization as well as sharing the risk.

- Hospital Y felt the pressure to expand its primary care base and, thereby, hoped to increase its referrals. A cornerstone of its strategy was to develop a network of urgent care centers providing low-cost, convenient care on evenings and weekends as well as weekdays. The hospital was the first in the market to develop such centers and hoped to reap the experience-curve effects of being a first mover. After 18 months, the financial results were disappointing, and the hospital divested three-fourths of its centers. The hospital failed to recognize the ease with which the urgent care center concept could be imitated by existing competitors. Rather than being first in the market, the urgent care centers represented a late entrant into a very crowded market that included not only the hospital's own emergency room (a case of service cannibalism) but numerous physician offices and clinics. It was relatively easy for these groups to compete by extending their own hours and emphasizing quality features that were not a part of the urgent care center marketing plan. The more successful centers did not rely on the experience-curve effect but rather on an explicit differentiation strategy focused on highly selected market niches not occupied by current physicians or treatment centers.

- A contrasting example is provided by Hospital Z, which was first in its market to develop an ambulatory surgery center. Other hospitals in the area were unable to react quickly enough because of an inability to secure needed physician agreement, as previously mentioned. Thus, Hospital Z was able to capture learning-curve effects by increasing volume over time, gaining experience, and lowering unit costs. The hospital was also able to take advantage of a changing reimbursement climate favoring outpatient surgery. By the time competitors were able to start their own centers, Hospital Z had established a stronghold in the market—a position that it maintains to the present.

Each of these scenarios illustrates the complexities involved in considering whether or not first mover experience-curve effects can be captured. Experience-curve effects are generally difficult to attain when there is rapid technological obsolescence, demand is unpredictable, the volume of output does not increase fast enough for the experience curve to provide sufficient leverage, demand is not price sensitive, the cost-reduction approach can be easily imitated by competitors, or there are strong competitors who are already following an experience-curve strategy or can easily do so (Ghemawat 1985).

Each of these criteria poses particular challenges for health care organizations because the industry is marked by rapid technological turnover—for example, in diagnostic imaging technology; unpredictable demand, particularly for less serious illnesses; low-volume service—for example, health promotion and lower back pain clinics; price inelasticity of demand due to third-party insurance coverage; cost reductions or service changes that can be easily imitated by others as in the case of Hospital Y; and sometimes strong competitors who are already following an experience-curve strategy such as in the case of Hospital X. While these criteria will not be equally relevant for each service, it is important that each service that is a candidate for diversification be carefully screened against these criteria to improve its chances for success. Particularly likely candidates include high-technology–oriented services with high-volume potential such as ambulatory surgery, diagnostic imaging, and renal dialysis.

Corporate executives frequently mentioned the importance of being the first or at least an early entrant into the market. This is due to the personal nature of health services that makes it very difficult to recapture market share after it is lost. People do not switch physicians or hospitals as quickly as they switch brands of beer or clothing. As a result, entering a market late is unlikely to result in recovering patients, although it may help prevent additional losses. Resources spent on late entry service strategies designed to prevent further erosion, as in the case of Hospital X, need to be balanced against resources that could be used for first mover advantages designed to increase market share in other areas. In making these decisons, we found that hospitals need to make inevitable trade-offs between the time needed to do thorough market and financial analyses and the opportunity to beat the competition to the punch. The old adage that analysis should not lead to paralysis has merit. Often more is learned from experimenting with an underanalyzed service than waiting for more desktop analysis while others preempt the opportunity.

While early entry strategies are important, there is also the need for sustaining a commitment to this strategy. The experience of the eight systems studied suggests that while losing ventures can generally be determined within two years, it often takes five years or longer before one is sure of a winner. The trick is in living with the uncertainty and ambiguity surrounding the third and fourth years. This requires a high degree of commitment from top management with sufficient financial strength to stay the course. As noted earlier, this often requires physician involvement and support and balancing physician needs for autonomy with the hospital's needs for some degree of control and accountability.

Working All Fronts

The lessons that have emerged from our inside look at hospital diversification suggest that the keys to success are the development of plans that are closely linked to physicians interests, strategically driven and strategically integrated in local markets, appropriately differentiated from acute inpatient care but building on acute care synergies where possible, and highly selective in regard to the timing of market entry. As suggested in Figure 2, these key success factors or "best practices" are related to each other. For example, without strong hospital-physician relationships it is not possible to integrate strategies locally, respond to different diversification requirements, nor move quickly to capture first mover advantages. At the same time, one cannot take advantage

Figure 2
Key Success Factors in Hospital Diversification

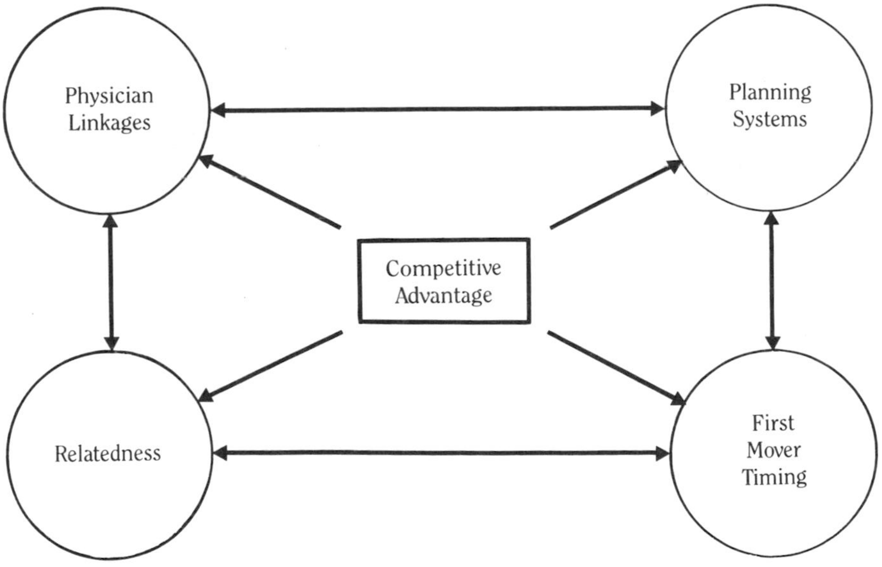

of strong local hospital-physician relationships by an overcentralization of strategy making at the corporate office. Lack of a combined adaptive centralized-decentralized approach to strategic planning also makes it more difficult to assess the degree of differentiation required by local diversification efforts. This, in turn, retards the local hospital's ability to launch new ventures in a timely fashion.

Because these lessons are based on the experiences of 570 hospitals located in 45 states over a period of three years, they have wide applicability to the industry in general. While differences of degree may exist by hospital and system size, ownership, and region, it is clear that hospital diversification in the future will have to demonstrate superior value in the local market. It will not fully protect nor make up for inpatient losses or weaknesses but, rather, should build on the strengths of the inpatient business. It will be characterized by a less restrictive adaptive approach to strategic planning that emphasizes flexibility and learning from mistakes. Diversification will need to be viewed as part, but only as a part, of a hospital's overall strategy to develop an integrated continuum of care in its market. Most importantly, it will need to be physician linked, reflecting the basic interdependence of hospitals and physicians.

Acknowledgments

The findings on which this article is based were supported by The National Center for Health Services Research and Health Care Technology Assessment (Grant #05159) and the Robert Wood Johnson Foundation, Princeton, New Jersey (Grant #9181 and #11451). This research would not have been possible without the active and ongoing support of the eight study systems: American Medical International, Evangelical Health Systems, Health Central (currently Health One), Hospital Corporation of America, Intermountain Health Care, National Medical Enterprises, Sisters of Mercy Health Care Corporation, and Southwest Community Health Services. We particularly acknowledge the contributions made by the advisory committee composed of representatives from each system. The support of the American Hospital Association is gratefully acknowledged. The article has also benefited from the comments of the reviewers. Appreciation is expressed to Alice Schaller and Cathy Ver Halen for their assistance in manuscript preparation.

Note

1.   Copies of the questionnaires may be obtained by writing to the authors.

References

Barney, Jay. "The Context of Formal Strategic Planning and the Economic Performance of Firms." Strategy Group Working Series, No. 88-005. College Station: Texas A&M University Department of Management, April 1988.

Burgelman, Rob A. "A Model of the Interaction of Strategic Behavior, Corporate Context, and the Concept of Strategy." *Academy of Management Review* 8 (1983a): 61–70.

———. "A Process Model of Internal Corporate Venturing in the Diversified Major Firm." *Administrative Science Quarterly* 28 (1983b): 223–44.

Clement, Jan P. "Does Hospital Diversification Improve Financial Outcomes?" *Medical Care* 25 (October 1987): 988–1001.

Coddington, Dean C., Lowell E. Palmquist, and William V. Trollinger. "Strategies for Survival in the Hospital Industry." *Harvard Business Review* 63 (May–June 1985): 129–38.

Fox, Wende L. *Vertical Integration Viewpoints.* Booz, Allen, and Hamilton, June 1988.

Ghemawat, Pankij. "Building Strategy on the Experience Curve." *Harvard Business Review* 63 (March–April 1985): 143–49.

Goldsmith, Jeff A. "A Radical Prescription for Hospitals." *Harvard Business Review* 68 (May–June 1989): 104–11.

Gray, D. H. "Uses and Misuses of Strategic Planning." *Harvard Business Review* 64 (January–February 1986): 90–97.

Gupta, Anil K. "SBU Strategies, Corporate-SBU Relations, and SBU Effectiveness in Strategy Implementation." *Academy of Management Journal* 30 (September 1987): 477–500.

Hill, Charles W., and Robert E. Hoskisson. "Strategy and Structure in the Multi Product Firm." *Academy of Management Review* 12 (April 1987): 331–41.

Lieberman, Marvin B., and David B. Montgomery. "First Mover Advantages." *Strategic Management Journal* 9 (Summer 1988): 41–58.

Mick, Stephen S., and Douglas A. Conrad. "The Decision to Integrate Vertically in Health Care Organizations." *Hospital & Health Services Administration* 33 (Fall 1988): 345–60.

Mintzberg, Henry. "Patterns in Strategy Formation." *Management Science* 24 (1978): 934–48.

Montgomery, Cynthia A. "The Measurement of Related Diversification: Some New Empirical Evidence." *Academy of Management Journal* 25 (1982): 299–307.

Porter, Michael E. *Competitive Advantage: Creating and Sustaining Superior Performance.* New York: The Free Press, 1985.

Roberts, Edward B., and Charles A. Berry. "Entering New Businesses: Selecting Strategies for Success." *Sloan Management Review* 26 (Spring 1985): 3–17.

Rumelt, Richard P. *Strategy, Structure and Economic Performance.* Boston: Division of Research, Graduate School of Business Administration, Harvard University, 1976.

Shortell, Stephen M., and Edward J. Zajac. "Internal Corporate Joint Ventures: Development Processes and Performance Outcomes." *Strategic Management Journal* 9 (November–December 1988): 527–42.

Shortell, Stephen M., Ellen M. Morrison, and Bernard Friedman. *Strategic Choices for America's Hospitals: Managing Change in Turbulent Times.* San Francisco: Jossey-Bass, 1990.

University of Chicago. "Does Diversification Make Health Care Organizations Healthier?" *Proceedings of the 29th Annual George Bugbee Symposium on Hospital Affairs.* Graduate Program in Health Administration and Center for Health Administration Studies of the University, May 1987.

Chapter 12

Competitive Strategy for Successful Hospital Management

William O. Cleverley
Roger K. Harvey

William O. Cleverley is Professor of Health Care Finance, Ohio State University, Columbus. He is a Faculty Associate of the College. Roger K. Harvey is Emeritus Associate Professor of Finance, Ohio State University, Columbus.

This article was published in *Hospital & Health Services Administration* 37, no. 1 (Spring 1992).

Today, more than at any other time in the past, competitive forces are shaping management strategy in the health care industry. In less than a decade the hospital industry has evolved from an industry that was virtually insulated from traditional market pressures because of entry regulation and cost reimbursement to one in which competitive factors influence virtually all strategic decisions.

Health care executives who fail to recognize competitive factors in their strategy formulation and implementation expose their organization to risk of financial losses and even failure. In a 1990 survey conducted by Deloitte & Touche, 43 percent of 1,765 responding hospital executives believed that their hospital could fail within five years (Nemess 1990). While the 43 percent represented a decline from 48 percent just two years previous, the primary conclusion still remains that many hospital executives, their boards, and medical staffs are legitimately concerned about corporate failure.

The central theme of this article is that hospital executives can create and maintain a competitive advantage for their hospital by formulating strategies that are linked to performance. Our method for identifying performance-based strategies is to study the actual experiences of successful and unsuccessful hospitals. It is our position that by comparing and contrasting the performance indicators of a large group of successful versus unsuccessful hospitals, we can show important relationships to strategies or actions that might be employed to enhance hospital competitive advantage.

The genesis for our approach may be found in the work of Buzzell and Gayle (1987). They used the PIMS (Profit Impact of Market Strategy) data base of over 450 firms and 3,000 business units to develop a set of empirically based strategic principles that help business executives understand and improve their performance. Their analysis has shown links between performance and market share, investment intensity, product or service quality, labor productivity, and vertical integration. We hope that the strategic principles reported herein will help hospital executives make better strategic choices that will enhance their performance and reduce the risk of failure.

What Is Successful Performance?

In this article empirical data will be used to determine successful and unsuccessful hospital strategy. The first question to be raised, however, is What is success? A hospital that one person might regard as highly successful may be categorized as unsuccessful by another. While we are not totally satisfied with our selection, we will use profitability as our criterion for success, recognizing that there are many other clinical and nonclinical definitions of success, and even acknowledging that there are financial measures other than "profit" that might define a successful hospital. We have chosen "profit" as our measure of success, however, because in today's competitive health care market, a hospital must have profits to survive. Without profits, a hospital will fail; with profits, a hospital has the opportunity to survive and to succeed. "Profit is like health. You need it, and the more you have the better. But it's not why you exist" (Peters and Waterman 1982).

Our specific measure of performance is Return On Asset Investment (ROI), defined as follows:

$$\frac{\text{Net Income} + \text{Interest}}{\text{Total Assets}}$$

Our measure of ROI adds back interest expense to neutralize the effect of financing: hospitals with the same operating and nonoperating income but with different proportions of debt in their capital structure will have the same ROI. With this measure, a hospital will not be classified as "successful" or "unsuccessful" because it is highly leveraged—success means the hospital has high operating and nonoperating income relative to its investment in assets.

Studies of performance in industry have used some ROI measure (Buzzell and Gayle 1987). Any business that over a sustained period of time is unable to generate an adequate ROI will find itself in one of three situations: (1) exiting the business through failure or closure; (2) resizing or repositioning itself within its market, or (3) seeking financial support from a third party, such as a governmental agency, to subsidize financial deficiencies.

Methods

For this investigation, empirical observations of successful strategies have been drawn from a data base of 1,025 hospitals that operate in the largest markets in the United States. All of the hospitals in our universe are defined as "large urban hospitals" under the Medicare prospective payment system. This means that they operate in metropolitan statistical areas that have populations exceeding one million.

The data presented is for 1988 only and was obtained using the Healthcare Financial Management Association's (HFMA) Medicare Cost Report (MCR+) data base. The HFMA extracts this data from the Health Care Financing Administration's Medicare cost reports. The MCR+ data base provides information on virtually every hospital in the United States operating in a large urban area during 1988. The comprehensiveness of this data base is a major advantage when discussing the generalizabilty of the findings because we are able to derive results from the entire universe of hospitals in large metropolitan areas rather than from a sample of those hospitals.

Hospitals operating in large urban areas were specifically selected to focus on successful competitive strategies. While competition may exist in rural and smaller urban areas, it may not be as important a force in those markets. Since the objective of our research was to examine successful competitive strategies, examining areas where competition was most likely to exist seemed important.

We performed two types of statistical analyses. First, our universe was split into high-performance and low-performance hospitals based on each hospital's ROI. High-performance hospitals were those hospitals in the upper-quartile group with respect to ROI, low-performance hospitals were in the lower-quartile group with respect to ROI. Since we segmented our high- and low-performance hospitals based on ROI quartiles (highest 25 percent versus lowest 25 percent of our sample of 1,025 hospitals), we identified 256 hospitals as upper-quartile hospitals and 256 hospitals as lower-quartile hospitals. For each group, we summed the 256 hospitals' balance sheet and income statement data accounts and then divided each account total item by 256. The result was a composite average for each account; these results are reported in Tables 1 and 2. We then computed composite average ratios from the values in Tables 1 and 2 and compared the ratios from the high- and low-performance groups. The results of these comparisons are reported below.

Second, a multiple regression equation was fitted to the entire data set (1,025 hospitals) using ROI as the dependent variable and a number of variables that were reflective of management strategy as the independent variables. Regression results are presented in Table 3. We use regression analysis to identify performance measures and then competitive strategies that significantly affect ROI. These results are reported below.

Cost Leadership

One of the three generic strategies cited by Michael Porter (1980) for dealing with competitive forces is cost leadership. While the advantages of lower costs have been cited for sometime in industries other than health care, only recently have health care executives expressed interest in the management strategies associated with lower cost. A 1990 article stated that cost control appeared to be critically related to improved financial performance in a small sample of 50 hospitals (Cleverley 1990).

Table 1
Balance Sheet and Income Statement Composite Averages for High- and Low-Performance Groups ($000)

	High-Profit Group ROI>9.21%	Low-Profit Group ROI<1.05%
Current assets	$14,644	$20,542
Net fixed assets	25,593	33,621
Other assets	9,235	13,405
Total assets	$49,473	$67,568
Current liabilities	$8,009	$13,616
Long-term debt	17,689	26,717
Equity	23,774	27,235
Total liability and equity	$49,473	$67,568
Inpatient revenue	$54,835	$60,795
Outpatient revenue	13,089	15,412
Total gross revenue	67,915	76,207
−deductions	20,240	21,609
Net patient revenue	47,615	54,597
+other operating revenue	1,753	4,975
Total operating revenue	49,428	59,572
−operating expenses	45,745	63,819
Net operating income	3,683	(4,247)
+nonoperating revenue	1,477	1,203
Net income	$5,160	$(3,044)
Average hospital beds	234	259
Average facility beds	256	295

Table 4 presents the composite averages found for selected cost indicators. These results, like the regression results reported in Table 3, clearly indicate that cost reduction is a critical factor in improving ROI. Furthermore, the data seem to suggest that four specific cost strategies have been used by high-ROI hospitals. First, strict attention to length of stay appears to be of paramount importance. The high-ROI average Medicare length of stay (LOS) after adjusting for case mix was 1.24 (7.79 minus 6.55) days lower than the low-ROI group. The regression results from Table 3 suggested that for every one-day reduction in Medicare case-adjusted LOS, ROI would increase by .738 percent.

How do hospitals control LOS? Very clearly reductions in LOS are made by physicians, but they may be facilitated by managers. A first step in this process is the sharing of information. Physician profiling should be initiated, and

189

Table 2
Profit per Adjusted Discharge Composite Average for High Low-Performance
Groups

	High-Profit Group ROI>9.21%	Low-Profit Group ROI<1.05%
Gross price	$6,438	$6,307
Less deductions	1,918	1,789
Net price	4,520	4,518
Costs		
Salary	1,892	2,477
Capital	421	397
Other	2,007	2,260
Total	4,320	5,134
Profit	$200	$(616)

results should be communicated with medical staff in an open environment. In many situations, a physician member of the management team would be an ideal choice.

Second, labor productivity appears to be critically related to financial performance. Since labor costs comprise such a large percentage of a hospital's total budget, this is not surprising. Much of the difference between the high- and low-ROI hospitals, however, can be attributed to LOS differences. The difference with respect to full-time equivalents (FTEs) per adjusted patient day is important, but combining shorter LOS and more efficient staffing per day creates sizable cost advantages.

Overhead cost control is the third strategy used by high-performance hospitals. General service costs per discharge, which represent costs from nonpatient care departments such as laundry, housekeeping, and administration, contribute a high-percentage of a hospital's total cost. High-ROI hospitals exert much greater control over nondirect patient care costs and therefore achieve significantly lower total costs.

Finally, our results confirm that hospitals should consider substituting capital for labor where possible. Hospitals that have higher capital expense ratios do have better ROI. As noted below in our discussion of investment strategy, this does not mean that hospitals should go on a buying binge to acquire new capital assets with debt. Results discussed later indicate that asset efficiency and financing do affect ROI values. The conclusion to be drawn from this is that acquiring labor-saving capital equipment whenever possible is an excellent strategy. The Medicare capital cost passthrough policy that existed in 1988 clearly supported this strategic recommendation.

Table 3
Multiple Regression Results

Strategy/Industry Factor	Sign	Statistical Significance
Cost leadership strategy		
Capital expense (percent)	.178	*
FTEs per adjusted patient	−1.271	*
Medicare case-adjusted length of stay	−.738	*
Market share factor		
Market share (percent)	.059	*
Pricing strategy		
Gross prices/cost	14.972	*
Product line/diversification strategy		
Medicare (percent)	−.053	**
Medicaid (percent)	−.191	*
Medicare case mix	−1.000	ns
Inpatient revenue (percent)	−.086	*
Nonoperating revenue/total operating revenue (percent)	.234	*
Investment strategy		
Revenue/fixed assets	.691	*
Revenue/current assets	−.002	ns
Financing factors		
Current ratio	.200	***
Long-term debt/equity	−.0005	*
Other factors		
Regulatory status	1.134	ns
Teaching status	.142	ns
Total facility beds	.003	**

*Significant at .01 or less.
**Significant at .05 or less.
***Significant at .10 or less.
ns=Not significant.

Market Share

Market share has been proposed by many to be a strategy or goal for success in business (Buzzell and Gayle 1987). Greater market share is believed to provide greater pricing liberty and better opportunities for economies of scale. Measuring market share is difficult in most empirical studies because defining the market is very complex. Buzzell and Gayle (1987) developed the concept of "served market." A served market represents the portion of the total market that the firm serves either because of production or marketing limitations. A

Table 4
Composite Averages

Cost Indicator	Successful ROI>9.21% n=256	Unsuccessful ROI<1.05% n=256
Cost per discharge	$4,320	$5,134
General service costs per discharge	$1,901	$2,445
FTEs per adjusted patient day	3.94	4.26
Labor hours per discharge	149.7	184.2
Medicare length of stay, case-mix adjusted	6.55	7.79
Capital expense/total expense (percent)	10.8	8.1

hospital's market area is very complex to define and it may vary for different services.

Market share for a hospital in this study was defined as the percentage of total net patient revenue, both inpatient and outpatient, to total net patient revenue in the county in which the hospital is located. We recognize that this measure is not always accurate, but we believe that it serves as a good proxy measure of market share for many large urban hospitals in the United States.

The regression results of Table 3 show that ROI is significantly associated with market share and in the expected direction. Increases in market share are associated with increases in ROI. The high-ROI group had a composite average market share of 20.1 percent, compared to 10.9 percent for the lower-ROI group. Those hospitals with larger market shares enjoyed the fruits of higher profitability.

Table 5 shows the relationship between cost and price and market share. The matrix depicts what one would normally expect in the nonhealth business world: lower prices and lower costs combine to produce greater market share. This may be akin to the chicken and egg: Does greater market share produce lower costs that can lead to lower prices, or do lower prices and costs capture greater market share? Our conclusion is that increasingly it will be lower costs and prices that will attract greater market share, especially in highly competitive urban markets.

One unexpected finding was the lack of a clear relationship between hospital size and market share. The largest hospitals in terms of bed size were not always the largest market share. Much of the rationale for this finding is related to the increasing importance of nonacute care dollars in the total health care market pie. Successful hospitals appear to be those that have successfully captured larger shares of the growing outpatient markets, a point that will be discussed later.

Table 5
The Impact of Price and Cost on Market Share Cell Values: Percentage of Market
Share

		Low	High
Group Prices	High	Market share 10.6	Market share 9.1
	Low	Market share 26.4	Market share 13.7
		Low	High

Cost per discharge

Table 6
Composite Averages

Revenue Indicators	Successful ROI>9.21% n=256	Unsuccessful ROI<1.05% n=256
Gross patient revenue/costs	1.52	1.27
Deductions from gross/gross revenue	.30	.28
Gross price per discharge	$6,438	$6,306
Net price per discharge	$4,520	$4,518

Pricing Strategy

Pricing is a critical strategy for hospital management to examine in its efforts
to formulate successful competitive strategies. The charging of premium
prices by market leaders, or those with high market share, may improve ROI,
but the charging of premium prices by firms with low market share may be a
dangerous strategy (Buzzell and Gayle 1987). Market leaders often have better
reputations or an image of higher quality that permits them to successfully
charge a higher price.

In the 1990 Cleverley study, hospitals that performed better financially were
more likely to have lower gross prices. Distinguishing between gross prices
and net prices is especially critical in the hospital industry, where different
buyers may pay different prices for the same service. Our composite average
results appear in Table 6.

193

In this study, which includes all hospitals located in large urban areas, prices appear to be very similar between high-performing and low-performing hospitals. The high-performing hospitals, however, have significantly higher markups (gross revenues to costs). This can be seen in Table 6 and the regression shown results in Table 3.

We have used markup as a quasi measure of pricing premium, although it also relates to cost control. Our analysis of the data suggests that cost control may be the dominant theme. While our high-ROI hospitals do have higher markups, their net prices are virtually identical. The major difference between this finding and the 1990 Cleverley study is that, while net prices are still virtually identical, the higher-ROI hospitals have slightly higher gross prices, and not lower gross prices, as the earlier study had found.

Product Line Selection/Diversification Strategy

There has been considerable discussion about the relative merits of diversification strategy within the hospital industry (Shortell, Morrison, and Hughes 1989). While it is difficult to define what diversification really means, most examples of diversification appear to include areas other than acute inpatient care, such as home health care, ambulatory surgery, and outpatient diagnostic clinics. One measure of diversification used in this study is the percentage of revenue derived from inpatient activity. Higher values would imply less diversification. In this study we will define product line/diversification strategy to broadly include both payer mix and intensity-of-care decisions.

There is some evidence to suggest that extensive product innovation and diversification by firms who are not dominant market share leaders will be counterproductive (Buzzell and Gayle 1987). Market leaders, on the other hand, are expected to benefit from increasing innovation and diversification. Table 7 illustrates that this hypothesis appears to be true in large urban hospitals. High–market share hospitals that also have high percentages of outpatient revenue (or low inpatient revenue percentages) have much higher ROI values. Interestingly, those hospitals with low market share and heavy outpatient revenue (our proxy for diversification) have very low values for ROI. This tends to support our earlier observation that diversification works best when the firm already has a large market share and it may hurt firms with low market share.

The composite averages for selected measures of product diversification strategies for the low- and high-ROI groups are presented in Table 8. At first glance, the data on inpatient revenue percentages may appear contradictory to

Table 7
The Effect of Market Share and Diversification on ROI Cell Values: ROI
Percentage

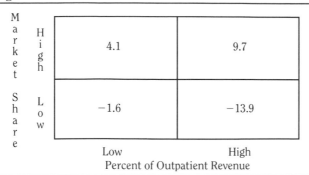

		Low	High
Market Share	High	4.1	9.7
	Low	−1.6	−13.9

Low   High
Percent of Outpatient Revenue

Table 8
Composite Averages

Product Diversification Strategy Measure	Successful ROI>9.21% n=256	Unsuccessful ROI<1.05% n=256
Inpatient revenue (percent)	80.7	79.8
Medicare case mix	1.314	1.299
Intensive care unit and cardiac care unit days (percent)	8.1	6.8
Medicaid (percent)	9.8	15.2
Medicare (percent)	29.6	28.4
Nonoperating revenue (percent)	2.9	2.0

earlier statements. While the higher-performing ROI hospitals do on the average have higher percentages of inpatient revenue, there is a negative association between this variable and ROI, as seen in Table 3. It might therefore be stated that the high-ROI hospitals achieved their increased performance in spite of higher inpatient revenue proportions.

Higher-ROI hospitals treat a slightly more severe and higher case-mix patient load as evidenced by a higher Medicare case-mix index and a higher proportion of intensive care and cardiac care patients. While the differences are not large, it further supports the cost-control programs of the high-ROI group. Even though the high-ROI hospitals treat patients who are more severely ill, they are able to accomplish this with lower costs.

Our conclusion that payer mix is related to ROI is not surprising. The regression results of Table 3 indicated that both Medicare and Medicaid revenue percentages have a negative effect on ROI. Again, the fact that the high-ROI group had a slightly higher Medicare percentage does not indicate that more Medicare is good, it merely indicates that these high-ROI hospitals were able to do well in spite of slightly higher Medicare percentages. Without question, however, Medicaid is the real culprit. The regression results suggest that the negative influence of increasing Medicaid volume is almost four times worse than a comparable Medicare increase.

The final product area under discussion is the amount of nonoperating revenue. Both Tables 3 and 8 show that increasing amounts of nonoperating revenue have a positive influence on ROI. These sources are most likely either contributions or investment income. Our results suggest that many hospital executives have forgotten that these sources of revenue represent a very effective way to achieve successful diversification that can support the core health care business.

Investment Strategy

An area that many executives and especially hospital executives often overlook is investment efficiency. From an accounting perspective, the more revenue that can be generated from a given level of investment, the better the firm's ROI. This is one of the basic concepts in the so called "DuPont Profit Model." Within the health care industry many executives believe that more capital, especially equipment, will attract new business because technology-hungry physicians will seek privileges at their hospitals. While there is clearly some truth in this concept, a hospital is much like any other business and must carefully evaluate the allocation of its scarce capital dollars.

Buzzell and Gayle (1987) concluded from their research that there is a positive association between both fixed capital and working capital intensity and ROI. Similar results were found in Cleverley's (1990) study of 50 hospitals. Table 9 clearly provides the relative importance of both fixed and working capital management. Hospitals with both high–fixed asset turnovers (revenues divided by fixed assets) and high–current asset turnovers (revenues divided by current assets) have very high ROI values.

The regression results of Table 3 are somewhat contradictory. While high–fixed asset efficiency is positively associated with ROI and is very significant, the sign for current asset efficiency is negative, which is the wrong direction, but the coefficient is not significant.

Data for the composite averages is presented in Table 10. The higher-ROI hospitals have significantly less fixed-asset investment per bed than the lower-

Table 9
The Effect of Investment Efficiency on ROI Cell Values: ROI Percentages

		Low	High
Current Asset Turnover	High	13.7	26.4
	Low	9.1	10.6
		Low	High

Percent of Fixed Asset Turnover

ROI group, which concurs with earlier results (Cleverley 1990) that had determined that not only was less investment used per bed, but that the investment was also newer. In other studies, new plant is frequently correlated with higher ROI. It would have been interesting to test also for this effect in our study, but no data was available on plant age. We can only conclude from these earlier studies that hospitals should balance low investment per bed with their needs for new physical facilities.

Financial Strategy

One competitive strategy that is often overlooked in many marketing-oriented strategy books and articles is financial strategy. The question to be answered is To what extent, if any, does the degree of financial leverage affect the firm's ROI? It should be emphasized that our measure of ROI is financing neutral because it relates profits before financing expenses to total assets.

The regression coefficient signs in Table 3 for both short-term debt policy as measured by the current ratio and long-term debt policy as measured by the long-term debt–to-equity ratio indicate that less rather than more debt is desirable. The composite average data presented in Table 11 also support this finding.

The major significance of this finding is not that hospitals should avoid debt, but rather that they should carefully compare the returns to be generated from debt-financed assets to the cost of financing. Many hospitals have historically used debt whenever they believed a financing need existed, without really evaluating the earnings to be derived from the project. Historical cost reimbursement may have permitted this luxury in the past, but it is no longer

Table 10
Composite Averages

Asset Efficiency Indicators	Successful ROI>9.21% n=256	Unsuccessful ROI<1.05% n=256
Fixed asset turnover	1.93	1.77
Current asset turnover	3.38	2.90
Net fixed asset per bed	$99,975	$113,969

Table 11
Composite Averages

Financial Leverage Indicators	Successful ROI>9.21% n=256	Unsuccessful ROI<1.05% n=256
Long-term debt to equity (percent)	74.4	97.7
Current ratio	1.83	1.51
Total debt to total assets (percent)	51.9	59.5
Long-term debt per bed	$69,097	$90,566

an option today. The loss of capital cost passthroughs in the future will make capital financing evaluation even more critical.

Before concluding this discussion of debt or leverage policy, it is important to emphasize that the use of less or no long-term debt is not suggested by our results. The actual value of the regression coefficient for the long-term debt–to-equity ratio suggests that a hospital increasing this ratio by 50 percent would experience a reduction in its ROI of only one-fourth of 1 percent. While debt policy has a statistically significant relationship to ROI, its influence is not major according to our regression results.

Other Factors

Based on the regression results in Table 3, note that three other factors are included—regulation, teaching status, and size, as measured by the number of facility beds.

Regulation was defined as a binary variable, that is, either present or absent. We defined regulation as present in only three states—Massachusetts, New Jersey, and New York. We realize that there are more states than these three that had rate regulation in 1988, but we subjectively defined these three states to be the most restrictive and burdensome. If the effects of regulation would

198

not be seen here, it seemed unlikely that regulation would be important in other states. When the regulation variable was included in the regression, it was not significant. To be sure, the average ROI in these three regulated states was far lower than the average in the other states. The failure of the regulatory variable to become significant surprised us, and we are not certain whether there might be some model specification error. However, if this is minimal, the results seem to suggest that strategic changes in productivity, market share, product diversification, and other areas might explain more of the variation in ROI than location in a regulated or nonregulated environment. This appears to be the conclusion for those hospitals operating in large urban areas.

Teaching status was also defined as a binary variable, but it did not have a significant influence on ROI. Again, this would suggest that factors and strategies other than teaching mission or location in a regulated state are more critically related to ROI.

Finally, the *number of facility beds* was included as a measure of scale. The results in Table 3 indicate that size does have a significant effect on ROI; however, the size of the regression coefficient is not large. We believe that our findings demonstrate that some advantages do result from the sheer size of the hospital, although these advantages do not result in lower costs. Larger hospitals have much higher costs that are not fully compensated for in higher prices.

Conclusions

We have attempted in this study to begin to build a set of strategic principles for effectively managing a hospital in a competitive environment. To this end, we have used a combination of statistical analysis and logical inference to find performance differences between successful and unsuccessful large urban hospitals. Our findings suggest these eight strategic principles.

1. *Cost control.* The single most important strategy discovered in this study is cost control. With such a high percentage of hospital revenue stemming from fixed-price payers such as Medicare, Medicaid, and other payers, attention to costs is clearly required. Our data simply reflects what many have already known. The two primary ways that cost control is exercised in successful hospitals is through enhanced labor productivity and reduced overhead costs. We believe that incentives may play an important role in both of these areas.

2. *Length of stay.* There is an important link between reduced costs and length of stay. Successful hospitals have much lower LOS even after

adjusting for case-mix differences. This reduced LOS most likely results from effective medical staff relationships and better communication.

3. *Market share.* Greater market share is positively associated with improved financial performance. One of the major benefits of a larger share may be the ability to price products and services at higher multiples above cost. This does not mean higher prices than competitors, but merely greater margins. Greater market share clearly provides greater market clout in establishing and recovering prices from that segment of the market that pays on the basis of internally set prices.

4. *Diversification.* In general, greater diversification appears to be an effective strategy for improving financial performance. There is an important qualification, however—low market–share hospitals should concentrate on their existing product lines before rushing into new product and market areas. Market share leaders need to aggressively pursue diversification to maintain their present positions of market dominance.

5. *Nonoperating revenue.* All hospitals should concentrate more on generating nonoperating income either from contributions or investment income from reserves. Hospitals clearly need to establish funded depreciation policies and to place more emphasis on development programs.

6. *Investment policy.* Hospitals that employ less investment per dollar of revenue generated have better financial performance. Hospitals should closely evaluate new capital expenditures to determine their desirability, but newer plants do appear to attract both medical staff and patients. There is also a clear directive to invest in capital projects that have the potential to reduce labor.

7. *Patient selection.* Where possible, it is desirable to limit both Medicare and Medicaid patient volumes, especially Medicaid. Heavy percentages of Medicaid patients will in most situations decrease profitability. Changes in payer mix are effected through medical staff recruitment and product line selections.

8. *Financing policy.* Poorer-performing hospitals appear to have more debt in their capital structures than higher-performing hospitals. It does not appear that the use of debt is to be avoided, however, but rather the excessive use of debt should be avoided. Hospitals should

carefully review new financings to ensure that returns from debt-financed assets are adequate to cover capital costs.

References

Buzzell, R., and B. Gayle. *Profit Impact of Market Strategy: Linking Strategy to Performance*. New York: Free Press, 1987.

Cleverley, W. "Improving Financial Performance: A Study of 50 Hospitals." *Hospital & Health Services Administration* 35, no. 2 (Summer 1990): 173–87.

Nemess, Judith. "Survey of Hospital CEOs Shows Fewer Fear Demise of Their Facilities." *Modern Healthcare* 65 (25 June 1990): 47–48.

Peters, T., and R. Waterman. *In Search of Excellence*. New York: Harper & Row, 1982.

Porter, Michael. *Competitive Strategy: Techniques for Analyzing Industries and Competitors*. New York: Free Press, 1980.

Shortell, Stephen, Ellen Morrison, and Susan Hughes. "The Keys to Successful Diversification: Lessons from Leading Hospital Systems." *Hospital & Health Services Administration* 34, no. 4 (Winter 1989): 471–92.

Chapter 13

Assessing Financial Outcomes of Not-for-Profit Community Hospitals

Thomas R. Prince

Thomas R. Prince is Professor of Accounting and Information Systems at the J. L. Kellogg Graduate School of Management, Northwestern University, Evanston, Illinois. He is a Faculty Associate of the College.

This article was published in *Hospital & Health Services Administration* 36, no. 3 (Fall 1991).

Problems with Intermediate Performance Measures

Operating-margin comparisons across community hospitals (Hadley, Zuckerman, and Feder 1989; Rosko 1989; Mennemeyer and Olinger 1989; Greene 1989) can result in erroneous inferences because of differences in financial reporting practice among various types of hospitals. Donations and contributions to a hospital with restricted funds can be transferred under certain conditions to the general fund and included as part of that hospital's operating margin. Gifts to hospitals without restricted funds must be reported as nonoperating revenue. Over 40 percent of government hospitals in this study received tax support awards unrelated to patient services that cannot be included in operating margin. These tax support awards of $781 million in 1988 were larger than the $607 million in operating margins for the study hospitals (see Table 1).

Differences in reporting practices for donations, contributions, gifts, and investment income among various types of community hospitals mean that the $1,683 million of nonoperating revenue in 1988 for the sample hospitals per Table 1 is only a portion of these revenues. The remainder is part of the $3,471 million of other operating revenue for hospitals with restricted funds that engaged in transfer activities. The "bottom line" of revenue over expenses and the "top line" of net patient revenue are two uniform measures across community hospitals.

Table 1
Statements of Revenue and Expenses for 1,297 Community Hospitals*

	1986	1987	1988
Net patient revenue	$63,816,631	$68,683,074	$75,867,404
Other operating revenue	2,658,347	3,071,386	3,470,607
Net operating revenue	66,474,978	71,754,460	79,338,011
Operating expenses	64,266,898	70,512,807	78,731,476
Operating margin	2,208,080	1,241,653	606,535
Nonoperating revenue	1,580,280	1,576,312	1,682,951
Tax support awards	616,750	729,592	780,745
Tax paid (unrelated business income)	(5,253)	(1,673)	(3,144)
Excess of revenue over expenses	$4,399,857	$3,545,884	$3,067,087

*Amounts in thousands.

Source: The specific information on individual hospitals is taken from the Merritt System®.

Selection of Six Panels

Financial measures of performance and capital structures of 1,297 community hospitals are examined for purposes of explaining revenue over expenses and classifying the overall financial outcomes. The six panels of study hospitals represent over 46 percent (see Table 2) of the net patient revenue and over 52 percent of revenue over expenses (see Table 3) for all community hospitals (about 5,500) per the American Hospital Association (AHA) (1990) reports.

The source of all data on selected community hospitals in this study was the Merritt System®, a credit analysis and database management system (DBMS) supporting comparative financial, operational, and bond issue data on not-for-profit hospitals.[1] Over 2,000 hospitals and 130 hospital systems are included as separate records in the Merritt System®. This DBMS runs on a personal computer and efficiently uses about six million characters of storage for the more than 2,150 health care entities within the database. Each hospital record

Table 2
Net Patient Revenue Comparison of Six Panels of Selected Hospitals with All Community Hospitals

Community Hospitals	Net Patient Revenue*		
	1986	1987	1988
All community hospitals per AHA	$137,939	$147,326	$161,062
5,533 hospitals in 1988			
5,611 hospitals in 1987			
5,678 hospitals in 1986			
Total for 1,297 community hospitals	$63,817	$68,683	$75,867
Percent of AHA total	46.26	46.62	47.10
Six panels			
Hospitals with restricted funds			
Panel A—110 government, nonfederal	$4,109	$4,552	$5,006
Panel B—158 church-operated	8,760	9,436	10,480
Panel C—623 independent community	34,614	37,142	40,998
Hospitals without restricted funds			
Panel D—88 government, nonfederal	2,763	2,984	3,324
Panel E—67 church-operated	3,520	3,863	4,302
Panel F—251 independent community	10,051	10,706	11,757

*Amounts in millions.

Sources: The AHA data are taken from Table 11, page 204 of 1987, 1988, and 1989–1990 editions of *Hospital Statistics*. The specific information on individual hospitals is taken from the Merritt System®.

Table 3

Net Income Comparison of Six Panels of Selected Hospitals with All Community
Hospitals

Community Hospitals	Excess of Revenue Over Expenses*		
	1986	1987	1988
Over 5,500 hospitals per AHA			
Net total revenue†	$148,548	$159,309	$174,558
Total expenses	140,654	152,585	168,723
Excess of revenue over expenses	7,894	6,724	5,835
Total revenue over expenses for 1,297			
community hospitals	4,400	3,546	3,067
Percent of AHA total	55.74	52.73	52.56
Six panels			
Hospitals with restricted funds			
Panel A—110 government, nonfederal	279	273	240
Panel B—158 church-operated	590	479	399
Panel C—623 independent community	2,339	1,867	1,538
Hospitals without restricted funds			
Panel D—88 government, nonfederal	219	166	140
Panel E—67 church-operated	302	211	255
Panel F—251 independent community	671	550	495

*Includes contributions, endowment revenue, government grants, and all other payments not
made on behalf of individual patients.
*Amounts in millions.

Sources: The AHA data are taken from Table 5A, page 21, and Table 11, page 204 of 1987, 1988,
and 1989–1990 editions of *Hospital Statistics*. The specific information on individual hospitals
is taken from the Merritt System®.

in the DBMS contains over 200 data elements, and there are annual entries for
over 100 financial and operational measures.

Six panels of not-for-profit community hospitals were drawn from the Merritt System's database with the stipulation that (1) the facility was classified in
the AHA *Guide to the Health Care Field* (1990) as Service Code 10 for general
medical and surgical services and (2) complete financial data were available for
the three years 1986–1988.[2] The three-years-of-data requirement excluded over
600 community hospitals with an AHA Service Code 10 in the Merritt System's®
database.[3]

The 1,297 not-for-profit community hospitals in the six panels selected for
this study are not a random sample of community hospitals. Each of the 50
states and the District of Columbia is represented in the selected facilities, but

all for-profit community hospitals are excluded. The credit-rating data source used for this study tends to exclude any freestanding community hospital with less than 60 beds. Twenty-one percent of not-for-profit community hospitals had less than 50 beds in 1985, and 45 percent were under 100 beds (Prince 1988). Small hospitals that are members of a system may be included in this study provided the institutions submit annual financial statements to commercial banks and investment firms because of long-term debt or line-of-credit requirements.

Ownership, legal, and organizational considerations were applied in partitioning the 1,297 study hospitals into six panels. Hospitals with restricted funds (Panels A, B, and C) can engage in fund transfers that are not available to hospitals without restricted funds (Panels D, E, and F). Government hospitals (Panels A and D) are different from church-operated hospitals (Panels B and E). Independent hospitals (Panels C and F) have a separate legal status from other health care entities per information in the AHA *Guide* (1990).

The logical partitioning of the 1,297 study hospitals into the six panels is supported by the median financial measures (see Table 4) and selected characteristics (see Table 5) for these hospitals. Panel B hospitals (church-operated with restricted funds) are larger in terms of net patient revenue, total assets, and revenues over expenses than the Panel C hospitals (independent with restricted funds), per Table 4. Panel E hospitals (church-operated without restricted funds) are smaller than Panel B and Panel C hospitals with respect to net patient revenue and net fixed assets; however, Panel E hospitals have the highest revenue over expenses of the six panels.

Panel A hospitals (government with restricted funds) are about half the size of Panel B hospitals in terms of assets and net patient revenue, per Table 4. Panel D hospitals (government without restricted funds) are smaller in assets and net patient revenues than Panel A hospitals; Panel D hospitals have higher operating margins than Panel A hospitals, but revenue over expenses favors Panel A hospitals. This difference in operating margins versus revenue over expenses between government hospitals (Panels A and D) is partially related to 48 percent of Panel A hospitals receiving tax support awards as compared with 31 percent for Panel D hospitals, as shown in Table 5.

Panels B and E have the most hospitals located in metropolitan statistical areas (MSAs) while Panels A and B have the most hospitals not located in MSAs. There are problems with the definition of rural hospital between the U.S. Department of Agriculture guidelines (Cordes 1989) and the Prospective Payment System (Cromwell et al. 1987; Ermann 1990); MSA and non-MSA locations are used in this study to facilitate understanding. Regional variations in hospital costs (Carter and Cromwell 1987) are outside the scope of this study.

Table 4
Comparison of 1986–1988 Median Values for the Six Panels*

Hospital Panels with Restricted Funds	Panel A 110 Government	Panel B 158 Church-Operated	Panel C 623 Independent
Net patient revenue 3 years	$71,325	$145,774	$135,180
Revenue over expenses 3 years	$ 3,298	$ 5,806	$ 5,604
Total unrestricted assets 1988	$34,575	$64,707	$59,287
Total assets 1988	$36,473	$66,520	$60,956
Net fixed assets 1988	$17,891	$32,654	$29,688
Long-term debt to equity 1988	80.8%	103.3%	83.6%
Operating margin 3 years	1.30%	3.05%	2.66%
1988 operating margin	0.75%	1.95%	1.80%

Hospital Panels without Restricted Funds	Panel D 88 Government	Panel E 67 Church-Operated	Panel F 251 Independent
Net patient revenue 3 years	$63,203	$123,262	$96,780
Revenue over expenses 3 years	$ 2,354	$ 6,445	$ 4,334
Total unrestricted assets 1988	$29,062	$ 61,081	$44,343
Net fixed assets 1988	$14,634	$ 29,308	$21,683
Long-term debt to equity 1988	90.0%	86.8%	82.6%
Operating margin 3 years	2.37%	3.35%	2.93%
1988 operating margin	2.14%	3.23%	2.16%

*Amounts in thousands.

Source: The specific information on individual hospitals is taken from the Merritt System®

The primary financial comparisons (see Table 4) were median values to avoid problems of variations in size of hospitals that highly influence the computations of arithmetic means. Using a trimmed mean excludes the 5 percent values on each end of the distribution, but this measure does not remove the variation in size problem for the remaining 90 percent of the distribution. The magnitude of these differences is illustrated in statistical measures for operating margins in Table 6. Panel A hospitals, for example, had a mean 1986–1988 operating margin of -4.94, a trimmed mean of $-.08$, and a median of 1.30. The 1988 operating margin for Panel D hospitals is another example where there is a negative mean ($-.46$), a positive trimmed mean (.93), and a substantial median (2.14). Using median values emphasizes the relative ranking of hospitals within the panel distribution without being influenced by size and extreme values.

Table 5
Selected Characteristics of Panel Hospitals

	Percent with Restricted Funds			Percent without Restricted Funds		
	Govern-ment Panel A (n = 110)	Church-Operated Panel B (n = 158)	Indepen-dent Panel C (n = 623)	Govern-ment Panel D (n = 88)	Church-Operated Panel E (n = 67)	Indepen-dent Panel F (n = 251)
Medical school affiliation	18	33	32	13	27	17
Member Council of Teaching Hospitals	11	13	16	3	7	6
Urban (metropolitan statistical area)	57	84	76	55	84	74
Receive tax support awards unrelated to patient services	48	1	2	31	0	2
Pay tax	3	1	1	1	1	1

Source: The specific information on individual hospitals is taken from the Merritt System®.

Explaining Revenue over Expenses

The concept of "revenue over expenses" is viewed by accountants from either a flow or stock position. The flow perspective emphasizes the bottom line results from net patient revenue. A flow perspective is especially applicable to a university teaching hospital that often has a much higher dollar volume of net patient revenues per fixed assets employed than that for other community hospitals, including those with membership in the Council of Teaching Hospitals (COTH).

The stock perspective views revenues-over-expenses-to-the-assets employed as the critical measure of return. There are problems with the stock perspective because not all hospitals have liquid board–designated funds (such as "funded" depreciation) and other unrestricted investments. A modified approach is to express revenue over expenses to net fixed assets, but this adjustment ignores investment incomes. In this study, both the flow and stock approaches are followed in explaining revenue in terms of 15 factors (see Tables 7 and 8).

The 15 factors used in partially explaining revenue over expenses do not include operational data on specific hospital departments. The American Institute of Certified Public Accountants (AICPA) old audit guide for hospitals

Table 6
Financial Measures of Hospitals within the Six Panels for 1986–1988

	Panels with Restricted Funds			Panels without Restricted Funds		
	A	B	C	D	E	F
	Govern- ment (n = 110)	Church- Operated (n = 158)	Indepen- dent (n = 623)	Govern- ment (n = 88)	Church- Operated (n = 67)	Indepen- dent (n = 251)
Operating margin 3 years						
Median	1.30	3.05	2.66	2.37	3.35	2.93
Mean	− 4.94	2.35	2.54	.21	3.61	2.16
Trimmed mean*	− .08	2.48	2.67	1.40	3.69	2.65
First quartile	− 3.46	− .04	.42	− 1.31	.75	.21
Third quartile	4.36	5.03	4.88	5.11	6.09	5.38
Operating margin 1988						
Median	.75	1.95	1.80	2.14	3.23	2.16
Mean	− 5.76	1.10	1.50	− .46	2.97	1.38
Trimmed mean*	− .60	1.56	1.77	.93	3.16	1.78
First quartile	− 4.69	− .88	− .52	− 2.16	.69	− 1.02
Third quartile	4.32	4.78	4.29	4.52	6.37	5.16

*The smallest 5 percent and the largest 5 percent of the values are trimmed. The middle 90 percent are then averaged as the trimmed mean.

Source: The specific information on individual hospitals is taken from the Merritt System[⑩].

(AICPA 1972) and the new guide for health care services (AICPA 1990; Kleiner, Garner, and Colbert 1989; Colbert 1990) do not contain a required reporting format for operational and statistical data.[4] More than 20 percent of the study hospitals did not include any statistical data on departmental areas, and there were many incomplete responses among the other 80 percent. This data limitation did not permit including study factors on hospital product and productivity (Long et al. 1987; Long, Chesney, and Fleming 1989), beds and services by department (Cromwell and Puskin 1989; Schlenker and Shaughnessy 1989), and continuing care arrangements (Welch and Dubay 1989).

Factor B1 expresses total restricted fund balance to total assets in the unrestricted fund. Legal limitations on the use of restricted funds are appreciated, and the actual cash transfers between the funds would be an ideal measure of this factor. AICPA's new audit guide (1990) includes this factor, but it has not become part of the Merritt System's database. In the case of Panel C hospitals, Factor B1 is significantly, negatively associated with increases of revenue over

Table 7

Prediction of Revenue over Expenses to Net Patient Revenue by Selected Characteristics of Community Hospitals

	Coefficients by Hospital Panels					
	With Restricted Funds			Without Restricted Funds		
	A	B	C	D	E	F
	110	158	623	88	67	251
Factors	Govern-ment	Church-Operated	Indepen-dent	Govern-ment	Church-Operated	Indepen-dent
B1 Restricted funds to unrestricted assets	.09	.02	− .06*	NA	NA	NA
B2 Long-term debt to unrestricted assets	.19*	.20*	.15*	.03	.13	.22*
B3 Equity balance to unrestricted assets	.27*	.20*	.14*	.06	.21†	.18*
B4 New investments	.03‡	− .01	.02*	.06	.03	.05*
B5 Age property plant and equipment	− .88*	− .64*	− .19†	− .50	− .45	− .10
B6 Capital cost	− .05	− .40*	− .12†	.10	.11	− .36*
B7 Cash flow to debt	− .01	.15*	.09*	.09†	.15†	.15*
B8 Liquid ratio	.14*	.08†	.10*	.19*	.13*	.10*
B9 Debt-service coverage	.33*	− .04	.03	− .10	− .31	.04
B10 Excess days in accounts receivable	− .00	.03‡	− .00	− .00	.00	.01
B11 Contractual allowances	.01	.01	− .01	.02	− .07	− .00
B12 Nonoperating revenue to net patient revenue	.02	.18	.52*	.09*	.79†	.42*
B13 Medical school affiliation	− .31	1.43‡	.51	1.49	− 1.60	.55
B14 Urban (MSA)	− 1.36†	− .20	− .00	.41	.84	1.29†
B15 Case-mix for Medicare	3.38	.00	2.50*	1.52	3.35	2.71
Constant	− 16.19*	− 7.71	− 12.14*	− 4.00	− 15.74‡	− 17.91*
R² (adjusted)	75.6%	56.9%	53.7%	48.0%	65.5%	52.2%
N cases	108	151	604	87	67	243

*Significant at 1 percent level.
†Significant at 5 percent level.
‡Significant at 10 percent level.

Table 8
Prediction of Revenue over Expenses to Total Unrestricted Assets by Selected Characteristics of Community Hospitals

	Coefficients by Hospital Panels					
	With Restricted Funds			Without Restricted Funds		
	A	B	C	D	E	F
	110	158	623	88	67	251
Factors	Govern-ment	Church-Operated	Indepen-dent	Govern-ment	Church-Operated	Indepen-dent
B1 Restricted funds to unrestricted assets	.09	.06	− .03*	NA	NA	NA
B2 Long-term debt to unrestricted assets	.12†	.12†	.11†	.05	.08	.10†
B3 Equity balance to unrestricted assets	.19†	.14†	.10†	.06	.09	.05‡
B4 New investments	.02	− .01	.01†	.03	.02	.04†
B5 Age property plant and equipment	− .80†	− .56†	− .09	− .48*	− .35	− .05
B6 Capital cost	− .23†	− .39†	− .19†	− .19	− .19	− .24†
B7 Cash flow to debt	.02	.13†	.10†	.06‡	.15†	.16†
B8 Liquid ratio	.08‡	.04	.05†	.11†	.07*	.06†
B9 Debt-service coverage	.04	− .06	.06‡	− .05	− .13	.13
B10 Excess days in accounts receivable	.01	.02	− .01	− .01	− .01	− .00
B11 Contractual allowances	.01	− .02	.00	− .01	− .05	− .00
B12 Nonoperating revenue to net patient revenue	− .01	− .00	.19†	− .10†	.26	.09
B13 Medical school affiliation	− .33	1.15*	.37	.96	− 1.52‡	.81*
B14 Urban (MSA)	− .82	− .49	.23	− .19	.82	.42
B15 Case-mix for Medicare	.68	− .84	.93	.43	2.79	1.20
Constant	− 4.73	.10	− 7.13†	1.20	− 5.35	− 6.44‡
R^2 (adjusted)	51.3%	49.4%	54.5%	50.1%	65.5%	63.5%
N cases	108	151	604	87	67	243

*Significant at 10 percent level.
†Significant at 1 percent level.
‡Significant at 5 percent level.

expenses under the flow approach (see Table 7) and the stock approach (see Table 8). A larger amount in the restricted fund balance means there is less total assets in the unrestricted fund versus a hospital that has transferred assets to the unrestricted fund.

Long-term debt to total unrestricted fund assets (Factor B2), equity (the unrestricted fund balance) to total unrestricted fund assets (Factor B3), and new (1987–1988) fixed asset investments to 1986 total unrestricted fund assets (Factor B4) are all significantly, positively associated with increases in revenue over expenses against a flow (net patient revenue per Table 7) or a stock (total assets per Table 8) for two or more of the panels. Factors B2 and B3 are capital structure measures, and increases in these ratios are influenced by prior period flows of revenue over expenses. A debt-to-equity ratio per Table 4 (Cleverley 1990a; Valvona and Sloan 1988) was not used because of the negative balances in some equity accounts and minimal balances in others; the combination of Factors B2 and B3 provides information on the same issue.

New investments (Factor B4) are expected to be directly related to increases in revenue over expenses during the following periods, and a lagged measure is typically used for Factor B4. The magnitude of downsizing operations in 1984–1986 requires that new investments data for this period must come from notes to the financial statements rather than from changes in the balance sheet account used in the current study. A detailed study of downsizing operations is the focus of a separate research project.

Age of property plant and equipment (Factor B5) is expressed by dividing accumulated depreciation by the current year's depreciation expense (Cleverley 1987a). Capital cost (Factor B6) is the relationship of depreciation and interest expense to total operating expenses. Both Factors B5 and B6 have significant negative associations with revenue over expenses in three or four of the panels under the flow and stock approaches. The negative association of Factor B5 is compatible with investments in medical technology and new equipment. Factor B6 suggests that there are certain required levels of salary (Pauly 1985; Cromwell 1989; Sloan, Morrisey, and Valvona 1988) and professional operating expenses in providing patient services; the difference between those levels of aggregate expenditures (Ashby 1984) and total revenues is divided between interest expense and depreciation (capital cost), and excess of revenue over expenses.

Cash-flow-to-debt (Factor B7) is the relative position against total debt (current liabilities plus other liabilities plus long-term debt) from current operating activities (revenue over expenses plus depreciation expense). Factor B7 expresses the time period required to satisfy all obligations from current cash flows generated by operating activities (Cleverley 1987b). The mix of total debt to equity and net fixed assets to total assets influences the impact of

Factor B7. The absence of any significant association for Panel A hospitals under either approach is of more interest than the positive findings for the other five panels.

Liquid ratio (Factor B8) relates cash plus marketable securities plus liquid board designated funds to total assets. The significant positive association between higher liquid ratio and increases in revenue over expenses for most of the panels show cash-related investments are superior to fixed assets in explaining annual returns. This ratio is based on the ending balance sheet position, and the significant findings for all six panels in Table 7 suggest that the relative cash position of a hospital on the balance sheet date is fairly constant over the year. The "window dressing" techniques near the balance sheet date employed by some industrial companies must not be widely practiced by not-for-profit community hospitals.

Debt-service-coverage ratio (Factor B9) measures the ability of the hospital to generate sufficient cash to cover short-term obligations (current portion of long-term debt plus interest expense). Revenue over expenses plus depreciation plus interest represent the cash flow (Cleverley 1988, 1990b) available for meeting these debt-related obligations. The significant positive finding for one of the panels under each approach shows some explanation of revenue flows from this measure. Factor B9 is also used in the next section of this study.

Excess days in accounts receivable (Factor B10) (Cleverley 1987b) and contractual allowances (Factor B11) show limited ability to explain the excess of revenue over expenses in this study. The ratio of nonoperating revenue plus tax support awards (see Table 1) to net patient revenue (Factor B12) shows some of the impact of financial reporting practices. The most interesting findings are the differences under both approaches for Panel B versus Panel C hospitals with the inference that financial reporting practices are not uniform among these hospitals with restricted funds.

Medical school affiliation (Factor B13), urban or MSA location (Factor B14), and case-mix index for the Medicare program (Factor B15) are significant measures for some panel hospitals in explaining revenue over expenses. The direction of the significant association is not constant among the panels, and this finding is not surprising given the mix differences among panels in selected characteristics (see Table 5). Medical school affiliation is a negative factor with Panel E hospitals and a positive factor with Panel B hospitals. It is possible that this finding may relate to differences in reporting practices where a church associated with Panel E hospitals may directly receive restricted gifts and donations. Table 9 shows that Panel E hospitals have higher median ratios for two revenue-over-expense measures than Panel B hospitals, and thus, they might be viewed by some individuals as having less "need" for receiving a gift. Other inferences can be made based on the additional cost of services for medical school–affiliated hospitals versus other hospitals within a panel. The combination of medical school affiliation and case-mix index (Factors B13 and B15) did not have as much influence as suggested by Medicare cost report studies (Friedman and Shortell 1988; Goldfarb and Coffey 1987; Welch 1987).

The overall findings show reasonable adjusted R^2 for the six panels under both the flow and stock approaches for explaining revenue over expenses. Four panels under the flow approach and two panels under the stock approach indicate that there are significant other factors explaining part of the revenue over expenses movement.

Combined Financial Ratings

Four financial measures are used in classifying the financial status of each study hospitals: (1) revenue over expenses to total unrestricted assets, (2) revenue over expenses to net patient revenue, (3) equity to unrestricted assets, and (4) debt-service coverage (see Table 9). These four measures are combined to create five financial status ratings: (1) critical, (2) warning, (3) average, (4)

Table 9
Financial Measures of Hospitals within the Six Panels for 1986–1988

	Percent with Restricted Funds			Percent without Restricted Funds		
	A	B	C	D	E	F
	Govern-ment	Church-Operated	Indepen-dent	Govern-ment	Church-Operated	Indepen-dent
	(n = 110)	(n = 158)	(n = 623)	(n = 88)	(n = 67)	(n = 251)
Percent of revenue over expenses to unrestricted assets	3.68	3.62	3.86	3.50	4.12	4.08
Percent of revenue over expenses to net patient revenue	4.85	4.57	4.90	5.13	5.53	5.19
Percent of equity to unrestricted assets 1988	45.64	41.44	44.87	45.17	45.23	44.24
Percent of debt-service coverage 1988	2.69	2.50	2.56	2.27	2.58	2.50
Omitted hospitals*	2	1	9	1	0	4

*17 hospitals without any long-term debt were excluded from the median computation of debt-service coverage.

excellent, and (5) outstanding. The critical rating is a narrow financial status assessment of hospitals in serious financial condition on at least three of the four financial measures. The warning rating is assigned to hospitals in serious financial condition on one or two of the financial measures, but the hospital has poor to average performance on the other financial measures. At the other end of the continuum, outstanding performance is assigned to hospitals with superior ratings on at least three of the four financial measures.

The two revenue measures are expressed by an index with values from 1 to 20, based on the relative ranking of a hospital for the given ratio within a panel. The 20-base index for each of these two revenue measures is then converted into a five-scale index to facilitate comparison with the other two financial measures and consolidation into a status rating. This procedure permits a distinction being made between a hospital at the 4 percent level and one at the 19 percent level on a revenue measure in the composite assessment of being in a "critical" condition.

Equity-to-total-unrestricted assets is expressed by an index with values from 1 to 5, based on percentage ranges that are uniform across panels (see Table 10). Hospitals with an equity ratio of less than 25 percent are classified as being critical; they have over a 300 percent total debt-to-equity ratio, and 142 hospitals across the six panels are in this layer, per Table 10. The ranges for the other four equity values are more flexible than suggested by some literature (Palm 1988; Johnsson 1990). The 1985 equity-asset ratio of 50.2 percent (Cleverley 1987b) is an excellent status, and another study's ratio of 33 percent (Cleverley 1990a) is an average status, per Table 10. The 1986–1989 median values for long-term debt to equity are 81.2–84.0 percent for all hospitals in the Merritt System[®] (Van Kampen Merritt 1990), and these values are not compatible with a standardized ratio of 30 percent (Cleverley 1987a). The 1,297 study hospitals had debt-to-equity ratios of 80.8 to 103.3 percent (see Table 4)[5].

Debt-service coverage is converted to a five-point index where a 1 designates a hospital that is unable to meet current debt obligations from cash flows (see Table 10). The other four levels of the debt-service index are more liberal than suggested by the literature (Solovy 1989; Cleverley 1990a). The 94 study hospitals (see Table 10) with a debt-service index of 1 includes only 36 of the 62 Panel C hospitals with negative revenue over expense flows for the three years.

The composite rating for the four financial measures shows 121 hospitals with a critical status, and this financial status condition is different from the use of that label in organization theory (Weitzel and Jonsson 1989). Many of the 203 hospitals with a warning status would have been classified as in a critical condition based on other ratios from the health care literature. The 462 hospitals in the top two groups were good to outstanding on most financial measures; a few were still going through downsizing activities but operating

Table 10
Financial Classification of Hospitals within the Six Panels for 1988

	Panels with Restricted Funds			Panels without Restricted Funds			
	A	B	C	D	E	F	
	Govern-ment	Church-Operated	Indepen-dent	Govern-ment	Church-Operated	Indepen-dent	Total
	(n = 110)	(n = 158)	(n = 623)	(n = 88)	(n = 67)	(n = 251)	(n = 1,297)
Debt-service coverage index by layer (1–5)							
1 — less than 1	11	13	36	11	2	21	94
2 — 1.0–1.70	13	30	93	15	10	43	204
3 — 1.71–3.00*	42	57	267	32	28	91	517
4 — 3.01–4.00	20	27	99	16	10	47	219
5 — 4.01 and over	24	31	128	14	17	49	263
Equity to unrestricted total assets (1988) index by layer (1–5)							
1 — less than 24 percent	8	21	54	13	5	41	142
2 — 25 to 29 percent	4	16	34	5	6	16	81
3 — 30 to 45 percent	38	53	186	27	24	80	408
4 — 46 to 59 percent	34	40	186	24	17	69	370
5 — 60 percent and over	26	28	163	19	15	45	296
Financial status							
1 — critical	8	20	44	11	4	34	121
2 — warning	16	24	91	13	13	46	203
3 — average	44	62	257	32	27	89	511
4 — excellent	33	35	160	21	15	48	312
5 — outstanding	9	17	71	11	8	34	150

*The 17 hospitals without any long-term debt are included in the middle layer (Index 3) in the above table.

from a strong financial base. The 511 hospitals with an average status are surviving the changes in health care delivery and investing in medical technology, but have not received any special financial returns from these efforts.

Conclusion

Financial comparisons of intermediate measures across community hospitals should be based on a peer group determined by legal, control, and organizational arrangements that also follow similar financial reporting practices. Otherwise, erroneous inferences may be drawn in these assessments. Hospitals with restricted funds may not be comparable in reporting practice to similar facilities without restricted funds.

The 1,297 study hospitals are separated into six panels to accommodate known differences in reporting practice. Revenue over expenses as related to net patient revenue and total unrestricted assets is partially explained by 15 factors using regression analysis. Some of the significant findings for factors in these regressions underscore differences between panels and demonstrate the impact of reporting practices with some financial measures.

An index is applied to four financial measures for the purpose of assigning a composite five-point financial status rating to the hospital. The results are (1) 121 hospitals in critical condition, (2) 203 hospitals in a warning status, (3) 511 hospitals with average outcomes, (4) 312 hospitals with an excellent rating, and (5) 150 hospitals with outstanding performance.

Information on the range of values for the five-point scales in Table 10 and median values in Table 9 by panel permit the application of this classification procedure by a health care executive to a given hospital. But the more important point of this article for the health care executive is to be certain across-hospital comparisons of intermediate measures are made with hospitals in the same panel so as to minimize differences in financial reporting practice.

Notes

1. The Merritt System® is the product of Van Kampen Merritt Investment Advisory Corp., ("VKM Advisory") a XEROX Financial Services Company, located in Lisle, Illinois. Copyright ® 1990 by Van Kampen Merritt Investment Advisory Corp.: All rights reserved.

2. The selection of community hospitals excludes all federal facilities and non federal psychiatric and long-term care hospitals. Nonfederal facilities for tuberculosis and respiratory diseases and short-term hospital units of institutions are also excluded by AHA's definition of a community hospital. The Service Code 10 designation excludes children's hospitals, women's hospitals, orthopedic facilities, and other special units.

3. Some of the 600 excluded community hospitals had financial data for only two of the three years in this study; a few hospitals had merged and used a new reporting entity (system) for the 1988 certified financial statement that was not identical to the entity used in prior years. Several church-operated hospitals had to be excluded from the study because the facilities failed to disclose all income statement items. The certified financial statements for the merged systems of church-operated hospitals were complete, but the supplementary reports for individual hospitals often stopped with the detailed disclosures of net income from operations. Donations and contributions were only reported for the merged entity.

4. Certified financial statements for hospitals changed significantly in format during 1988 after the AICPA issued the proposed audit guide (AICPA 1988). Many community hospitals that were issuing securities prepared revised financial statements for 1986 and 1987 based on the proposed audit guide. There are some additional changes in the final version (AICPA 1990) that will affect the 1991 financial statements for community hospitals.

5. The Merritt System's® database includes financial information on many health care entities that are not hospitals but are separate legal entities that contain the long-term debt of related hospitals. The 600 excluded hospitals for this study included many in this category. The financial statements for many hospitals stop before including donations with this information only reported on the health care system's certified financial report. A few hospitals have all the fixed assets and long-term debts only in the system's report.

References

American Hospital Association. *Guide to the Health Care Field.* Chicago: The Association, 1990.

———. *Hospital Statistics.* Chicago: The Association, 1987, 1988, 1989–1990.

American Institute of Certified Public Accountants. Committee on Health Care Institutions. *Hospital Audit Guide.* New York: The Institute, 1972.

———. Health Care Committee and the Health Care Audit Guide Task Force. *Audits of Providers of Health Care Services.* New York: AICPA, 1990.

———. Health Care Committee and the Health Care Audit Guide Task Force. *Exposure Draft; Proposed Audit and Accounting Guide; Audits of Providers of Health Care Services; March 15, 1988.* New York: The Institute, 1988.

Ashby, John L., Jr. "The Impact of Hospital Regulatory Programs on Per Capita Costs, Utilization, and Capital Investment." *Inquiry* 21, no. 1 (Spring 1984): 45–59.

Carter, Carol, and Jerry Cromwell. "Variations in Hospital Malpractice Costs, 1983–1985." *Inquiry* 24, no. 4 (Winter 1987): 392–404.

Cleverley, William O. "Improving Financial Performance: A Study of 50 Hospitals." *Hospital & Health Services Administration* 35, no. 2 (Summer 1990a): 173–87.

———. "Is a Leveraged ESOP a Possibility for the Voluntary Hospital?" *Hospital & Health Services Administration* 33, no. 3 (Fall 1988): 385–405.

———. "Promotion and Pricing in Competitive Markets. *Hospital & Health Services Administration* 32, no. 3 (August 1987a): 329–41.

———. "ROI: Its Role in Voluntary Hospital Planning." *Hospital & Health Services Administration* 35, no. 1 (Spring 1990b): 71–82.

————. "Strategic Financial Planning: A Balance Sheet Perspective." *Hospital & Health Services Administration* 32, no. 1 (February 1987b): 1–20.

Colbert, Robert G. "The New Health Care Audit and Accounting Guide." *Topics in Health Care Financing* 16, no. 4 (Summer 1990): 14–23.

Cordes, Sam M. "The Changing Rural Environment and the Relationship between Health Services and Rural Development." *Health Services Research* 23, no. 6 (February 1989): 757–84.

Cromwell, Jerry. "An Analysis of the Prospective Payment System's Labor-Nonlabor Share by Diagnosis-Related Group." *Health Services Research* 24, no. 2 (June 1989): 213–36.

Cromwell, Jerry, and Dena Puskin. "Hospital Productivity and Intensity Trends: 1980–87." *Inquiry* 26, no. 3 (Fall 1989): 366–80.

Cromwell, Jerry, Janet B. Mitchell, Kathleen A. Calore, and Lisa Iezzoni. "Sources of Hospital Cost Variation by Urban-Rural Location." *Medical Care* 25, no. 9 (September 1987): 801–29.

Ermann, Dan A. "Rural Health Care: The Future of the Hospital." *Medical Care Review* 47, no. 1 (Spring 1990): 33–73.

Friedman, Bernard, and Stephen Shortell. "The Financial Performance of Selected Investor-Owned and Not-for-Profit System Hospitals Before and After Medicare Prospective Payment." *Health Services Research* 23, no. 2 (June 1988): 237–67.

Goldfarb, Marsha G., and Rosanna M. Coffey. "Case-Mix Differences Between Teaching and Nonteaching Hospitals." *Inquiry* 24, no. 1 (Spring 1987): 68–84.

Greene, Jay. "Negative Margins to Hurt Access to Capital." *Modern Healthcare* 19, no. 24 (16 June 1989): 42.

Hadley, Jack, Stephen Zuckerman, and Judith Feder. "Profits and Fiscal Pressure in the Prospective Payment System: Their Impacts on Hospitals." *Inquiry* 26, no. 3 (Fall 1989): 354–65.

Johnsson, Julie. "S&P: Anatomy of Four Recent Hospital Bond Defaults." *Hospitals* 64, no. 15 (5 August 1990): 56–60.

Kleiner, Richard G., Martha Garner, and Robin G. Colbert. "A Preview of the New Healthcare Audit Guide." *Journal of Accountancy* 168, no. 3 (September 1989): 32–44.

Long, Michael J., James D. Chesney, Richard P. Ament, Susan I. DesHarnais, Steven T. Fleming, Edward J. Kobrinski, and Brenda S. Marshall. "The Effect of PPS on Hospital Product and Productivity." *Medical Care* 25, no. 6 (June 1987): 528–38.

Long, Michael J., James D. Chesney, and Steven T. Fleming. "Were Hospitals Selective in Their Product and Productivity Changes? The Top 50 DRGs after PPS." *Health Services Research* 24, no. 5 (December 1989): 615–41.

Mennemeyer, Stephen T., and Lois Olinger. "Selective Contracting in California: Its Effect on Hospital Finances." *Inquiry* 26, no. 4 (Winter 1989): 442–57.

Palm, Kari Super. "Credit Ratings at Nation's Hospitals Slipping." *Modern Healthcare* 18, no. 4 (22 January 1988): 18–28.

Pauly, Mark V. "Policy Lessons from Studying Hospital Costs." *Business and Health* 2, no. 9 (September 1985): 22–26.

Prince, Thomas R. "Community Hospital Statistics by Ownership and Bed-Size Group: 1962–1985." *Journal of Health Administration Education* 6, no. 1 (Winter 1988): 85–108.

Rosko, Michael D. "Impact of the New Jersey All-Payer Rate-Setting System: An Analysis of Financial Ratios." *Hospital & Health Services Administration* 34, no. 1 (Spring 1989): 53–69.

Schlenker, Robert E., and Peter W. Shaughnessy. "Swing-Bed Hospital Cost and Reimbursement." *Inquiry* 26, no. 4 (Winter 1989): 508–21.

Sloan, Frank A., Michael A. Morrisey, and Joseph Valvona. "Effects of the Medicare Prospective Payment System on Hospital Cost Containment: An Early Appraisal." *Milbank Quarterly* 66, no 2 (1988): 191–220.

Solovy, Alden. "Health Care in the 1990's: Forecasts by Top Analysts." *Hospitals* 63, no. 14 (20 July 1989): 34–46.

Valvona, Joseph, and Frank A. Sloan. "Hospital Profitability and Capital Structure: A Comparative Analysis." *Health Services Research* 23, no. 3 (August 1988): 343–57.

Van Kampen Merritt. *The Merritt Roll.* Lisle, IL: Van Kampen Merritt, 1990.

Weitzel, William, and Ellen Jonsson. "Decline in Organizations: A Literature Integration and Extension." *Administrative Science Quarterly* 34, no. 1 (March 1989): 91–109.

Welch, W. P. "Do All Teaching Hospitals Deserve an Add-on Payment Under the Prospective Payment System?" *Inquiry* 24, no. 3 (Fall 1987): 221–32.

Welch, W. P., and Lisa C. Dubay. "The Impact of Administratively Necessary Days on Hospital Costs." *Medical Care* 27, no. 12 (December 1989): 1117–32.

Chapter 14

Improving Financial Performance: A Study of 50 Hospitals

William O. Cleverley

William O. Cleverley is Professor of Health Care Finance, Ohio State University, Columbus. He is a Faculty Associate of the College.

This article was published in *Hospital & Health Services Administration* 35, no. 2 (Summer 1990).

Most, if not all, hospital executives are very interested in management policies or strategies that will improve their firm's performance. Even in the current depressed financial environment, there are many examples of hospitals that have continued to prosper and grow. This article assesses whether there are any significant strategic differences between high-performing and low-performing hospitals. If such differences exist, can hospital executives adopt these strategies to improve their firm's performance?

Definition of High Performance

A variety of methods can assess performance in a hospital. In this article a rather narrow but extremely important measure, return on equity (ROE),[1] will be used. Ultimately, any firm's ability to remain viable is directly linked to its capacity to generate capital for both replacement of existing assets and new growth.

High-ROE firms are able to increase their total pool of available funds for new investment for two reasons. First, high-ROE firms are generating greater growth in equity capital, which is one major source of asset financing. Second, with greater growth in equity capital comes an ability to borrow more debt. Debt capacity is defined in several ways, but one measure often used is the relationship of debt to equity, or a "leverage multiplier." High-ROE firms are able to use their profitability to attract more debt financing when needed.

ROE is also a traditional measure used to evaluate the investment attractiveness of taxable firms. ROE is just as important for voluntary hospitals.[2]

From a purely accounting perspective, ROE can be defined as the product of four financial indicators (Cleverley 1987):

$$ROE = \frac{Operating}{Margin} \times \frac{Total}{Asset\ Turnover} \times \frac{1}{1 - Nonoperating\ Revenue} \times \frac{1}{Equity\ Financing}$$

Where

$$Operating\ margin = \frac{Net\ operating\ income}{Operating\ revenue}$$

$$Total\ asset\ turnover = \frac{Operating\ revenue}{Assets}$$

$$Nonoperating\ revenue = \frac{Nonoperating\ revenue}{Excess\ of\ revenues\ over\ expenses}$$

$$Equity\ financing = \frac{Fund\ balance}{Assets}$$

224

This framework suggests that ROE can be affected by changing operating margins, total asset turnover (capital intensity), nonoperating revenue, and debt financing (financial leverage). This accounting identity is very useful for analysis, but it does not directly suggest actual strategies for effecting change. For example, how do managers change their operating margins?

Financial performance in general, and ROE in particular, is often described as a function of three basic market/strategic factors: market structure, competitive position, and firm strategy (see Figure 1) (Buzzell and Gayle 1987). Market structure encompasses such variables as market differentiation, entry conditions, unionization, and growth rates. Competitive position includes market share, relative cost, and quality. Strategy includes pricing, new product introductions, marketing, vertical integration, and other variables.

In this study the accounting identity and the market/strategic framework will be used to analyze and discuss differences between high-performance and low-performance hospitals. Many of the differences that exist are suggestive of possible strategic actions.

Figure 1
PIMS Competitive Strategy Paradigm

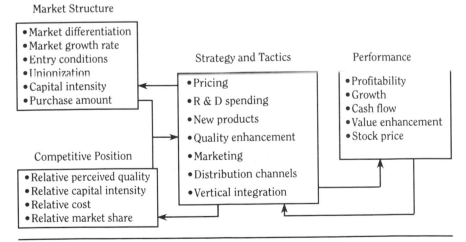

Source: R. Buzzell, and B. Gayle, *The Profit Impact of Market Strategy Principles: Linking Strategy to Performance.* (New York: Free Press, 1987), 28.

Data for the Study

The sample of hospitals used in this study was taken from the set of hospitals that were subscribers to the Healthcare Financial Management Association's Data Plus Financial Analysis Service (FAS) and Strategic Operating Indicators (SOI) in 1988. Ideally, it would have been desirable to draw a sample from more than one year to assess trends, but the SOI data set was only started in late 1987, and data prior to 1988 for both FAS and SOI were limited.

The FAS data set encompasses 30 key financial ratios that are derived from audited financial reports. This creates a very high degree of data reliability and validity that is not possible within other hospital financial data sets. The SOI data set consists of 30 operating indicators that are partially related to audited data but based on subscriber-submitted data forms.

From this set of all hospitals subscribing to both services, the highest 50 and lowest 50 firms in terms of ROE were selected. The sample was further reduced to remove extreme outliers. For example, firms with extraordinary gains or losses were eliminated because of their dramatic nonrecurring effect of ROE. Firms with extremely high financial leverage (more than $4.00 of long-term debt per $1.00 of equity) were also eliminated. Other circumstances creating removal from the sample included negative fund balance values, initial start-up operations, and transfers of equity from government entities. Some additional hospitals were also excluded because of missing data that prevented the calculation of some indicators considered critical. The final sample consisted of the top 25 and bottom 25 ROE hospitals that remained. All of these hospitals were voluntary not-for-profit firms.

Only 50 firms were selected to permit more individual analysis of specific cases. In this initial exploratory study statistical analysis of a larger data set that was not carefully screened could be very misleading. Therefore, in some respects, this article is a case study with a larger number of cases than is usual.

Tables 1, 2, and 3 show weighted average financial information for the lowest 25 and highest 25 hospitals in the study. For example, total assets was derived by adding the individual values for all 25 hospitals and then dividing by 25. Table 4 presents some summary demographic information on the sample. Tables 5 and 6 contain basic financial statements for the excluded hospitals that match the data in Tables 1 and 2. It was not possible to develop a table for the excluded hospitals that matched the data in Table 3 because of missing data.

Operating Profitability

One of the most striking differences between the high-ROE and low-ROE hospitals is in the area of operating profitability. The weighted average operat-

Table 1
Balance Sheets of High- and Low-ROE Composite, 1988 (hundreds)

	Low-ROE Hospitals	High-ROE Hospitals
Assets		
Cash and short-term investments	$ 2,462	$ 6,136
Accounts reservable	7,542	8,454
Inventory	714	916
Other current assets	667	940
Total current assets	11,385	16,446
Gross fixed assets	42,097	48,895
Less accumulated depreciation	15,876	19,705
Net fixed assets	26,221	29,190
Replacement funds	3,979	12,014
Other assets	4,625	12,562
Total assets	$46,210	$70,212
Liabilities and Fund Balance		
Current liabilities	$ 7,101	$ 6,307
Long-term debt	23,070	26,557
Other liabilities	711	702
Fund balance	15,328	36,646
	$46,210	$70,212

Table 2
Income Statement of High- and Low-ROE Composite, 1988 (hundreds)

	Low-ROE Hospitals	High-ROE Hospitals
Gross patient revenue	$56,308	$66,255
Less deductions	23,483	15,318
Net patient revenue	32,825	50,937
Plus other operating revenue	987	1,815
Total operating revenue	$33,812	$52,752
Less depreciation	2,315	3,109
Less interest	1,786	1,753
Less other operating expense	31,064	43,412
Operating income (loss)	(1,353)	4,478
Plus nonoperating revenue	536	1,691
Excess of revenues over expense	($ 817)	$ 6,169

Table 3
Profit Per Case Weighted Discharge

	Low-ROE Hospitals	High-ROE Hospitals
Revenue		
Gross price	$ 6,293	$4,263
Less contractual allowances	2,360	764
Less bad debt and charity	270	253
Net price	$ 3,663	$3,246
Costs		
Salaries and wages	$ 1,700	$1,393
Fringe benefits	314	207
Capital costs	456	312
Professional liability	77	40
Other costs	1,306	1,092
Direct medical education	73	40
Total	$ 3,926	$3,078
	$ (263)	$ 168
Inpatient profit (hundreds)	$(1,965)	$2,160
Outpatient profit (hundreds)	(375)	503
Other revenue (hundreds)	1,523	3,506
Excess of revenues over expenses (hundreds)	$ (817)	$6,169

ing margin for high- and low-ROE hospitals was .085 and − .040, respectively. While not unexpected, this information is very useful in discussing the factors that led to this difference. In fact, some of the differences here are quite large.

Pricing

It is generally agreed that pricing is one managerial strategy that may be employed to affect financial performance. Table 3 presents differences between our high- and low-ROE hospitals. First, the gross or "sticker" price per case-mix weighted discharge is $2,030 higher in the low-ROE group. This difference most likely indicates little if any opportunity to raise prices further and may already be adversely affecting the ability of these firms to attract payers who are sticker-price sensitive. In short, to attract new business, enormous discounts might be required.

While sticker prices are much higher in the low-ROE group, differences in net-realized prices per case weighted discharge are much smaller. The high-ROE group has a net price per case weighted discharge of $3,246 compared to

Table 4
Sample Characteristics

	Low-ROE Hospitals	High-ROE Hospitals
Average bed size (percent)	219	305
Rural	40	32
Urban	60	68
Teaching	8	8
Nonteaching	92	92
Church operated	28	16
Government nonfederal	12	12
Nongovernment nonprofit	60	72
Number of Hospitals by State		
Alabama	1	0
Arizona	1	0
California	0	1
Colorado	0	1
Florida	0	2
Georgia	1	1
Illinois	5	2
Kansas	1	0
Kentucky	1	0
Louisiana	1	0
Michigan	1	1
Missouri	0	2
Montana	0	1
North Carolina	0	1
North Dakota	0	1
Ohio	1	0
Oregon	0	3
Pennsylvania	4	5
South Carolina	1	1
Tennessee	2	0
Texas	0	1
Virginia	1	0
Washington	2	0
West Virginia	0	1
Wisconsin	2	1
Total	25	25

$3,663 in the low-ROE group. Since bad debts and charity care allowances are fairly close in each group, $253 per case weighted discharge in the high-ROE group versus $270 in the low-ROE group, the best explanation is clearly related to contractual write-offs, as Table 3 shows.

Table 5
Balance Sheets of High- and Low-ROE Composite for Excluded Hospitals, 1988
(hundreds)

	Low-ROE Hospitals	High-ROE Hospitals
Assets		
Cash and short-term investments	$ 2,393	$ 2,688
Accounts receivable	9,790	7,957
Inventory	576	650
Other current assets	1,214	925
Total current assets	13,973	12,220
Gross fixed assets	44,406	40,101
Less accumulated depreciation	16,952	15,807
Net fixed assets	55,910	48,321
Replacement funds	6,632	5,976
Other assets	7,851	5,831
Total assets	55,910	48,321
Liabilities and Fund Balance		
Current liabilities	7,911	5,689
Long-term debt	23,030	17,986
Other liabilities	1,590	664
Fund balance	23,379	23,982
	55,910	48,321

High prices in the low-ROE group were not effective in creating a major improvement in net-realized prices. The presence of fixed-price payers, such as Medicare and other major discounted payers, have unquestionably created this situation. It is important to note, however, that there is very little difference in the Medicare patient loads between the high- and low-ROE groups. The low-ROE group had 32.9 percent of its discharges coming from Medicare while the high-ROE group actually had slightly more, 34.7 percent. Heavy reliance on Medicare patients does not appear to be a significant factor associated with excellence in this study.

The major conclusion with respect to pricing strategy is that any difference in operating profitability between the two groups does not appear to be due to pricing. The high-ROE group actually had a lower realized net price per case-adjusted discharge than the low-ROE group. The difference is thus clearly related to cost.

Table 6
Income Statement of High- and Low-ROE Composite for Excluded Hospitals, 1988
(hundreds)

	Low-ROE Hospitals	High-ROE Hospitals
Gross patient revenue	$58,459	$55,378
Less deductions	12,337	13,151
Net patient revenue	46,122	42,227
Plus other operating revenue	1,736	1,194
Total operating revenue	$33,812	$43,421
Less depreciation	2,895	2,177
Less interest	1,727	1,207
Less other operating expense	42,964	37,528
Operating income (loss)	272	2,509
Plus nonoperating revenue	536	749
Excess of revenues over expenses	853	3,258

Cost Control

Net prices per case weighted discharge are $417 higher in the low-ROE group, but costs are significantly higher. The average cost per case mix–adjusted discharge was $3,926 in the low-ROE group compared to $3,078 in the high-ROE group. The presence of teaching programs or relative differences in cost of living between the two groups do not account for much of the difference. Both groups had two teaching hospitals and the high-ROE group had a higher percentage of urban hospitals (68 percent) than the low-ROE group (60 percent).

One factor creating some of the cost difference is volume related. The high-ROE group had an average occupancy of 63.6 percent, compared to 50.9 percent in the low-ROE group. High-ROE hospitals also generated 35.3 discharges per bed per year while the low-ROE hospitals generated 29.9. Length of stay per case mix–adjusted discharge was about the same, 5.17 in the low-ROE group versus 5.22 in the high-ROE group.

Greater volume in the high-ROE group has clearly permitted these hospitals to spread some of their fixed costs over a greater number of units to produce a lower cost per discharge. To speculate, if the low-ROE hospitals had generated 35.3 discharges per bed as the high-ROE group did, they would have realized an average increase of 1,183 additional discharges per hospital. At their existing net price per discharge this would have produced $4,332,864 of additional patient revenue. If, and this is the speculative part, incremental costs would have increased only 50 percent or $1,963 per discharge, the total increase in cost would have been $2,322,229, the net improvement in operating profit would have been $2,009,633, and the average operating margin would have changed from − .040 to .017. Whether the incremental cost increase is 50 or 70 percent, added volume would be very beneficial to the low-ROE hospitals.

Why do the low-ROE hospitals have lower volume? High prices and costs may have restricted their competitive position with respect to negotiated contracts. In addition, market position and dominance is clearly an important issue, as shown in Table 7.

The high-ROE urban hospitals are slightly larger than the low-ROE urban hospitals, but they have a much larger market share. The high-ROE hospitals are much more likely to be the dominant player in their markets than the low-ROE hospitals, which may mean that they are more able to attract medical staff and competitive contracts. The result may be greater volume with reduced fixed costs per unit of service. The low-ROE hospitals have not been able to attract sufficient volumes for economical operations. As a result they must raise prices to cover higher unit costs, but since they are the "small fish in the pond," they cannot find enough payers willing to pay those higher rates so their contractual allowances and discounts widen further.

Aside from volume and market share, some other factors have also led to higher costs for the low-ROE group. The low-ROE hospitals have higher salaries, $23,500 compared to $21,600 in the high-ROE group. Their fringe benefit programs are also higher. The low-ROE group pays 18.5 percent of salaries in additional fringe benefits while the high-ROE group pays only 14.8 percent. Total compensation costs then are $27,848 per full-time employee (FTE) in the low-ROE group compared to $24,797 in the high-ROE group. This difference adds $197 to the cost per case weighted discharge in the low-ROE hospital compared to the high-ROE group.

Staffing is another causal factor. The low-ROE group requires 150.25 hours of work per case weighted discharge while the high-ROE group required only 134.19. At their average compensation per FTE of $27,848, this additional

Table 7
Competitive Position of High- and Low-ROE Hospitals

	Low-ROE Hospitals	High-ROE Hospitals
Number of urban hospitals	14	17
Average bed size in urban area	285	321
Market share of beds in the urban area	6.5 percent	25.2 percent

staffing adds $215 to the cost per case weighted discharge in the low-ROE group.

Capital costs are also higher in the low-ROE group by $144 per case weighted discharge. The difference, which is discussed in greater detail later, is due to both greater debt and higher interest rates. The low-ROE group had $105,381 debt per bed while the high-ROE group had $87,089 debt per bed. As would be expected, the low-ROE hospitals paid more for their debt, an average of 7.74 percent in the low-ROE group compared to 6.61 percent in the high-ROE group. The low-ROE group also has a greater investment per bed, $119,774 compared to $95,717 in the high-ROE group. Since the low-ROE group has a lower level of discharges per bed, the combination of higher debt, higher interest rates, and greater investment pushes the fixed capital costs (interest and depreciation) skyward. The three other cost areas (professional liability, other, and direct medical education) also show higher costs (see Table 3).

Asset Efficiency

The overall level of asset efficiency as measured by the total asset turnover ratio (total operating revenues divided by total assets) is fairly close. The high-ROE group generates $.75 of revenue per dollar of assets while the low-ROE group generates $.73. While the difference is in the direction expected, it does not appear to be too large. When examining the individual categories however, some critical strategic differences emerge. First, the high-ROE hospitals carried 61 days in accounts receivable compared to 84 days in the low-ROE group.

The high-ROE hospitals generated $1.81 of revenue per $1.00 of investment in fixed assets while the low-ROE group generated only $1.29, which is the result of not only low volume but also higher investment in fixed assets— $119,774 per bed in the low-ROE group versus $95,717 in the high-ROE group. This difference would be even larger if the investment were stated in current dollars. The high-ROE group had an average age of plant ratio of 6.4 years, compared to 6.9 years for the low-ROE group.

If the high-ROE hospitals are so much more efficient in the areas of plant and receivables, why are the total asset turnover ratios so similar? Very simply, the high-ROE hospitals carry much more cash and investments: they had 50 days cash on hand compared to 27 days cash on hand in the low-ROE group. Even more striking is the level of replacement funds: high-ROE hospitals had $12,014,000 on the average in replacement funds while low-ROE hospitals had only $3,979,000.

In sum, the high-ROE hospital groups have been reserving funds from prior profits. As we will soon see, these retained profits have provided another significant advantage in additional nonoperating income.

Nonoperating Income

The high-ROE hospitals are generating significantly more nonoperating and other operating revenue. While we cannot be certain of the actual source, the lion's share of the nonoperating income appears to be derived from investment income. As just shown, the high-ROE hospitals have much larger balances or replacement funds. These funds are producing a very nice addition to already good levels of operating income. Some key characteristics of the two groups' revenue composition are presented in Table 8.

On average the high-ROE hospitals generated $3,506,000 in other operating revenue and nonoperating income while the low-ROE hospitals generated only $1,523,000 (see Table 2). These additional funds padded operating profits in the high-ROE group to create an average net income of $6,169,000 while they reduced the loss from patient operations in the low-ROE group to an average loss of $817,000.

Leverage

The last area affecting ROE is the use of debt or financial leverage. The initial ROE formula suggests that the use of debt will raise a firm's ROE; however for this to be true, the firm must earn a return on borrowed funds in excess of the cost of those borrowed funds.[3]

The low-ROE group has made much greater use of debt, both short term and long term. The indicators in Table 9 summarize the leverage position.

The low-ROE group is very highly leveraged, but returns from its debt-financed assets are less than interest costs, which results in a further reduction in profitability. Debt service coverage is also at a point where the future viability of the low-ROE hospitals may be a problem. The high-ROE hospitals have made effective use of debt financing. The average age of their plant is younger than the low-ROE group, indicating less need for new capital in the

Table 8
Characteristics of Revenue Composition in High- and Low-ROE Hospitals

	Revenues (percent)	
	High-ROE Hospitals	Low-ROE Hospitals
Inpatient	76.2	80.1
Outpatient	17.4	15.4
Other operating	3.3	2.9
Nonoperating	3.6	1.6
Total	100.0	100.0

Table 9
Leverage Position of High- and Low-ROE Hospitals

	High-ROE Hospitals	Low-ROE Hospitals
Equity/assets	.52	.33
Long-term debt/equity	.73	1.51
Current liabilities/current assets	.38	.62
Debt service coverage	4.46	1.29
Long-term debt/bed	$87,084	$105,381

future. Should opportunities arise for new investments through acquisitions, these high-ROE firms not only have sizeable cash reserves but also significant additional debt capacity. They stand ready to acquire rather than to be acquired.

Conclusions

Given this initial case study of high-ROE and low-ROE firms, what general conclusions result regarding strategic directions that should be pursued by hospitals interested in improving financial performance? The following eight strategies appear to be important.

1. *Market share.* For hospitals operating in reasonably competitive environments, obtaining reasonable market share appears to be very important. Market shares based on beds for urban hospitals in the high- and low-ROE groups were 25.2 and 6.5 percent, respectively.[1] How do you build market share if you are a small hospital in a big market? One popular strategy is merger. While this is clearly a rather dramatic step, there do appear to be sizeable benefits available to those hospitals that can be significant players in their market areas.

2. *System affiliation.* While market share appears to be critical, joining a system does not appear to provide any guarantee of improved financial performance. Twelve hospitals in the high-ROE group and 11 in the low-ROE group were members of a system. Two key differences in system affiliation did however appear to be present. Of the 12 high ROE–system hospitals, only four were part of a religious system. This is in sharp contrast to the low-ROE group where nine of the 11 hospital system members were part of a religious system. The high-ROE hospitals also appeared to be affiliated with local or regional systems that

had a multiple presence in their market area. For example, one hospital in the high-ROE group that was in a major urban area had only 3.3 percent of the available beds. However, it was affiliated with a nonreligious system that had another hospital in that same market. Together the two hospitals had 12.1 percent of the available beds. If these results can be generalized, it strengthens the argument for increasing market share within defined markets. Large national or regional systems that do not concentrate hospitals within given markets do not appear to provide any major advantages.

3. *Pricing.* Setting prices at levels far above costs may appear necessary to meet financial requirements but may have a negative effect on volume. Our high ROE–hospital group set prices at $4,263 per case weighted discharge, a 38.4 percent markup from costs of $3,078. The low-ROE group set prices at $6,293 per case weighted discharge, a 60.3 percent markup above costs of $3,926. Payer mix in the two groups appeared to be similar. The high-ROE group actually had a slightly larger Medicare load while bad debts and charity care were fairly similar. While the data do not permit verification of this point, some of these high-priced hospitals may have lost volume because of a noncompetitive price structure. This loss of volume appears to be a major factor explaining higher costs.

4. *Cost control.* The higher-ROE group appeared much better able to control costs than the low-ROE group. In addition, staffing patterns were much better: the average high-ROE hospital used only 134.2 hours of work per case weighted discharge while the low-ROE hospital used 12 percent more labor, 150.3 hours of work per case weighted discharge. Costs in all areas were uniformly higher.

5. *Excessive debt.* High-ROE hospitals use debt, but they use less than low-ROE hospitals. The high-ROE hospitals had $87,084 in long-term debt per bed while the low-ROE hospitals had $105,381 long-term debt per bed. This additional debt at a higher interest rate has increased their level of fixed costs that must then be spread over fewer units.

6. *Capital intensity.* The low-ROE hospitals appear to have overspent on plant assets. Their average investment in plant and equipment per bed is $120,000, compared to $96,000 per bed in the high-ROE hospitals. Initially, greater investment may be expected to attract more medical staff and therefore greater volume. In this limited sample, this does not appear to be the case. Volumes are lower in the high-investment low-ROE group. Because volumes are not greater, the excess invest-

ment adds another layer of fixed cost that further serves to weaken the competitive posture of the low-ROE hospitals.

7. *Accounts receivable investment.* The low-ROE hospitals carry 23.3 more days in accounts receivable than the high-ROE hospitals, which translates into $2.1 million dollars of excess investment on the average. Quicker collection could help the low-ROE hospitals increase their relatively weak levels of replacement funds.

8. *Revenue diversification.* High-ROE hospitals derive greater absolute and relative amounts of revenue from nonoperating and other operating sources. Much of this difference results from greater retention of prior profits in cash and replacement reserves, which is easier to accomplish when profits are higher. High-ROE hospitals also appeared to derive slightly greater amounts of patient revenues from outpatient sources, which may indicate greater expansion into these areas. Outpatient operations are, however, profitable for the high-ROE hospitals; they are not in the low-ROE group.

Notes

1. ROE is defined as the excess of revenues over expenses divided by ending equity or fund balance.

2. There are some voluntary hospitals that may continue to thrive with low-ROE values because they receive new equity funding from either contributions, tax support, or other sources.

3. In the ROE formula as equity/assets gets smaller, a multiplier effect results since the inverse of equity/assets is multiplied by the other terms.

4. It should be emphasized that using a beds percentage is not an ideal measure of market share. Without additional data however, it was the best measure available.

References

Buzzell, R., and B. Gayle. *Profit Impact of Market Strategy: Linking Strategy to Performance.* New York: Free Press, 1987.

Cleverley, W. O. *FAS-Plus Users Guide.* Westchester, IL: Healthcare Financial Management Association, 1987.

Part IV

Quality Management

In the wake of the obsession with cost control for the past two decades, a passion for quality has been revived out of a recognition that the public interest must be served through better measurement and surveillance. Just as "excellence" was the normative condition of success in business management in the 1980s, Total Quality Management (TQM) and Continuous Quality Improvement (CQI) have become the watchwords for health care organizations in the 1990s.

Perceptions of quality will obviously differ among managers, physicians, and consumers, with one likely to place a high value on the prudent use of resources, another on technical prowess, and the third on the personal aspects of care. Complicating the issue is a sphere of unacceptable quality, urged on by rising expectations of health care providers. While the concept of quality may be narrow or wide depending on the researchers, the fundamental questions are: Was the right thing done—and was it done right? Was the patient treated in a humane manner? Did it produce a good outcome? But we may come to realize that quality, like excellence, is neither object nor law that awaits discovery, but a scientific enterprise in which progress is influenced by individual, professional, and cultural values.

In Chapter 15, Joyce A. Lanning and Stephen J. O'Connor suggest that health care managers assist purchasers in developing quality measures that include patient perceptions in addition to technical competence, and simultaneously construct a managerial philosophy that places a high value on quality.

Susan M. C. Payne and her colleagues write in Chapter 16 that hospitals are currently under enormous pressure to improve the efficiency of operations without sacrificing quality of care. Often overlooked is useful information that already exists—data routinely collected as part of the utilization review (UR) process. The article describes a system using UR data for management purposes. Information derived from UR in a study hospital is discussed, as well as factors that should be considered in adapting some or all of the system's components.

239

A report by Joseph A. Boscarino (Chapter 17) expands on earlier findings reported in *Hospital & Health Services Administration* as to how the public perceives the quality of hospital care. This study examines the public's overall quality ratings of 155 short-term, medical and surgical hospitals. These are analyzed by type, size, staff ratio, mortality rate, case mix, and location of hospital. The hospitals represented a national cross-section of institutions, with results based on 20,000 adults surveyed in 40 U.S. market areas. Initial analysis shows that the facilities rated highest by the public tend to be: larger, nonrural, tertiary care, teaching, well-staffed, and have higher patient census and lower mortality.

Jane C. Linder argues in Chapter 18 that improved information, especially outcomes information, is part of the solution to the health care crisis. The article explores whether implementing an outcomes measurement system would compel significant change in the hospital environment. It examines the experiences of 31 hospitals that implemented a market-leading outcomes measurement system.

Chapter 15

The Health Care Quality Quagmire: Some Signposts

Joyce A. Lanning
Stephen J. O'Connor

Joyce A. Lanning is a health care consultant and holds adjunct appointments in the schools of Public Health and Health Related Professions, University of Alabama at Birmingham. Stephen J. O'Connor is Assistant Professor of Health Care Management, School of Business Administration, University of Wisconsin—Milwaukee. He is a Faculty Associate of the College.

This article was published in *Hospital & Health Services Administration* 35, no. 1 (Spring 1990).

The late Supreme Court Justice Potter Stewart was once asked to define pornography. He answered, "I can't define pornography, but I know it when I see it!" (Bendiner 1983). The concept of quality also resists precise definition, but the health care industry is caught up in controversial efforts to identify operational measures. The fact that this is an issue is a sign of changing times. Where professional autonomy is intact, the profession remains the undisputed guardian of quality. But we are moving from an era of trust in professional judgment to a new position where either the market or the government as regulator will define accountability.

Consultants such as Walter McClure (1987) are urging purchasers to "buy right" by identifying cost-efficient, high-quality providers and sending them more business. The "buy right" challenge would be easier for firms to accept if it were not for the current quandary over how to identify the right providers. How health care management finds its way through this health care quality quagmire to an acceptable definition of "good care" will have far-reaching consequences.

Many groups are trying to map the territory. Before the Health Care Financing Administration (HCFA) was forced to release hospital death rate statistics in 1986, private firms were already trying to pool and analyze their own health care data, and 17 states had mandated some kind of health data/cost information program. Consumer groups such as the American Association of Retired Persons (AARP) and the People's Medical Society (PMS), a consumer group organized to provide feedback on patient perceptions, have their own approaches.

There is no turning back from the effort to rate providers for effectiveness as well as efficiency. It will either be done poorly or well, but the journey has begun in spite of the absence of adequate road signs. What follows is a description of the signposts at important intersections—the specific directional signals are still under development.

The first section provides a conceptual overview of services quality, and the following two sections describe what is being done to measure aspects of technical competence and patient perceptions. A fourth section draws some alternative maps, and finally, suggestions are offered for health care managers working to meet the challenges of quality care.

Quality: How Will I Know It When You See It?

The concept of quality in any environment can vary depending on who defines the term. In the health care system, the definers are practitioners, patients, payers, and society. A model for conceptualizing quality health care and a distillation of some of the definitions offered by the various health care constituencies are presented in Figure 1.

All systems include inputs, processes, and outputs. In health services, human and capital resources and the patient population serve as the inputs. These inputs are combined with health services processes (what is done to patients) to produce changes in patient health status as outputs (Brewster and Bradbury 1988). This definition overlaps the classic categories of structure, process, and outcome developed over 20 years ago by Donabedian (1966).

System component linkages are identified as efficiency, appropriateness, and effectiveness. Efficiency is achieving a desired result at a minimum cost; it links resource inputs with hospital service processes. Appropriateness considers service suitability with respect to a patient's specific health requirements and links the patient inputs with hospital service processes. Effectiveness links the hospital service processes with outputs—improved or maintained health status (Donabedian 1973). Incentives that reward both *efficiency and effectiveness* are required for a proper quality control system to exist.

Traditional health care quality models have focused on health status as the end result, but more recent models (Lehtinen 1983; Longest 1977) have also considered the human interaction and consumer perceptions of quality. In this approach, structure still relates to physical facilities, personnel, and organization, but process deals with the *interaction* between provider and consumer. The interactive view of process focuses on how well the service employee delivers functional quality (how care is experienced by the consumer) as well as technical quality (competence in what is done). How well the service interaction meets consumer expectations is of primary importance as an outcome measure. Thus, outcomes in Figure 1 refer to the consequences of service delivery both in terms of health status (technical aspects) and patient perceptions (interpersonal aspects) in judging quality (Donabedian 1980).

Two realities about health care have downplayed the role of consumers (patients, governments, payers) in determining what constitutes quality. First, if the core definition of quality is that health benefits outweigh health harms, a health care organization's first responsibility is to the clinical/medical needs that comprise this prerequisite core (Kelman 1976; Kotler and Clarke 1986). Second, lay consumers are not qualified to determine what truly constitutes quality with respect to the scientific and technical aspects of their clinical/medical needs (Demby 1985; Donabedian 1980). Now, however, functional or interpersonal needs are increasingly recognized.

Donabedian (1980) classifies the definitions used by providers in the past as absolutist and those used by patients as individualized. The societal definition is an aggregate one, and the newest—the payer's definition—is statistical. The

---

Figure 1
Definitions of Quality Health Care

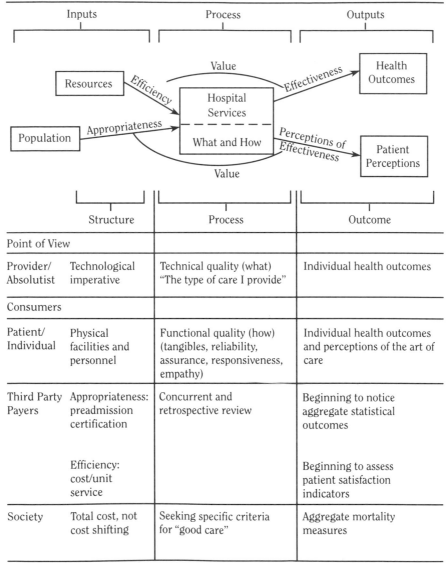

Point of View	Structure	Process	Outcome
Provider/ Absolutist	Technological imperative	Technical quality (what) "The type of care I provide"	Individual health outcomes
Consumers			
Patient/ Individual	Physical facilities and personnel	Functional quality (how) (tangibles, reliability, assurance, responsiveness, empathy)	Individual health outcomes and perceptions of the art of care
Third Party Payers	Appropriateness: preadmission certification	Concurrent and retrospective review	Beginning to notice aggregate statistical outcomes
	Efficiency: cost/unit service		Beginning to assess patient satisfaction indicators
Society	Total cost, not cost shifting	Seeking specific criteria for "good care"	Aggregate mortality measures

---

Adapted in part from *The New Healthcare Market* by P. Boland (ed.), page 720, with permission of Aspen Publishers, Inc. ©1988.

absolutist definition is the province of professionals, scientists, and technocrats, since they alone are deemed to have the extensive training and knowledge necessary to know what constitutes quality. This definition depends on the nature of the specific health problem as well as on the current state of medical art, science, and technology (Donabedian 1980).

The individualized (consumer/patient) definition takes into account the large variation in patients' desires, values, expectations, and means. The social definition, from the viewpoint of the community, state, or nation, is an aggregate of the net utility gained by individuals and interpreted as the benefits accrued to society (Donabedian 1980).

Payers of health services provide an increasingly important perspective on the definition of quality. Payers are comprised of insurance companies, governments, employers, and a variety of competitive health plans that include such organizational models as health maintenance organizations (HMOs) and preferred provider organizations (PPOs). Their emphasis on cost per unit of service, or efficiency, is now being tempered with concerns for value—what they are receiving per dollar spent.

The payer perspective contains elements of the individual and the social definitions. It is based, in part, on monitoring individual encounters with the health care system—through preadmission certification, concurrent review, measures of cost per unit of service—to assure appropriateness and efficiency of service. In addition, payers are working with aggregate data to find variations from a statistically defined norm of acceptable care.

Defining Technical Quality: Where Are We?

In the past, definitions of technical quality were left to professionals. However, in systems in which health care is allocated, components of quality (as defined by professionals or any other group), access, and cost will prompt a certain amount of tension. The passage of Medicare and Medicaid legislation in the 1960s increased access in the 1970s without much intrusion on professional decision making about quality, though costs increased. This led to new limitations on access as the focus changed to containing costs.

Now issues of access are demanding attention along with issues of cost. Massachusetts recently passed the first universal health insurance bill, and three proposals for a national insurance scheme were announced in the first month of 1989. The provider's autonomy to determine quality is increasingly being challenged. Major purchasers and funders (government, insurers, employers) are finding themselves forced into the quality-definition gap.

Structural measures, such as those used by the Joint Commission on the Accreditation of Healthcare Organizations (JCAHO), continue to be used.

These include the qualifications of the staff, the age and capabilities of the physical structure, and the administrative organization. Practitioner training, continuing education, membership in professional societies, and participation in medical staff activities are considered important for the hospital medical and nursing staff.

For the institution, licensure, accreditation, availability of the latest technology, nurse/patient staffing ratios, administrator credentials, and the institution's academic affiliations are stressed. Major assumptions in this approach to quality are that providers know what "better" means when it comes to staff, facilities, and organization, and that good care is more likely when the desired structural characteristics are present.

Although subjective peer review of physician diagnosis and treatment has always been a part of medical care, such process measures took on new importance when the prospective payment system (PPS) based on diagnosis-related groups (DRGs) prompted the necessity of keeping expenditures per case below allowed reimbursable amount. Extensive work has been done to develop criteria for objective measurement of the "right" treatment, that is, correct application of previously defined diagnostic and treatment approaches, as well as appropriate response to complications. These vary in their validity, their importance to case management and case outcomes, their adaptability to variations in cases, and the level of deviation they consider acceptable (see Donabedian 1986 for examples).

Outcome measures, however, are currently receiving the most attention (Winslow 1989). In December 1989, HCFA released the third round of diagnosis-specific mortality data comparing expected deaths for Medicare patients to observed deaths (percentage of Medicare patients who died anywhere and of any cause within 30 days of admission). Although HCFA does not tout these results as measures of quality, it does appear to believe that public scrutiny will result in increasingly better measures of outcomes that can be used to discriminate among hospitals on the basis of quality.

Several efforts are underway to adjust these death rates for severity of illness, condition on admission to the hospital, and socioeconomic status. Which, if any, of these case-mix adjustments will be adopted is unclear, but there is definitely a "comparability signpost" awaiting patient classification measures to make it possible to compare hospital results.

Among the patient classification systems being marketed as aids to quality assurance are (Jencks and Dobson 1987; Fifer 1987)

1. APACHE (acute physiology and chronic health evaluation) developed by Knaus and his colleagues (1985) to predict the risk of death in intensive care units

2. Computerized Severity Index, developed by Horn and Averill, which uses the discharge diagnosis to provide severity ratings within the DRG (Horn and Horn 1986)

3. Disease Staging (from local disease to death) developed by Gonnella, marketed by SysteMetrics, and based on the uniform hospital discharge data set (UHDDS) (Coffee and Goldfarb 1986)

4. MedisGroups (medical illness severity grouping system), based on Key Clinical Findings from evidence in the medical record, and developed by Brewster et al. (1985)

5. Patient Management Categories developed by Young (1984) at Blue Cross of Western Pennsylvania.

There is pressure on hospitals to adopt such a classification system, partly to prove that their results are as good or better than competitors. However, these systems are undergoing rapid change. Some require collection of primary data from the patient record, making them costly to implement. Even after severity adjustments, some medically appropriate variation in outcomes is likely to remain, so that differences still cannot be completely attributed to quality. Iezzoni (1987) suggests that hospitals resist the pressure to choose a system as long as possible. This may be difficult in the face of the government dictating the use of quality control approaches, such as the mandate by the state-established Health Care Cost Containment Council that Pennsylvania hospitals use the MedisGroups system.

Peer review organizations (PROs), successors to the professional standards review organizations of the 1970s, are looking at a limited set of outcome measures. They must screen a sample of Medicare discharges to see that appropriate follow-up has been planned and that the patient was medically stable prior to discharge. The PROs review charts for unexpected deaths, any deaths during or following elective surgery or return to a special care unit. In addition, they check the record for nosocomial (hospital-acquired) infections, unscheduled return to surgery, and trauma suffered in the hospital. Depending on their findings in individual institutions, they may also add hospital-specific indicators. Peer review organizations have recently added the responsibility of ambulatory care review.

It is even more difficult to develop outcome guidelines for ambulatory care quality due to the infrequency of occurrence or reporting of complications, such as stroke as a result of hypertension. Consequently, greater reliance will continue to be placed on process measures for tracer conditions as a proxy for outcomes. An example would be the proportion of patients with diabetes who have yearly eye examinations.

Seventeen states have adopted legislation requiring the reporting of health care cost and/or quality data that they and other purchasers can use as a base for statistical analysis of variations in cost and use of care. Iowa was one of the first states to use Wennberg and Gittlesohn's (1982) analysis of small-area variations in rates of surgical procedures to awaken both providers and consumers to the need for more information about physician practice patterns and their impact on quality of care.

In the absence of a uniform hospital discharge data set mandated by the state, business purchasers of care have joined together through coalitions or common carriers of insurance to analyze claims data. There is still a need for comparable data dealing with a complete episode of care (inpatient and outpatient), as well as measures of functional status that would help in assessing the impact of treatment. There is definitely a "data" signpost demanding attention.

Consumer groups are less actively involved in defining the information needed to make "buy right" decisions about health care. However, the AARP Public Policy Institute has prepared model specifications for state health care data collection, which recommends that states establish a distinct entity within state government to collect indicators of quality as well as price and utilization data for hospitals, ambulatory surgery centers, physicians, HMOs, nursing homes, and home health agencies.

Of 14 quality indicators suggested for hospitals, seven fall in the area of structure. The following measures are considered by AARP to be health outcome and satisfaction measures:

- Procedures in which the hospital specializes and annual number of procedures performed
- Morbidity and mortality rates by DRG at discharge and in 30 days post discharge
- Hospital infection rates by service
- Cesarean section rates as a percentage of deliveries
- Rates of readmission within 30 days
- Malpractice suits lost by physicians and hospitals per year
- Number of patient care recommendations and citations arising from licensure, certification, and accreditation surveys.

Quality indicators recommended for physicians include board certification, official licensure actions and disciplinary records in any state, and malpractice suits lost per year (Tilly 1987).

In the past, the JCAHO has asked whether staffing, facilities, organization, and procedures at the hospital were such that it *could* deliver quality health care. In 1987, an effort to look at results or outcomes was begun. Although progress in developing clinical outcome indicators has been slower than expected, indicators of hospitalwide anesthesia and obstetrical care are being tested in 12 hospitals now. Trauma and cardiovascular disease are next, and long-term care is being considered. Implementation of continuous data collection and feedback as part of accreditation is targeted for the 1990s.

Organized medicine is not unaware of the need for quality indicators. In the final report of the American Medical Association's undertaking entitled "The Health Policy Agenda for the American People," 34 of the 195 recommendations dealt with ensuring quality. Appropriate concern for the patient's physical, psychological, and social needs is mentioned, but not evaluation of the patient's satisfaction or perception of quality.

Defining Functional Quality

Although most efforts at examining health care quality have focused on the technical competence (what is being provided) of health professionals and institutions, the functional considerations (how it is provided) are receiving increased attention in the new market-oriented environment.

Parasuraman, Zeithaml, and Berry (1986) derived a purified set of five quality dimensions believed important to consumers of service businesses.

1. Tangibles—Physical facilities, equipment, and appearance of personnel

2. Reliability—Ability to perform the promised service dependably and accurately

3. Responsiveness—Willingness to help customers and provide prompt service

4. Assurance—Knowledge and courtesy of employees and their ability to convey trust and confidence

5. Empathy—Caring, individualized attention the firm provides to its customers.

These functional or caring aspects of quality—reliability, responsiveness, assurance, empathy—become more important to the patient as the technical aspects of medical care become more difficult to understand, as consumers assume the majority of practitioners to be equally competent, and in cases where technical quality is considered satisfactory (Friedman 1986).

249

Several provider and consumer groups as well as a few state governments have attempted to integrate patients' perceptions of quality into an overall assessment of health care quality. The Voluntary Hospitals of America (VHA), a provider coalition consisting of over 500 voluntary hospitals, has also recognized the importance of how consumers perceive quality in the health care marketplace. Peoples' Medical Society, based in Allentown, Pennsylvania, has developed a questionnaire for its members to fill out and send in regarding the "caring" aspects of their health care. The AARP guidelines also include some indicators of functional quality in addition to the technical aspects mentioned above (James 1987), and the Group Health Association of America has developed a patient satisfaction instrument for use by payers and providers.

Government legislation in several states has mandated requirements for providers to disseminate information on technical and functional quality to consumers. An early example of this is incorporated as a major component of Pennsylvania's Health Care Cost Containment Act, which became law in July 1986 (James 1987). Paul Ellwood is pushing his own approach to "Outcomes Management" through Quality Quest, which would analyze patient experiences over time in terms of quality of life measures, clinical information, disease-specific outcome measures, and patient satisfaction information (Faltermayer 1988).

Some Alternative Routes

Meeting the Expectations of Consumers/ Purchasers

In the past, a health care facility that undertook a comprehensive assessment of quality "exposed itself to liability and incurred a cost that competitors, who weren't measuring quality, didn't" (McClure in Sandrick 1986). Now, health care organizations are pressured to prove that their care is as good or better than their competitors, both technically and from the perspective of consumers (patients, payers, government). No longer will the quality dimension remain the sole purview of practitioners; it will be shared increasingly with other consumer/purchaser groups and become a more homogenous blend of professional and consumer input, with consumer expectations as a primary component (Donabedian 1980, 1985).

Because large group purchasers of health care have come to exercise such enormous leverage, what they consider to be important quality considerations will have portentous implications for quality in the future United States health care delivery system. Will these groups purchase based on value (efficiency, appropriateness, and technical and functional effectiveness) or will they become "price mad" buyers, bent on purchasing only the cheapest health care that providers have to offer? Walter McClure (1987) notes that the answer to this question will reveal if good medicine will drive out bad, or whether bad medicine will drive out good.

The federal government, through HCFA, has initiated a seminal attempt to quantify health care quality through hospital mortality rates—information that has been made available to the public. Ostensibly, these crude measures should provide a vehicle for determining those organizations that need improvement so performance can be upgraded to result in better health outcomes and to furnish a "scorecard" for consumers. Is this what will occur?

The HCFA tactic is one that concentrates on cases of wrongdoing. It offers no rewards for good performers and no information as to how an organization can improve in cases of substandard performance. This punitive approach is most likely to result, not in better health outcomes, but in greater defensive behavior on the part of health care providers (Rosen and Green 1987). As Berwick (1987) points out, "If quality measurement is valued primarily by purchasers only to catch miscreants in the act of misdeed, that will assure only bad measurement, not good quality."

The clear delineation, explication, and meeting of customer expectations will be extremely vital as quality becomes a competitive element for hospitals. The identification of segments based on consumer/purchaser expectations of health services quality can serve as a valuable tool for the manager of health services (Clifford and Plomann 1985; Sacks 1985). However, it should be cautioned that health care organizations could emphasize comfort and amenities as a substitute for technical quality in order to please patients (Donabedian 1986).

Quality in a Service System

A service system consists of the service package, the process by which it is produced and delivered, and its quality (Lehtinen 1983). When working properly, this service system develops a service culture that helps to communicate institutional quality to the external environment, in part through consumer/patients.

Consumers can easily sense and communicate their experiences with a service organization, and for this reason, it is important to develop a quality culture (Lehtinen 1983; Schneider 1973). To do so, the focus on quality and quality control should be directed not only at the specific aspects of output, process, or structure, but at the entire health service organization as a pervading general philosophy that values quality (Berry, Zeithaml, and Parasuraman 1985; Kume 1987; Wolfe 1986).

Advice for Managers

> We are forced, therefore, to speak of it through myth—that is, through special metaphors, analogies, and images which say what it is *like* as distinct from what it *is*. . . .Yet "myth", in this second sense is not to be taken literally. . . .Thus in using myth one must take care not to confuse image with fact, which would be like climbing up the signpost instead of following the road. (Watts 1966)

Watts is not describing the efforts to define quality of health care, but the image behind his message is applicable, especially if we take the liberty of substituting the word "indicators" for "myth." Dedication to perfecting quality standards has probably never been more important in the health care industry. However, overzealous promotion of these standards as the destination itself could, indeed, be climbing the signposts rather than following the road. Instead, a thorough dedication to quality detection and improvement built into the organization will be the most effective strategy in the long run.

The responsibility for the assessment and control of quality is often diffuse and spread through the organization in such areas as risk management, peer review, medical audit, and utilization review. Quality assurance should have a high-level position within the health care organization (Rosen and Affisco 1985) and should be complemented by the marketing and strategic management functions to help ensure that quality is the responsibility of each employee.

Standardized procedures (programmed decisions and set protocols), vertical integration, and a fully integrated management information system can help reduce variation and improve the quality of the services offered. However, defective functional or technical delivery of services is not always due to specific causes like poor worker performance. Management practices, such as those leading to high worker turnover, may be more important to quality care than daily variations in individual employee performance.

This is the major message from Deming (1986), the guru of the Japanese turnaround in quality and productivity (Gartner and Naughton 1988). Rather than exhortations and work quotas, he suggests that management break down the barriers between different levels of workers and departments and reduce the fear of failing to live up to standards. He sees the main responsibility for quality as management's. Management should not only use statistical methods to analyze carefully collected management information to identify and remove any special causes of low quality, but also should adopt a philosophy and create a system that allows employees to minimize waste, delays, and mistakes.

One of the best examples of implementation of Deming's philosophy in the health care system is the Department of Quality-of-Care Measurement at the Harvard Community Health Plan (HCHP), a large HMO in New England. This program goes far beyond the classic utilization review measures of proper process or even health status outcome measures like mortality rates for lung cancer or obstetrical morbidity.

The quality program has a budget of one-half of 1 percent of premium revenues, spending it to develop and implement methods to measure and track quality and identify and regularly report problems. Fixing them is everybody's job. The department measures coordination of care, patient and staff satisfaction, ambiance, interpersonal relationships, and has five indicators for access alone (Berwick and Knapp 1987; Berwick 1987).

Another excellent example of the Deming philosophy is the patient judgment system developed by Hospital Corporation of America (HCA), which uses 11 scales to obtain patient feedback (admission, daily care, information, nursing care, physician care, auxiliary staff, living arrangements, discharge, billing, total process, and allegiance). After thorough testing for reliability, validity, and representativeness, the results of these questionnaires have been used in a consistent framework to target specific processes for improvement—for example, use of signs in the hospital or steps to streamline admissions. Part of the problem involves training hospital leaders in the theory and techniques of continuous quality improvement, which is seen as everyone's responsibility (Nelson et al. 1989).

"Made in Japan," once a pejorative statement, is now a recognition of quality, partly due to the successful adoption of Deming's techniques by organizations such as HCHP and HCA. What the health care industry needs now is the development of agreed-upon measurement techniques and procedures for using the information they provide to become better. This will require a systematic rethinking of the philosophy of quality in health care in place of the current obsessive quest for standards. Anything else would be climbing the signposts rather than following the road.

References

Bendiner, R. "The Law and Potter Stewart." *American Heritage* 35, no. 1 (1983): 98–104.

Berry, L. L., V. A. Zeithaml, and A. Parasuraman. "Quality Counts in Services, Too." *Business Horizons* 28, no. 3 (1985): 44–52.

Berwick, D. M. "Monitoring Quality in HMOs." *Business and Health* 5, no. 1 (1987): 9–12.

Berwick, D. M., and M. G. Knapp. "Theory and Practice for Measuring Health Care Quality." *Health Care Financing Review* Annual Supplement (1987): 49–55.

Brewster, A. C., B. G. Karlin, L. A. Hyde, C. M. Jacobs, R. C. Bradbury, and Y. M. Chae. "MEDISGRPS: A Clinically Based Approach to Classifying Hospital Patients at Admission." *Inquiry* 22 (Winter 1985): 377–87.

Brewster, A. C., and R. C. Bradbury. "Hospital Quality Control—A Key to Competitive Health Plans." In *The New Healthcare Market*, edited by P. Boland. Rockville, MD: Aspen Publishers, 1988.

Clifford, L. A., and M. P. Plomann. "Cost and Quality: Two Sides of the Coin in Cost Containment." *Healthcare Financial Management* 39, no. 9 (1985): 30–32.

Coffee, R. M., and M. G. Goldfarb. "DRGs and Disease Staging for Reimbursing Medicare Patients." *Medical Care* 24, no. 9 (1986): 814–29.

Demby, N. "Quality Assurance and Marketing." *Dental Clinics of North America* 29, no. 3 (1985): 605–14.

Deming, W. E. *Out of the Crisis.* Cambridge, MA: MIT Press, 1986.

Donabedian, A. *Aspects of Medical Care Administration: Specifying Requirements for Health Care.* Cambridge, MA: Harvard University Press for the Commonwealth Fund, 1973.

———. "Criteria and Standards for Quality Assessment and Monitoring." *Quality Review Bulletin* 12, no. 3 (1986): 99–108.

———. "Evaluating the Quality of Medical Care." *Milbank Memorial Fund Quarterly* 44, no. 3, Part 2 (1966): 166–203.

———. *Explorations in Quality Assessment and Monitoring. Volume I: The Definition of Quality and Approaches to Its Assessment.* Ann Arbor, MI: Health Administration Press, 1980.

———. *Explorations in Quality Assessment and Monitoring. Volume III: The Methods and Findings of Quality Assessment and Monitoring.* Ann Arbor, MI: Health Administration Press, 1985.

Faltermayer, Edmund. "Medical Care's Next Revolution." *Fortune* (10 October 1988): 126–27, 130, 132–33.

Fifer, W. R. "Quality Assurance in the Computer Era." *Quality Review Bulletin* 13, no. 8 (1987): 266–70.

Friedman, E. "What Do Consumers Really Want?" *Healthcare Forum* 29, no. 3 (May–June 1986): 19–22, 24.

Gartner, W. B., and M. J. Naughton. "The Deming Theory of Management" (Book review). *The Academy of Management Review* 13, no. 1 (1988): 138–42.

Horn, S. D., and R. A. Horn. "The Computerized Severity Index: A New Tool for Case-Mix Management." *Journal of Medical Systems* 10, no. 1 (1986): 73–78.

Iezzoni, L. I. "Case Classification and Quality of Care: Issues to Consider before Making the Investment." *Quality Review Bulletin* 13, no. 4 (1987): 135–39.

James, F. E. "Controversy Mounts over Efforts to Measure Quality of Health Care." *Wall Street Journal* (17 December 1987): 33.

Jencks, S. F., and A. Dobson. "Refining Case-Mix Adjustment: The Research Evidence." *New England Journal of Medicine* 317, no. 11 (1987): 679–86.

Kelman, H. "Evaluation of Health Care Quality by Consumers." *Journal of Health Services* 6, no. 3 (1976): 431–40.

Knaus, W., E. Draper, D. Wagner, and J. Zimmerman. "APACHE II: A Severity of Disease Classification System." *Critical Care Medicine* 13, no. 10 (1985): 818–29.

Kotler, P., and R. N. Clarke. "Creating the Responsive Organization." *Healthcare Forum* 29, no. 3 (May–June 1986): 26–32.

Kume, H. "Quality Control in Japan's Industries." *Journal of the San Francisco State University School of Business* (Winter 1987):60–67.

Lehtinen, J. R. "Asiakasohjautuva Palvelujarjestelma—Kassitteisto ja Empiirisia Sovellutuksia." ["Customer Oriented Service System."] *Acta Universitatis Tamperensis* 160, Series A (1983): 295–316.

Longest, B. B. "Productivity in the Provision of Hospital Services: A Challenge to the Management Community." *Academy of Management Review* 2, no. 3 (1977): 475–83.

McClure, W. *Assuring Quality of Care in a Competitive Environment.* Paper presented at Public Health Update, Birmingham, AL, December 1987.

Nelson, E. C., R. D. Hays, C. Larson, and P. B. Batalden. "The Patient Judgment System: Reliability and Validity." *Quality Review Bulletin* 15 (June 1989): 185–91.

Parasuraman, A., V. Zeithaml, and L. L. Berry. *SERVQUAL: A Multiple Item Scale for Measuring Customer Perceptions of Service Quality.* Cambridge, MA: Marketing Science Institute, 1986.

Rosen, H. M., and B. A. Green. "The HCFA Excess Mortality Lists: A Methodological Critique." *Hospital & Health Services Administration* 32 (February 1987): 119–27.

Rosen, H. M., and J. G. Affisco. "Strategies for Managing Quality Assurance." *Health Management Quarterly* (Spring 1985): 6–8.

Sacks, J. G. "Definitions of the Quality of the Medical Care: A Strategy for Segmentation of the Health Care Market." *Health Marketing Quarterly* 3, no. 1 (1985): 11–18.

Sandrick, K. "Quality: Will It Make or Break Your Hospital?" *Hospitals* 60, no. 13 (1986): 54–58.

Schneider, B. "The Perception of Organizational Climate: The Customer's View." *Journal of Applied Psychology* 57, no. 3 (1973): 248–56.

Tilly, J. *Model Specifications for a State Health Data Collection System.* Washington, DC: Public Policy Institute, American Association of Retired Persons, 1987.

Watts, A. *The Book: On the Taboo Against Knowing Who You Are.* New York: Vintage Books, 1966.

Wennberg, J. E., and A. Gittlesohn. "Variations in Medical Care among Small Areas." *Scientific American* 246, no. 4 (1982): 120–34.

Winslow, R. "Patient Data May Reshape Health Care." *Wall Street Journal* (17 April 1989): B1.

Wolfe, N. S. "Quality, Leadership, and Culture." *Healthcare Executive* 1, no. 6 (1986): 36–39.

Young, W. W. "Linking Financial Analysis and Quality Assurance Using Patient Management Categories." *Journal of Quality Assurance* (Fall–Winter 1984): 17–21.

Chapter 16

Using Utilization Review Information to Improve Hospital Efficiency

Susan M. C. Payne
Joseph D. Restuccia
Arlene Ash
Michael Shwartz
Lillian Tarr
Brian Williams

Susan M. C. Payne is Research Assistant Professor, Health Services Department, School of Public Health, Boston University. Joseph D. Restuccia is Associate Professor and Chair, Operations Department, Graduate School of Management, Boston University. Arlene Ash is Adjunct Associate Research Professor of Medicine and Public Health, Boston University. Michael Shwartz is Associate Professor of Operations Management, Graduate School of Management, Boston University, and Director, Institute of Urban Health Policy Research and Education, Department of Health and Hospitals, City of Boston. Lillian Tarr and Brian Williams are Vice Presidents, Utilization Management Associates, Wellesley, Massachusetts.

This article was published in *Hospital & Health Services Administration* 36, no. 4 (Winter 1991).

In the increasingly competitive health care environment, hospitals are under great pressure to improve the efficiency of internal operations without sacrificing quality of care. Sophisticated new hospital management information systems and severity-of-illness measurement systems are being implemented to support management efforts to better control operations. In the rush to do this, hospitals often overlook an extremely useful source of information already available—data routinely collected by the utilization review department.

Hospitals are required to perform utilization review (UR) for accreditation by the Joint Commission on Accreditation of Healthcare Organizations and to be eligible to provide care under many third party payer programs, including Medicare, most Blue Cross plans, health maintenance organizations, preferred provider organizations, and other managed care systems. Because UR has been externally mandated, it has been implemented and supported by hospitals only to the extent necessary to meet the letter of the law; hospital administrators often view UR activities as "nuisance" requirements. As a result, UR information tends to languish in basement filing cabinets, used only to support the claim for reimbursement for a particular patient and to confirm compliance with the UR process. However, the advent of prospective payment provides a new *internal* incentive for hospitals to manage utilization and to support the departments that can contribute to improving efficiency and reimbursement. Reliable and valid UR data, effectively analyzed and presented, can help managers to identify inefficiencies in hospital operations and clinical practice (Restuccia et al. 1987; Payne, Ash, and Restuccia, 1991).

Utilization review information can help answer questions such as: Which services and physicians are exceptionally efficient in their practice patterns? Which need to be more efficient? What are the obstacles to improving efficiency? How can UR be focused on the types of patients more likely to be admitted prematurely or to have unnecessarily long stays? How effective are management interventions designed to improve efficiency?

Knowing the answers to these questions allows one to take informed, constructive action. For example, one large teaching hospital in New England provided informational feedback on the percentages of inappropriate admissions and days of care to physicians in its medical, but not its surgical, service. The "treated" group reduced inappropriate patient days from 30.0 to 14.6 percent over a nine-month period, during which inappropriateness rates in the surgical service did not change (Restuccia et al. 1986).

Because reviews are expensive, the value of focusing them on patients, physicians, or hospital services with higher rates of medically unjustified (that is, inappropriate) utilization has been recognized since at least the early 1970s (McClain and Riedel 1973). However, there has been no *systematic* method for focusing reviews on patients most likely to experience inappropriate utilization.

As part of a study to develop improved methods of UR (Restuccia et al. 1989), we developed a system for systematically collecting, analyzing, presenting, and using review data. The complete system has three components: (1) data collected by trained reviewers applying the Appropriateness Evaluation Protocol (AEP); (2) software for data collection using inexpensive, highly portable computers; and (3) formats for reporting UR findings to hospital administrators and physicians.

We describe here the purpose and design of the components, the process of implementing a computerized system to collect UR data, the uses of the data to improve hospital efficiency, and the implications of the project for administrators and UR directors in other hospitals.

The Appropriateness Evaluation Protocol: Explicit Review Criteria

The foundation of any review system is the method of identifying problematic cases for further examination. In our project, the AEP, a UR instrument initially developed by Gertman and Restuccia in the mid-1970s (1981) and recently modified by Restuccia and his colleagues (1986), was used. However, any valid and reliable UR instrument incorporating explicit criteria could be used to identify problematic cases.

The AEP consists of a set of generic criteria to assess the appropriateness of the timing and level of care of hospital services provided. The criteria are used to evaluate whether a patient's stability and illness severity or the specific services received justify inpatient care. The information used to assess appropriateness is taken from the medical record, including the history and physical examination findings, progress notes, nurses' notes, consultation notes, and information from other providers. The AEP is designed to be used by nonphysician reviewers with recourse to physician consultation in ambiguous cases.

The AEP has two parts: one evaluates the appropriateness of the timing and level of care of an admission and the other, the appropriateness of subsequent individual days of stay. The instrument is used as follows: if one or more of 16 admission criteria is met, the admission is deemed appropriate; if one or more of 25 day-of-care criteria is met, the day is deemed appropriate (see Table 1). This determination can be overridden (generally after referral to a physician advisor) when the criteria do not accurately capture a patient's situation.

Table 1
Appropriateness Evaluation Protocol: Adult Medical/Surgical Day-of-Care Criteria*

A. Medical Services
    1. Procedure in operating room that day
    2. Scheduled for procedure in operating room the next day, requiring preoperative consultation or evaluation
    3. Cardiac catheterization that day
    4. Angiography that day
    5. Biopsy of internal organ that day
    6. Invasive central nervous system diagnostic procedure (e.g., lumbar puncture, cisternal tap, ventricular tap, pneumoencephalography) that day
    7. Any test requiring strict dietary control, for the duration of the diet
    8. New or experimental treatment requiring frequent dose adjustments under direct medical supervision
    9. Close medical monitoring by a doctor at least 3 times daily (observations must be documented in record)
    10. Postoperative day for any procedure covered in numbers 1, or 3–6 above

B. Nursing/Life Support Services
    1. Respiratory care—intermittent or continuous respirator use and/or inhalation therapy (with chest physical therapy, intermittent positive pressure breathing machine) at least thrice daily
    2. Parenteral therapy—intermittent or continous intravenous fluid with any supplementation (electrolytes, protein, medications)
    3. Continuous vital sign monitoring, at least every 30 minutes, for at least 4 hours
    4. Intramuscular and/or subcutaneous injections at least twice daily
    5. Intake and output measurement
    6. Major surgical wound and drainage care (e.g., chest tubes, T-tubes, hemovacs, Penrose drains)
    7. Close medical monitoring by nurse at least 3 times daily, under doctor's orders

C. Patient Condition
    Within 24 hours on or before day of review
    1. Inability to void or move bowels (past 24 hours) not attributable to neurologic disorder

    Within 48 hours on or before day of review
    2. Transfusion due to blood loss
    3. Ventricular fibrillation or electrocardiogram (ECG) evidence of acute ischemia, as stated in progress note or in ECG report
    4. Fever at least 101 degrees rectally (at least 100 degrees orally), if patient was admitted for reason other than fever
    5. Coma—unresponsiveness for at least 1 hour
    6. Acute confusional state, not due to alcohol withdrawal
    7. Acute hematologic disorders, significant neutropenia, anemia, thrombocytopenia, leukocytosis, erythrocytosis, or thrombocytosis, yielding signs or symptoms
    8. Progressive acute neurologic difficulties

---

*See Ash et al. 1990 for a list of the AEP admission criteria.

The AEP provides a list of potential reasons for inappropriate admissions and days. The reasons for inappropriate admissions can be classified as either *level of care* (the patient did not need hospital-level care) or *premature admission* (the patient was admitted too far in advance of a procedure or treatment) (see Table 2). The reasons for inappropriate days of care can be grouped into two categories: those for *patients who need continued stay on medical grounds* (that is, the patient did not receive needed acute-level services on the specific day reviewed but was waiting to receive services on a later day and was not ready for discharge), and those for *patients who do not need continued stay on medical grounds*. The latter category is subdivided into three areas of responsibility: *hospital/physician* (e.g., failure to initiate discharge orders on a timely basis), *patient/family* (e.g., the family was not ready or willing to take the patient home), and *environmental* (e.g., unavailability of a skilled nursing facility–bed). On the average, completing an AEP medical/surgical admission and day-of-care review takes ten minutes.

AEP criteria sets have been developed for many categories of patients (e.g., elective surgery, obstetrics, pediatrics, and psychiatry). We used the Adult Medical/Surgical AEP.

The AEP has several strengths. It is easy and reliable to apply; it is based on objective and explicit criteria; information required for review is known to be well documented in medical records; it can be applied retrospectively or concurrently; and it is "generic" or independent of diagnosis so that the results are not influenced by errors of classification. The AEP has been extensively tested, validated, and used by a variety of other researchers and practitioners (Borchardt 1981; Studnicki and Stevens 1984; Siu et al. 1986; Rishpon, Lubacsh, and Epstein 1986; Wakefield et al. 1987; Strumwasser et al. 1990).

Collection of Utilization Review Data

Before beginning to collect the data, members of the UR committee in the project hospital examined the review criteria and agreed that the AEP was an acceptable instrument to measure appropriateness of utilization. Utilization review personnel from the hospital were then trained by an expert AEP nurse reviewer. Training included review of the criteria and the AEP Adult Medical/ Surgical Training Manual (which provides detailed explanations and examples of application of the criteria), application of the criteria to abstracted medical records, application to currently hospitalized patients, and reliability testing.[1]

The AEP reviews were performed on all adult medical/surgical admissions to the study hospital between October 1986 and December 1987. Day-of-care reviews were performed, subject to reviewer availability, on every third day of a hospital stay. The outcome of each review was a determination as to whether the admission or day of stay was appropriate or not, based on the AEP criteria.

261

Table 2

AEP List of Reasons Used to Categorize Inappropriate Days of Care*

A. For patients who need continued hospital stay on medical grounds
    1. Problem in hospital scheduling of operative procedure
    2. Problem in hospital scheduling of tests or nonoperative procedure
    3. Premature admission
    4. Patient "bumped" because of operating room problems
    5. Delay due to "40-hour week" problem (i.e., procedures not done on weekend)
    6. Delay in receiving results of diagnostic test or consultation, needed to direct further evaluation/treatment
    7. Other—specify

B. For patients who do *not* need continued hospital stay on medical grounds
    Hospital or physician responsibility
    1. Failure to write discharge orders
    2. Failure to initiate timely hospital discharge planning
    3. Physician's medical management of patient overly conservative
    4. No documented plan for active treatment or evaluation of patient
    5. Other—specify

    Patient or family responsibility
    1. Lack of family for home care
    2. Family unprepared for patient's home care
    3. Patient/family rejection of available space at appropriate alternative facility
    4. Other—specify

    Environmental responsibilities
    1. Patient from unhealthy environment—patient kept until environment becomes acceptable or alternative facility found
    2. Patient convalescing from an illness, and it is anticipated that his/her stay in an alternative facility would be less than 72 hours
    3. Unavailability of alternative facility
    4. Unavailability of alternative nonfacility-based treatment (e.g., home health care)
    5. Other—specify

---

*See Ash et al. 1990 for a list of AEP reasons for categorizing inappropriate admissions.

All cases judged inappropriate using the criteria were referred to physician advisors on the hospital UR committee for the final determination of appropriateness.

Development of the UR Data Base

In developing a focused review system it is essential that the characteristics of the patient or the hospital stay that are associated with inappropriateness be determined and that this information be readily accessible. We therefore merged the AEP data with information routinely collected by the hospital upon admission and stored on the hospital's mainframe computer. These data included patient's age, sex, admitting diagnosis, date of admission, zip code of residence, admission source (e.g., home, nursing home, hospital), admission type (e.g., emergency, urgent, elective), admitting physician, and admission service.

Software Development for Direct Data Entry

A computerized system for entering UR data is essential if the data are to be used to support timely management decision making. The two features of the software system developed are (1) direct entry of review data into portable laptop computers by UR personnel on the hospital floor and (2) routine merging of UR information with existing administrative information on the patient and the hospital stay to create information that can readily be analyzed.

The software development process had three phases:

1. *Testing, acquiring, and programming lap-top or portable computers.* Hospital UR coordinators worked with a software development consultant to identify an inexpensive portable computer with adequate memory capacity for data entry and storage. This resulted in the purchase of NEC® 8300™ hand-held computers for use in data entry by the coordinators. Programs were then written to facilitate data entry and downloading to a full-sized personal computer in the UR department.

2. *Downloading data from the hospital mainframe to the UR system.* Programs were also written to capture information on the patient and the hospital stay from the hospital mainframe computer and to merge it with information on the UR department's personal computer.

3. *Training of UR personnel in the use of the system.* Hospital UR personnel were trained to enter data into the lap-top computers and perform downloading to the department's computer. Manual data collection was continued during the initial period of training and "debugging" the computerized data entry system.

Development and implementation of the computerized system took approximately nine months.

Development of the Report Formats

Feedback from a previous study indicated a need for reports that provide systematic, concise, focused, and easily understood information for hospital managers (Restuccia et al. 1986). In this project, we worked with the hospital's UR committee and with UR and data processing personnel to develop report formats responsive to the perceived needs of the users. The report system we developed features

- Physician- and service-specific information on rates of appropriate admissions and days of care

- Information by service on the reasons for inappropriate admissions and days of care, separated into those that are under hospital or physician control and those that are not

- The capability of producing medical record numbers of patients with inappropriate admissions or days of care, for use by UR committee members and admitting or attending physicians who wish to review individual cases.

We did not analyze or present information by diagnosis-related group (DRG) for two reasons. First, there were too few cases in most DRGs to yield meaningful rates. Second, we wanted to focus on patterns in patient management (such as premature admissions or delays in discharge planning) that affected patients regardless of diagnosis and procedure.

We prepared reports describing both the admissions and the days of care reviewed. For simplicity and because of the importance of reducing length of stay for hospitals operating under the Medicare prospective payment system, we focus here on the day-of-care data.[2]

In developing our reports and predictive models, we emphasized the outcome of the initial review based on the AEP criteria (the "criteria-based" or "objective" decision) instead of the outcome of the final review performed by the physician reviewers (the "override" decision). The criteria-based outcomes are objective and replicable, whereas physician overrides reflect the particular philosophy at an individual hospital and may be influenced by individual physicians' practice patterns, experiences, or biases. The AEP criteria-based decisions thus provide a better basis for comparison with systems in use elsewhere. The reports are produced using simple statistical procedures (percentages, t-tests, and chi-square tests of significance).

Description of the Reports

The final report formats are presented in Tables 3–5 and Figure 1. For illustrative purposes, we have included information on the discharges reviewed in the study hospital. The rates of inappropriate days of care and the types of cases with high levels of inappropriateness can be expected to differ in other hospitals. Each hospital should use its own data in designing management strategies.

The first report presents information on the number of patients and days of care reviewed and the rates of nonacute days of care by service (see Table 3). For example, in the study hospital 580 cardiology-service patients (11.2 percent of the total number of patients included in the data base) had at least one day reviewed and 1,065 (9.3 percent of the total) days reviewed were from that service. The third column presents the rates of inappropriate days, as determined from AEP criteria. In the cardiology service, 10.2 percent of the days reviewed were judged to be inappropriate.

The wide variation in rates of nonacute use across the services is striking. For example, note the range in rates from close to 0.0 percent in plastic surgery, stomatology, and vascular medicine to over 16 percent in endocrinology, geriatrics, and rheumatology.

In the second report, the criteria-based rate of nonacute days is repeated, and four general categories of reasons or responsibilities for inappropriate days are listed: continued stay necessary, hospital/physician, patient/family, and environmental (see Table 4).

In several services, over half of the inappropriate days were attributed to the hospital or physician; in others, environmental factors (probably post-discharge placement problems) played an important role in extending stays unnecessarily. As an example, in cardiology almost half of the inappropriate days (48.4 percent) were attributed to actions, or rather inaction, of the hospital or physician; two-fifths (42.0 percent) were due to patients needing continued stay, which can indicate scheduling problems leading to delays in treatment; and the remaining 4.8 percent were due to environmental factors.

In the next report, information on the patient and the hospital stay are presented for variables that were significantly related to inappropriate days of care (see Table 5). The patient aged 65 or older, female, living less than 36 miles from the hospital, or having insurance coverage under Medicare or "other" were all associated with higher levels of inappropriate use. The inappropriateness rate for Medicare patients may be high due to the age factor or to delays in discharge due to living alone. Medical cases had a higher inappropriateness rate than surgical cases. The probability that a day would be inappropriate was much higher if the admission had been inappropriate due to

265

Table 3
Number of Patients and Days Reviewed and Rates of Inappropriate Days

Service	Number (Percent) of Patients, at Least 1 Day Reviewed	Number (Percent) of Days Reviewed	Percent Days Inappropriate, Criteria-Based Decision
Cardiology	580 (11.2)	1,065 (9.3)	10.2
Endocrinology	41 (0.8)	59 (0.5)	25.4
Gastroenterology	78 (1.5)	165 (1.4)	12.1
Geriatrics	253 (4.9)	637 (5.5)	16.8
Gynecology	58 (1.1)	82 (0.7)	1.2
Hematology	146 (2.8)	305 (2.6)	6.2
Hypertension	20 (0.4)	40 (0.4)	10.0
Medical oncology	211 (4.1)	547 (4.8)	13.7
Medicine	850 (16.4)	1,792 (15.6)	14.1
Neurology	359 (6.9)	781 (6.8)	9.4
Neurosurgery	225 (4.4)	488 (4.2)	5.3
Opthalmology	39 (0.8)	62 (0.5)	9.7
Orthopedics	252 (4.9)	537 (4.7)	13.2
Otolaryngology	52 (1.0)	118 (1.0)	5.9
Plastic surgery	17 (0.3)	42 (0.4)	0.0
Pulmonary medicine	101 (2.0)	304 (2.6)	3.6
Renal medicine	117 (2.3)	227 (2.0)	7.0
Rheumatology	19 (0.4)	34 (0.3)	23.5
Stomatology	12 (0.2)	17 (0.2)	0.0
Surgery	925 (17.9)	2,256 (19.6)	4.7

continued

Table 3   (continued)
Number of Patients and Days Reviewed and Rates of Inappropriate Days

Service	Number (Percent) of Patients, at Least 1 Day Reviewed	Number (Percent) of Days Reviewed	Percent Days Inappropriate, Criteria-Based Decision
Thoracic surgery	535	1,357	6.0
	(10.3)	(11.8)	
Urology	243	467	2.8
	(4.7)	(4.1)	
Vascular medicine	41	112	0.9
	(0.8)	(1.0)	
Total	5,174	11,494	8.9
	(100.0)	(100.0)	

a level-of-care problem or if a preceding day in the stay had been judged to be inappropriate.

Many of these categories overlap, such as age and payer. Multivariate analysis, if available, could be used to explore interactions among the variables and to identify key variables to focus the review further.

Figure 1 presents the numbers of physicians with specified levels of inappropriate days of care, using medical services as an example. Similar figures for surgical services and for all services (medical and surgical combined) can be produced. Information that can be produced for each physician is presented in Table 6.

Using UR Information

There are many important ways in which UR information can be used, especially when it is merged with other routinely collected data. Utilization reviews can be concentrated on the types of patients most likely to experience inappropriate days of care, thus improving the efficiency of the review process. Interventions to improve the efficiency of admitting or discharge procedures can be focused on the hospital services, the types of patients, or the physicians with high rates of inappropriate admissions and days of care. Information on the reasons for inappropriate use can be used to design interventions.

In discussing potential uses of UR information, we will use, as an example, the patterns of inappropriate use found in the study hospital. Services with high rates of inappropriate days of care *and* high patient volume are good candidates for focused review and corrective action. For example, cardiology, geriatrics, medical oncology, medicine, and orthopedics each had more than

Table 4

Rates of Inappropriate Days of Care and Reasons/Responsibilities for Inappropriate Days

| Service | Percent Days Inappropriate | Reasons/Responsibilities (Percent of Inappropriate Days) | | | |
		Continued Stay	Hospital/ Physician	Patient/ Family	Environ- mental
Cardiology	10.2	42.0	48.4	0.0	4.8
Endocrinology	25.4	0.0	60.0	10.0	30.0
Gastroenterology	12.1	20.0	20.0	0.0	55.0
Geriatrics	16.8	6.2	39.6	2.1	51.0
Gynecology	1.2	0.0	0.0	0.0	100.0
Hematology	6.2	11.8	70.6	17.6	0.0
Hypertension	10.0	0.0	0.0	100.0	0.0
Medical oncology	13.7	7.3	56.1	0.0	31.7
Medicine	14.1	8.1	60.3	1.9	28.2
Neurology	9.4	15.6	75.6	0.0	8.9
Neurosurgery	5.3	0.0	66.7	0.0	20.0
Ophthalmology	9.7	0.0	100.0	0.0	0.0
Orthopedics	13.2	4.3	53.2	0.0	40.4
Otolaryngology	5.9	0.0	75.0	0.0	25.0
Plastic surgery	0.0	0.0	0.0	0.0	0.0
Pulmonary medicine	3.6	12.5	25.0	0.0	62.5
Renal medicine	7.0	0.0	55.6	0.0	44.4
Rheumatology	23.5	0.0	100.0	0.0	0.0
Stomatology	0.0	0.0	0.0	0.0	0.0
Surgery	4.7	18.4	47.4	1.3	31.6
Thoracic surgery	6.0	77.6	16.4	1.5	4.5
Urology	2.8	58.3	16.7	0.0	8.3
Vascular medicine	0.9	0.0	100.0	0.0	0.0
Total	8.9	18.8	50.3	1.7	27.1

200 patients with at least one day reviewed and a rate of inappropriate days of more than 10 percent (see Table 3). Services with fewer cases reviewed that have high rates (such as endocrinology with 25.4 percent inappropriate days among 41 patients reviewed and rheumatology with 23.5 percent inappropriate days in 19 patients) can be monitored to determine if the high rates persist and, thus, warrant corrective action.

In the study hospital, 50.3 percent of the inappropriate days detected were directly attributable to the hospital or the physician (see Table 4), and 18.8 percent of the patients had delays in service delivery that added unnecessarily to their length of stay (the "continued stay" patients). In some services (hematology and neurology), these two categories account for over 80 percent of the

Table 5
Rates of Inappropriate Days of Care by Characteristics of the Patient and the Hospital Stay

Variable	Distribution	Rate of Inappropriate Days of Stay	P-value*
Patient characteristics			
Age			.000
Young (age<65)	46.2	6.8	
Old (age≥65)	53.8	10.6	
Sex			.001
Male	49.2	8.0	
Female	50.8	9.8	
Residence			.027
Metro (residence<36 miles from hospital)	84.4	9.1	
Nonmetro (residence>36 miles from hospital)	15.6	7.5	
Payer			.000
Medicare	58.8	10.5	
Medicaid	8.2	6.5	
Blue Cross/commercial	28.4	6.4	
Self-pay	3.1	7.9	
Other	1.5	9.5	
Hospital stay characteristics			
Type of case†			.000
Medical	37.9	12.3	
Surgical	40.2	5.1	
Not assigned	21.9	10.1	
Appropriateness of admission			.000
Appropriate	89.7	7.4	
Inappropriate, premature	1.4	10.3	
Inappropriate, level of care	9.0	23.7	
Appropriateness of prior days reviewed			.000
One or more prior days inappropriate	5.4	39.8	
No prior days inappropriate	94.6	7.1	

*Based on the chi-square test.
†Based on the DRG assigned by the hospital.

inappropriate days. This indicates the need for concerted action by both physicians and hospital administrators to identify the sources of the problems in those services so that plans for corrective action to reduce them can be designed and implemented.

Figure 1
Distribution of Physicians by Rates of Inappropriate Days of Care: Medical
Services

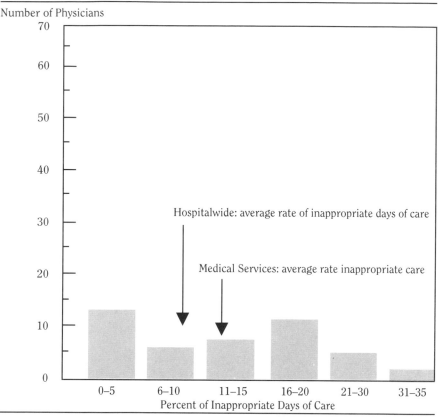

Number of Physicians

Hospitalwide: average rate of inappropriate days of care

Medical Services: average rate inappropriate care

Percent of Inappropriate Days of Care

Inappropriate utilization under the control of the hospital or the physician
can often be influenced by administrative action. This is true whether the days
were inappropriate because the patient was waiting to receive tests or services
delayed by inaction (the "continued stay" category) or because discharge was
indicated but was delayed by inaction (the "hospital/physician" category). Depending on the specific reasons for inappropriate days, management can intensify concurrent review, identify and resolve scheduling bottlenecks for lab
or other services, or initiate discharge planning earlier. In contrast, the hospital may not be able to reduce inappropriate days due to environmental or
patient/family reasons, although timely initiation of discharge planning may
be of some help in such cases.

Table 6
Simulated Data: Number and Percent of Inappropriate Days of Care with Reasons for Inappropriate Admissions, Fourth Quarter 1986–First Quarter 1987

Physician: Dr. Doe
Service: Surgery

Review Information	Physician		Physician's Service	
Number of days reviewed	75		370	
Percent (number) inappropriate				
Based on AEP criteria	9.3	(7)	4.0	(15)
Incorporating reviewer override	8.0	(6)	3.2	(12)
Percent (number) inappropriate days by reason*				
Continued stay necessary	16.7	(1)	16.7	(2)
Continued stay not needed on medical grounds	0.0	(0)	0.0	(0)
Hospital/physician	66.7	(4)	58.3	(7)
Patient/family	0.0	(0)	8.3	(1)
Environment	16.7	(1)	16.7	(2)

*The denominator used here is the number of inappropriate days incorporating the reviewer override.

In the study hospital, 128 of the 264 physicians studied had rates of inappropriate days of care of 5 percent or less and the majority (181 of 264 or 68.6 percent) of the physicians had rates of inappropriate days near the hospital average of 8.9 percent (see Figure 1). However, 46 physicians had rates of inappropriate days of 15 percent or more, and 14 had rates of 30 percent or more. Suitable interventions can be formulated based on the reasons for these high rates of inappropriateness. For example, if the physicians with higher rates have a large proportion of discharges that are delayed due to environmental factors (such as lack of available nursing home beds), the hospital could initiate intensified or earlier discharge planning. "Overly conservative medical practice" (physicians keeping the patient in the hospital beyond the time required for receipt of acute-level care) is the most frequent reason found in AEP reviews (Payne 1987). If days are deemed to be nonacute for that reason, the practice patterns of physicians with high and low rates of inappropriate use for similar types of patients could be compared by a physician committee, with a goal of developing a consensus regarding clinically acceptable, more efficient practice.

In addition, the results of the appropriateness review, especially the reasons for unnecessary days of care, can be used in discussions between administrators and clinicians and in medical grand rounds on the hospital's efficiency and quality of care (Griner and Brideau 1987). Utilization review

271

information can be valuable in promoting productive problem solving between clinicians and administrators because it is specific to the hospital, based on explicit criteria and an objective review process, and inclusive—identifying problems caused by physicians, administrative processes, and other factors.

The UR data-collection and reporting system described in this article is useful in itself. It also lends itself to more sophisticated extensions, including the development of multivariate models for predicting inappropriate use. Predictive models can be used to implement probability-based sampling of cases for review, so that cases more likely to include inappropriate use are more likely to be reviewed. Over time, the models can be run again with more recent data to detect changes in the types of patients or stays in which problems are occurring and to refocus reviews to new areas that could benefit from more reviewer attention. Such a Self-Adapting Focused Review (SAFR) system is described in Ash et al. (1990). Although the SAFR system offers great potential for improving the efficiency of UR activities, it requires the integration of hospital administrative records and the UR information system, something not easily achievable in most hospitals at this time.

Conclusions

There are many levels at which hospitals can use UR data to generate management information. Hospitals with limited data processing and analytical capabilities can produce reports like those described here for presenting and understanding UR or quality assurance results. They can also identify the characteristics of the patient, physician, hospital service, or hospital stay that are associated with higher levels of inappropriate use through calculating simple percentages.

Hospitals with access to more sophisticated tools for data management, analysis, and presentation may aim for more sophisticated uses, such as multivariate analysis or the SAFR system, which can improve the efficiency of the review process through targeted sampling.

Whatever the level at which a hospital is able to participate, the message is clear—a hospital's UR information is the raw material from which useful management information can be extracted at relatively low marginal cost. The reports described here are only simple examples of how such information can be used. Once the data are computerized and the information used, other benefits will surely present themselves.

Acknowledgment

Funding for this project was provided by the Robert Wood Johnson Foundation.

Notes

1. In retrospect, including the physician advisors in the formal training sessions with the nurse reviewers would have facilitated the implementation of the project and the uniformity of the review results. Our later experience indicates that joint physician-nurse training increases physicians' familiarity with the interpretation, purpose, and application of the criteria and the use of the override provision, as well as increasing a sense of interdisciplinary teamwork among those involved in the UR process.

2. Information on the results related to admissions are presented in Ash et al. (1990).

References

Ash, A., M. Shwartz, S. Payne, and J. Restuccia. "The Self-Adapting Focused Review System: Probabilistic-Based Sampling of Medical Records to Monitor Utilization and Quality of Care." *Medical Care* 28 (November 1990): 1025–39.

Borchardt, P. J. "Non-acute Profiles: Evaluation of Physicians' Non-acute Utilization of Hospital Resources." *Quality Review Bulletin* 7 (November 1981): 21–26.

Gertman, P., and J. Restuccia. "The Appropriateness Evaluation Protocol: A Technique for Assessing Unnecessary Days of Hospital Care." *Medical Care* 19, no. 8 (August 1981): 855–71.

Griner, P. F., and L. P. Brideau. "Academic General Internists and Managers of Teaching Hospitals: An Agenda for Collaboration." *Journal of General Internal Medicine* 2, no. 3 (May–June 1987): 204–5.

McClain, J. O., and D. C. Riedel. "Screening for Utilization Review: On the Use of Explicit Criteria and Non-Physicians in Case Selection." *American Journal of Public Health* 63, no. 3 (March 1973): 247–51.

Payne, S. M. C. "Identifying and Managing Inappropriate Hospital Utilization." *Health Services Research* 22, no. 5 (December 1987): 709–69.

Payne, S. M. C., A. Ash, and J. D. Restuccia. "The Role of Feedback in Reducing Medically Unnecessary Hospital Use." *Medical Care* 29, no. 8 (August 1991 Supplement) AS91–AS106.

Restuccia, J. D., S. M. C. Payne, C. H. Welge, S. J. Dayno, B. E. Kreger, S. Reamer, and P. Gertman. "Reducing Inappropriate Use of Inpatient Medical/Surgical and Pediatric Services." Report on HCFA Contract No. 18C-98317/1-02. Boston: Health Care Research Unit, Boston University Hospital, 1986.

Restuccia, J. D., S. M. C. Payne, G. M. Lenhart, H. P. Constantine, and J. Fulton. "Assessing the Appropriateness of Hospital Utilization to Improve Efficiency and Competitive Position." *Health Care Management Review* 12, no. 3 (Summer 1987): 17–28.

Restuccia, J. D., S. M. C. Payne, M. Shwartz, and A. Ash. "Final Report: The Self-Adapting Utilization Management System." Prepared for the Robert Wood Johnson

273

Foundation. Boston: Health Care Research Unit, Boston University School of Medicine, January 1989.

Rishpon, S., S. Lubacsh, and L. M. Epstein. "Reliability of a Method of Determining the Necessity for Hospital Days in Israel." *Medical Care* 24, no. 3 (March 1986): 279–82.

Siu, A. L., F. A. Sonnenberg, W. G. Manning, G. A. Goldberg, E. S. Broomfield, J. P. Newhouse, and R. H. Brook. "Inappropriate Use of Hospitals on a Randomized Trial of Health Plans." *New England Journal of Medicine* 315, no. 20 (13 November 1986): 1259–66.

Strumwasser, I. S., N. V. Paranjpe, D. L. Ronis, D. Share, and L. J. Sell. "Reliability and Validity of Utilization Review Criteria: Appropriateness Evaluation Protocol, Standardized Medreview Instrument, and Intensity-Severity-Discharge Criteria." *Medical Care* 28, no. 2 (February 1990): 95–111.

Studnicki, J., and C. E. Stevens. "The Impact of a Cybernetic Control System on Inappropriate Admissions." *Quality Review Bulletin* 10, no. 10 (October 1984): 304–10.

Wakefield, D. S., M. A. Pfaller, G. Hammons, and R. M. Massanari. "Use of the AEP for Estimating the Incremental Costs Associated with Nosocomial Infection." *Medical Care* 25, no. 6 (June 1987): 481–88.

Chapter 17

The Public's Perception of Quality Hospitals: Implications for Patient Surveys

Joseph A. Boscarino

Joseph A. Boscarino is President, The Boscarino Consulting Group, Inc., Chicago, Illinois.

This article was published in *Hospital & Health Services Administration* 37, no. 1 (Spring 1992).

Hospital administrators, trustees, and medical staffs have always been concerned about the images of their hospitals. Increased competition and the focus on quality-care provision have accelerated this concern. Hospitals that have better quality images among their publics often have had better prospects for development of alternative delivery systems, ambulatory care facilities, and other strategies designed to the ensure long-term viability (Gregory 1986). In the past, hospitals with better images often, but not always, were in a position to translate these into increased utilization and market share. During the 1980s, hospital administrators increasingly engaged the services of marketing research firms to understand how local publics rated their facilities (Steiber and Boscarino 1985). This type of information was often important for planning efforts and developing marketing programs. The data presented in this report represent an extension of an earlier research effort on how the public perceives a "quality" hospital (Boscarino 1988b).

Evaluating "quality" in health care delivery presents a difficult challenge today (Cleary and McNeil 1988; Graham 1987; Lohr, Yordy, and Thier 1988; U.S. Congress 1988). Currently, there is no consistent agreement as to the standards for assessing quality care. This study presents findings related to the public's perception of quality, which in some form or another will likely be a component of evaluating health care delivery in the future (Davies and Ware 1988; Nelson et al. 1989; Stewart et al. 1989; Ware et al. 1983). The aspect of quality assessed in this study is measured by means of the public's overall evaluation of local hospitals on a scale of the "best" to "worst" quality. This type of quality perception is related to, although it is a more global measure of, how patients rate their satisfaction with the hospital care they have recently received (Inguanzo and Harju 1985).

Many of the components that form the basis of the public's perception of hospitals and the motivation for hospital choice have been documented (Boscarino and Steiber 1982; Jensen 1987; Smith and Clark 1990). In the 1980s, Voluntary Hospitals of America commissioned large-scale national research measuring the public's perception of hospital care (Arnwine 1987; Hays 1987). This research documented that the majority of the adult public believes it can discern high-quality hospitals from low-quality ones. In addition, the public indicates that it would pay more for care from the higher-quality institutions. Generally, the research shows that the public perceives patient relations, medical staff, nursing staff, convenience, and technology as key in defining a quality hospital. Normally "patient relations" is very high on the public's quality list.

If current trends continue, efforts to develop viable indicators of quality hospital care will intensify (Robinson 1988). The implications of defining the quality of care provided by hospitals are far-reaching. Clearly, quality will be one of the most important health care issues (next to cost) in determining the survival of hospitals in the 1990s, and most likely tied to payment differentials in some form. The findings presented in this article contribute to our knowledge in this area. Previous research analyzed the public's ratings of only 65 hospitals in terms of limited facility variables—hospital size, patient census, hospital location, geographic region, care level, and death rate (Boscarino 1988b). This initial study found the most important factor related to the public's overall rating was the tertiary care level of the hospital, followed by its patient census (both positively related to quality). The public also rated larger hospitals to be of higher quality, but this was not significant when tertiary care level was taken into consideration because the two are interrelated.

The Data Base

The data base for this current study was developed from community surveys conducted between 1984 and 1988. It consists of the compilation of hospital-area marketing surveys conducted in 40 separate service areas spanning 20 states.[1] Specific facilities that had conducted community surveys during the targeted time frame were primarily identified (by the author) through the professional activities and membership lists of the American Marketing Association's Academy for Health Services Marketing. Each survey was conducted with approximately 500 adult household heads. Survey participants were contacted anonymously (i.e., the sponsoring hospital was not revealed) by professional telephone interviewers working from central telephone room facilities. Standard random-digit-dialing procedures and multiple callbacks were used in the surveys to prevent biases resulting from contacting only listed telephone households or easy-to-reach adults (Frey 1989). In addition, geographic, gender, and age quotas (matched to local demographics) were used in the studies as a final control over potential survey biases. Altogether, data were collected on 155 short-term, nongovernment medical and surgical hospitals. Government, nonacute, and nonmedical/surgical facilities were excluded from the study. The 155 hospitals represented a comprehensive national cross-section of institutions, including urban, suburban, and rural facilities. Study results are based on data collected from approximately 20,000 adult household heads.

Respondents in these surveys were polled on a range of health care issues, with each interview lasting about 10–15 minutes. It is important to emphasize that the surveys were conducted among the general public, not just past patients. Past-patient households were included in the surveys insofar as they were represented in the general population. However, this figure is not insignificant, considering that a recent national survey found that 40 percent of

U.S. households have had a household member hospitalized in the past two years alone (Steiber 1989). In each survey included in this study, the same attitude-rating question on the quality of local hospitals was presented to all respondents. This question was designed as a standard five-point Likert scale (Oppenheim 1966) and was presented, for each major hospital in their service area, to respondents in the following general format: "Based on experience or what you may have heard, how would you rate the following hospital overall? would you say that '_____' Hospital was much worse, somewhat worse, the same, somewhat better, or much better than other area hospitals overall?"

The five-point Likert scale is widely used in social science and marketing research conducted by telephone because of its accuracy and practicality. Other scaling methods are normally too difficult to administer by telephone or provide less useful information. Using this five-point method, the "average" hospital in the United States receives a collective community rating of 3.54 (scale values are scored so that much better = 5 and much worse = 1).[2] The overall median score received is 3.56. Low-quality rating scores (25th percentile or below) are 3.26 or lower. High-quality ratings (75th percentile or above) are 3.87 or higher. The distribution of these scores closely approximates a normal distribution.

Study Results

Previous research found that the public's perception of overall hospital quality was associated with basic facility characteristics, such as size and type (Boscarino 1988b). The current study analyzes the public's perception with a much broader range of variables. Altogether 16 variables were used in the analysis. These factors are classified into four general groups—community, institutional, quality and cost, and control.

Community variables relate to the neighborhood in which the hospital is located. For example, some older hospitals in the United States are located in deteriorating inner-city neighborhoods. It is reasonable to expect that this may influence the public's perception of care at these facilities. Community variables include socioeconomic status (SES INDEX), urbanization level (URBAN LEVEL), percent black in the community (BLACK), and percent Hispanic in the community (HISPANIC).[3] Institutional variables relate to the type and size of the facility. These include number of beds (BEDS), patient-census level (CENSUS), level of tertiary care (CARE LEVEL), and teaching status (TEACHING). Quality and cost variables include number of employees per occupied bed (EMPL/BED), religious affiliation status (AFFILIATION), Medicare mortality rate (MORTALITY), cost per admission (COST/ADM), and average employee salary (AVG. SALARY). Religious affiliation status was included under quality because it is often suggested that hospitals with strong religious ties provide more humane and compassionate care. In terms of the public's perception, it is reasonable to expect this variable could have an impact. Finally, control variables are included in the analysis to potentially adjust for other "outside factors," which could be related to the public's perception. These included geographic region (REGION), hospital case-mix index (CASE-MIX), and statewide bed average (STATE BED AVG.). Geographic region and the statewide average bed size are important control variables because these could be related to facility variables that in turn are related to the public's perception. If this is the case, inclusion in the analysis permits statistical adjustments for these factors. Hospital case mix was included for the same reason. While case mix is probably related to such factors as care level and cost per admission, inclusion in the analysis as a statistical control permits adjustment for this variable.

Table 1 shows the bivariate results for all 16 factors, based on the conservative two-tail t-test for statistical significance. Noteworthy is that urban level is the only community variable significantly related to the quality rating. Somewhat expected, rural hospitals receive a lower average quality rating than nonrural ones. The institutional variables are all significantly related to perceived quality in the expected direction. That is, hospitals that are larger, have higher census, more tertiary care services, and are teaching facilities receive higher scores. Also noteworthy are the results for quality and cost factors. Facilities with better staffing ratios and lower patient mortality rates receive higher-quality ratings, as do those with higher employee salaries. Although not quite significant at $p<.05$, more costly hospitals receive better ratings too. (If the one-tail t-test was used, this would, of course, be significant.) With respect to the control variables, hospitals in the Midwest and West receive higher ratings, as do those with higher case-mix indices (see Table 1).

While useful for exploratory purposes, bivariate analyses can be misleading when variables are interrelated. For example, as shown in Table 1, the public rates larger hospitals better than smaller ones, tertiary care hospitals better than nontertiary care ones, and higher-census hospitals better than lower-census ones. However, larger hospitals are more likely to be tertiary care and higher-census facilities (Boscarino 1988b). In this context, multivariate analyses can more accurately uncover the impact of the these variables on the public's perception of quality. For this reason, multiple regression analysis is used in the next analysis phase (Cohen and Cohen 1983). The purpose of this analysis will be to determine the relative importance of these variables on the public's perception.

Table 2 shows the results of a linear multiple regression, in which all 16 variables were used simultaneously to predict the public's quality rating. Note-

Table 1

Average Rating Score by Key Background Factors with Mean, Standard Deviation, and Significance Level

Background Variable	(n)	Group Means	Standard Deviation	Value of t of F	Two-Tail Significance
SES INDEX					
99 or <	(76)	3.51	.482		
100 or >	(79)	3.57	.354	−.89	NS
URBAN LEVEL					
Rural	(33)	3.30	.410		
Suburban	(83)	3.59	.362		
Urban	(39)	3.65	.474	8.23	.001
BLACK					
19% or <	(113)	3.52	.415		
20% or >	(42)	3.60	.437	−1.07	NS
HISPANIC					
4% or <	(124)	3.53	.426		
5% or >	(31)	3.60	.403	−.84	NS
BEDS					
200 or <	(45)	3.30	.403		
201–400	(65)	3.50	.326		
401 or >	(45)	3.85	.380	26.33	.001
CENSUS					
69% or <	(66)	3.40	.397		
70% or >	(89)	3.65	.409	−3.80	.001
CARE LEVEL					
Primary	(59)	3.33	.381		
Secondary	(52)	3.53	.365		
Tertiary	(44)	3.86	.339	27.05	.001
TEACHING					
No	(121)	3.44	.376		
Yes	(34)	3.90	.386	−6.14	.001
EMPL/BED					
4.8 or <	(95)	3.48	.388		
4.9 or >	(60)	3.65	.453	−2.51	.05
AFFILIATION					
Secular	(111)	3.51	.430		
Nonsecular	(44)	3.62	.391	−1.45	NS
MORTALITY					
13% or <	(119)	3.59	.426		
14% or >	(36)	3.40	.374	2.37	.05
COST/ADM					
$3,800 or <	(76)	3.48	.397		
$3,801 or >	(79)	3.61	.436	−1.92	.06

continued

Table 1   (continued)
Average Rating Score by Key Background Factors with Mean, Standard Deviation,
and Significance Level

Background Variable	(n)	Group Means	Standard Deviation	Value of t of F	Two-Tail Significance
AVG. SALARY					
$20,300 or <	(70)	3.44	.424		
$20,301 or >	(85)	3.63	.400	−2.96	.01
REGION					
North	(52)	3.43	.403		
South	(30)	3.49	.521		
Midwest	(68)	3.64	.373		
West	(5)	3.75	.267	3.12	.05
CASE MIX					
Low	(83)	3.41	.404		
High	(72)	3.69	.392	−4.39	.001
STATE BED AVG.					
230 or <	(59)	3.57	.431		
231 or >	(96)	3.53	.417	.52	NS

NS=not significant.

worthy are the variables that still remain statistically significant. The most important predictor variable in the regression is level of tertiary care (beta = .353). The second most important is patient census level (beta = .241). Unexpectedly, average employee salary is third (beta = .232), followed by teaching status (beta = .187). Cost per admission (beta = − .220) and percent black (beta = − .155), although not quite significant, are both negatively related to perceived quality, which is interesting and will be further analyzed and discussed below. Altogether, the 16 variables explain 50 percent of the variance ($R^2 = .503$) of overall perceived quality (Table 2), which is substantial ($p < .001$). It is clear from Table 2 that tertiary care level, census level, teaching status, employee salary, costs, and percentage of the community that is black contribute the most to this prediction. (In fact, when these six variables are used alone to predict quality, they account for 40 percent of the variance.) It should be noted, however, that the interrelationship between some of these variables can be complex. For example, when a regression was done predicting quality without the variable of geographic region, employee salary was not significant, suggesting a classic suppression effect (Cohen and Cohen 1983). A more detailed analysis of these more complex interrelationships is not within the scope of this article.

Table 2
Multiple Regression of Hospital Rating Score by Hospital Background Factors

Background Variable	Regression Coefficient	Beta Weight	Two-Tail Significance
SES INDEX	.0009	.061	NS
URBAN LEVEL	.0180	.038	NS
BLACK	−.0028	−.155	.10
HISPANIC	.0028	.045	NS
BEDS	.0002	.122	NS
CENSUS	.0082	.241	.01
CARE LEVEL	.0509	.353	.01
TEACHING	.1902	.187	.05
EMPL/BED	.0622	.144	NS
AFFILIATION	−.0190	−.020	NS
MORTALITY	−.0026	−.016	NS
COST/ADM	−.0627	−.220	.08
AVG. SALARY	.0291	.232	.05
REGION*			
North	−.1730	−.195	NS
South	.1072	.101	NS
Midwest	−.0137	−.016	NS
CASE MIX	−.1435	−.042	NS
STATE BED AVG.	−.0010	−.141	NS
(INTERCEPT)	2.3517	—	—

R=.709
R^2=.503
Standard error of estimate=.316

F=7.648
Significance $p<.0001$

*Region is coded as a dummy variable with "West" as the reference category (see Cohen and Cohen 1983).
NS=not significant.

Identifying High-Quality Hospitals

Using all 16 independent variables, a discriminant function analysis was conducted to "classify" high- and low-quality hospitals. This multivariate statistical method is useful to relate a set of categorical information (such as high-quality versus low-quality hospitals) to a battery of predictor variables. By taking the mathematical combinations of predictor variables, this statistical technique forms one or more linear functions that create maximum separation between the discrete "criterion groups"—in this case, high- versus low-quality hospitals. Technically, this method can be understood as a special type of factor analysis that extracts orthogonal factors from a measurement battery to statistically maximize the separation in "measurement space" between the criterion groups (Cooley and Lohnes 1971; Boscarino 1981). For this analysis the criterion groups were defined as follows: high-quality hospitals were those with a rating score of 3.90 or higher; low-quality hospitals were those with a rating below 3.90. Clearly, hospitals with a 3.90 rating or better were among a unique group of facilities (above the 75th percentile). Thus, the purpose of this analysis phase was to discover how these perceived quality leaders might be differentiated.

The results of this analysis are presented in Tables 3 and 4. Table 3 shows the discriminant function coefficients in standardized and unstandardized form. The unstandardized coefficients are similar to the regression weights derived in calculating a multiple regression. The standardized coefficients are similar to beta weights in regression. However, they can be interpreted similar to the factor loadings in factor analysis, with the main difference being that here they represent the relative magnitude and direction of variables in separating the criterion groups, not simply defining a factor. Similar to factor analysis, the + .30 or − .30 level can be used to identify noteworthy standardized coefficients and interpret a meaningful pattern among them.

As seen in Table 3, care level has the largest standardized coefficient (.610), followed by the South (.456). Case mix is next (− .431), followed by employees per occupied bed (.424), teaching status (.421), urban level (.420), cost per admission (− .402), census level (.387), and percent black in the local community (− .372). The direction of the coefficient (+ or −) is important because it indicates the group membership to which the coefficient contributes. As the bottom of Table 3 indicates, the group centroid (center point) for "low quality" is − .474; for "high quality" it is 1.624. Thus, as perceived by the public, high-quality hospitals (defined as those with a rating of 3.90 or greater) tend to have more tertiary care, are in the South, have a lower case-mix index, have more employees per occupied bed, are teaching facilities, are located in more urban areas, have lower costs, have higher censuses, and have fewer blacks residing in the local community. This is an interesting pattern because it appears to identify the major suburban medical center.[4] This finding, although speculative at this point, is in line with the demographic trend of shifting resources (as well as the perception of such) from the United States' older inner cities and Rust Belt, to the newer suburbs and Sun Belt.

The most important feature of the discriminant function method is its classification aspect, and Table 4 presents the results of this final phase. Classification is achieved by multiplying each independent variable in the analysis by its respective (unstandardized) discriminant function, summing the results for each variable and adding a constant. Based on the results of

Table 3
Discriminant Function Analysis Predicting Group Membership by Background
Factors

Background Variable	Unstandardized Discriminant Function Coefficients	Standardized Discriminant Function Coefficients
SES INDEX	−.0029	−.085
URBAN LEVEL	.4880	.420
BLACK	−.0161	−.372
HISPANIC	−.0157	−.106
BEDS	.0014	.272
CENSUS	.0325	.387
CARE LEVEL	.2416	.610
TEACHING	1.1391	.421
EMPL/BED	.4506	.424
AFFILIATION	−.4247	−.193
MORTALITY	−.0989	−.264
COST/ADM	−.2854	−.402
AVG. SALARY	.0070	.024
REGION		
North	−.4435	−.207
South	1.1475	.456
Midwest	.4415	.218
CASE MIX	−3.6733	−.431
STATE BED AVG.	−.0010	−.061
(Constant)	.2362	—

Eigenvalue=.7790.
Canonical Correlation=.6617.
Wilks' Lambda=.5621.
$p<.0001$.

Group 1 (low quality) discriminant centroid = −.474.
Group 2 (high quality) discriminant centroid = 1.624.

this, each case is classified into a specific group. However, before this classification can be evaluated, it is important to test for the equality of the covariances between the discriminating group variables. When this was done (using Box's M) the covariances were found to be significantly unequal. As a result, the classification is based on separate group covariances, which is the standard procedure for this (Cooley and Lohnes 1971). A comparison of results using pooled covariances, however, found that they were virtually the same as those obtained with separate covariances.

Table 4
Discriminant Function Classification Results

Actual Group Membership	Number Cases Classified	Group 1: Predicted Lower Rating (percent)	Group 2: Predicted Higher Rating (percent)
Lower rating (3.89 or <)	(120)	86	14
Higher rating (3.90 or >)	(35)	20	80

Box's M=322.11.
$p<.0001$.
Percent cases correctly classified = 85.

Examination of Table 4 indicates that the 16 variables used in the analysis could separate high- and low-quality hospitals extremely well, with a total correct classification rate of 85 percent. Lower-quality hospitals are slightly more likely to be correctly classified than higher-quality ones (86 versus 80 percent). To test for a potential biased estimate of group classification, the sample was cross-validated in the following manner (Cooley and Lohnes 1971). The sample was randomly split in half, with all the discriminant functions derived from the first sample half only. Next, the cases in the second sample half, which were not used in deriving the discriminant functions, were classified using the functions derived from the first sample half. The results of this cross-validation were virtually the same as the results using the whole sample. It is therefore concluded that the classification is statistically unbiased.

Implications and Recommendations

As was shown, the public's perception of quality hospital care is positively associated with a facility's tertiary care level, census level, teaching status, and employee salaries. In addition, hospitals that stand out as the "quality leaders" in the public's mind are not only tertiary care, higher census, and teaching facilities, they also are better staffed, are located in the South, have lower case-mix indices, are located in nonrural areas, have lower costs, and are situated in predominantly white neighborhoods.

Some of these variables—such as staffing ratios—can be associated with quality care; however, some—such as geographic location—may not. While it is recognized that some of the facility variables in this analysis are interrelated, and the public's awareness of some of them may be limited (e.g., awareness of facility mortality rates), it is suggested that the public's perception of quality hospital care is associated with factors not related to quality. Since there is growing reliance on using the patient's perception and patient surveys in defining quality hospital care, this suggestion has special significance. (The public's perception of the facility variables used in this analysis will be discussed below.) As was seen, basic facility-level variables can account for much of the public's perception of overall hospital quality. Rarely in the social and behavioral sciences does one find this much of the variance explained. Furthermore, using these same variables, the hospitals that are the perceived quality leaders can be correctly predicted a high percentage of the time. Again, rarely is this found. These findings are especially noteworthy because this study was derived from a large data base of surveys of adult household heads from across the United States. Many of these households, as was noted, have had recent hospitalization experiences occur among family members within the past several years. Thus, many household heads, similar to recently hospitalized patients, provided ratings based on actual facility experiences.

Use of Patient Surveys

It is recognized that the health care field is a dynamic and evolving one. As a result, definitions of quality will change. Thus, no matter how researchers attempt to operationally define quality, whether in terms of distinct outcome, process, or even simple patient satisfaction, it will be elusive (Lohr, Yordy, and Thier 1988). This is the nature of a field that is constantly changing, and a definition that cross-cuts many dimensions. It is suggested, nevertheless, that the "state-of-art" is sufficiently developed in the patient survey area to measure quality care. A way to do this, minimizing potential biases, is discussed below. This assertion is made possible because of the growing precision of patient, special population, and general public surveys in measuring medical outcome and health status (Fowler 1989; Centers for Disease Control 1988; Stewart et al. 1989; Tarlov et al. 1989). These developments make less relevant the classic distinction (Lanning and O'Connor 1990) between technical quality as defined by experts and information gathered from patients. If properly conducted, surveys of patients can provide important data on the technical quality of health care services, although other methods, such as controlled clinical trials, physician surveys, and medical chart reviews, may also be required (Salive, Mayfield, and Weissman 1990).

First and foremost, the patient survey items used must be psychometrically valid and reliable in terms of the dimensions measured (Ley 1973). Currently, there are survey instruments available that measure key dimensions of patients' medical outcomes (Stewart, Hays, and Ware 1988), as well as key dimensions of the perceived hospital experience (Nelson et al. 1989). If a hospital's administration wishes to monitor the quality of its care, including medical outcomes, then both of these (or key components of them) should be used, preferably by qualified researchers. If the administration, for management purposes, is more interested in simply monitoring "patient satisfaction," then there are a broader range of useful and less stringent approaches available to achieve this objective (Steiber and Krowinski 1990).

In addition to the issues of reliability and validity, patient "nonresponse" is often a serious problem in measuring quality by means of patient surveys. For example, if less than 50 percent of patients surveyed actually complete the interview, there is almost no way to determine if the data collected represents the patient population studied (Gallagher 1989). Nonresponse bias is not only a problem in patient surveys, but is a serious problem with most population surveys as increasing numbers of individuals refuse to complete interviews (Bradburn and Sudman 1988; Fowler 1988). Thus, if accurate data on quality care are to be derived from patients, in addition to originally selecting a representative group of patients for surveys, the majority of those surveyed must complete the interview.[5] This normally means substantially increased survey costs because some patients must be contacted three (or more) times to obtain their participation. However, this is necessary because patient surveys with low response rates (i.e., high nonresponse) are extremely misleading (Gallager 1989).

Measurement of Quality

Another issue—to which the research findings in this report allude—is that a patient's perception of quality may not be an absolute factor, but a relative one. As was shown, overall quality perceptions can vary greatly by facility variables such as hospital type, size, and location. These may or may not be related to quality care, but the patient's perception of it. Thus, it is important when using patient data to address the question of quality relative to *what*? The solution to this third issue can be complex because many of the "nonquality" factors that can affect the public's (and the patient's) perception of care are not known at this time. It is suggested, nevertheless, that reliable and valid normative data can be effectively used as a baseline to evaluate individual hospital results, control biases and, thus, gauge quality care.[6]

Figure 1 shows a possible quality standard for a hypothetical "City Hospital." These minimum data standards would permit the monitoring of quality care at City Hospital using patient survey data. Based on the current state of knowledge (U. S. Congress 1988), it is recommended that data be collected in at least six general patient information areas, including, but not limited to, medical outcome, medical staff, nursing staff, patient relations, support services, and patient demographics.[7] Support services are broadly defined here to potentially include food service, housekeeping, admitting, discharge, and ancillary services, such as radiology and laboratory. Medical outcome (Stewart, Hays, and Ware 1988) is defined in terms of perceived functional health status (e.g., pain, mobility, mood state, role functioning, etc.). There are numerous survey items currently in use that cover the key medical staff, nursing staff, patient relations, and support services issues. It is recommended that the items not use the "satisfaction" versions of these questions, but rather those that are more behaviorally specific. For example, a question about whether nurses responded to the patient's call button should be worded so the response categories are something like "always," "mostly," "seldom," "never," rather than in terms of "satisfaction" (i.e., "good," "fair," "poor").

Figure 1 also suggests a general reporting format. Note that there are five subscales plus an overall quality score. The subscales would be the summed results of individual questionnaire items, with perhaps 5–15 items for each subscale. For cost and research reasons, there is a limit to questionnaire length so that the number of items and subscales are restricted to the most important ones (i.e., those with the best predictive validity for the dimensions measured). For ease of interpretation, the subscale results should be standardized to range from 0 to 100. For example, if a subscale had five items, each with a series of individual response category values ranging from 1 to 5, the results should be reweighted to range from 0 to 100, rather than 5 to 25 (Ley 1973).

In addition to the subscale results, it is important to provide an indication of overall quality. Many patient studies do this but base it on only one questionnaire item, such as an overall rating. This is easy to do but can be misleading. The best approach is to provide a weighted composite index of all the key subscales, again, standardized to range from 0 to 100 (see Figure 1). This will provide more stable and reliable results than a single-item index. The issue then is determining how much each of the subscales should contribute to the overall quality score. The answer to this can be straightforward: It depends on how overall quality is to be defined or "operationalized." For example, the previously discussed study of the Voluntary Hospitals of America (Hays 1987) suggests that physicians would put more emphasis on medical outcome and medical staff, the public on nursing and patient relations, and employers on cost. Although not part of this study, hospital administrators would probably put more emphasis on support services than these other groups. Most health care researchers would probably suggest giving more weight to the medical outcome, medical staff, and nursing staff in defining overall quality. It is

Figure 1
City Hospital Quality (hypothetical example)

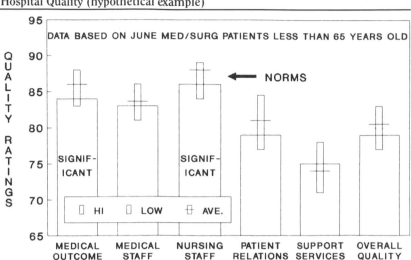

DATA BASED ON JUNE MED/SURG PATIENTS LESS THAN 65 YEARS OLD

← NORMS

SIGNIF-ICANT   SIGNIF-ICANT

□ HI   □ LOW   ⊟ AVE.

QUALITY RATINGS

MEDICAL OUTCOME   MEDICAL STAFF   NURSING STAFF   PATIENT RELATIONS   SUPPORT SERVICES   OVERALL QUALITY

NORMS BASED ON MEDICAL AND SURGICAL
PATIENTS LESS THAN 65 YEARS OLD IN
URBAN TEACHING HOSPITALS.

suggested that as long as there is a defensible rationale for the overall composite quality weighting (i.e., stressing the physician, public, or administrator's view) and this is explicit to the users of these data, then it is of value in evaluating and defining quality care. Identifying the actual quantitative weighting scheme that *best* defines overall quality can be complex and is beyond the scope of this study. Until this issue is sufficiently addressed by researchers in the future, it is suggested that a qualitative approach be used to weight specific quality dimensions based on "end-user" criteria, as discussed here.

Use of Quality Norms

Perhaps the most important component required to monitor hospital quality from the patient's perspective is the provision of norm data. Thus, in addition to City Hospital's results (large bars), Figure 1 shows the results for comparable hospitals and patients (small bars) from a hypothetical data base.[8] Three basic types of information are recommended for norm comparison—the highest, the lowest, and the average scores. In addition, statistical significance is shown for any City Hospital results above or below the norm. In this case, City Hospital is shown to be statistically below the norm on medical outcome and nursing staff, but not on the overall composite average. In addition to this type of subscore information, it would also be useful (especially to a hospital's administrative team) to examine the individual results for some survey questions using a similar normative report format. This detailed information should be part of a hospital's quality monitoring system although it is not presented here because of space limitations.

It is important that any norm data base used in evaluating an individual hospital's care provide comparison results for similar hospitals based on facility type and size. In addition, given current knowledge, it is recommended that norm comparisons only be made between similar groups of patients segmented on, at the very least, service type and patient age (see Figure 1). For example, it would be misleading to compare or group patients from teaching facilities with nonteaching ones, obstetrical patients with medical/surgical ones, or elderly patients with younger ones. This means it may be difficult to provide an unbiased comparison of a hospital's overall care using patient surveys—that is, unless it can be assured that the norm data base contains a similar overall patient mix. It also means that a major teaching hospital will have a different questionnaire than a nonteaching one. For example, a teaching hospital will probably need questionnaire items related to its medical residents, which is not applicable to a nonteaching hospital.

Future Quality Issues

At this time, studies that have longitudinally documented the public's perception of quality of care at specific institutions, especially after institutions have implemented quality improvements, are limited. One exception is in the more focused quality area of patient satisfaction. Recently, Fisk et al. (1990) provided a detailed description of a patient satisfaction–monitoring system used at a major teaching hospital in Philadelphia and documented how this system is used to address quality issues. Key components of this system include the use of ongoing patient surveys, the commitment and support of administration, a strong "guest relations" effort, and measurable goals for patient satisfaction. (An obvious deficiency of this system was the absence of a comprehensive norm data base—something that can be added as other facilities use this system in the future.) Measuring medical outcomes by means of patient surveys, such as recently reported by Stewart et. al (1989), is a new endeavor. This approach has its direct research origins as recent as the RAND Corporation's Health Insurance Studies of the late 1970s (Stewart et al. 1978). At this point, the public's current perception of quality hospital care—similar to the industry in the recent past—is often based on satisfaction, convenience, cost, and anecdotal medical information. Detailed studies of the medical outcomes of different institutions will be available to the public in the near future. The impact of this type of information on the public (in terms of both perception and behavior) will be of great interest to the health care industry and researchers.

Given recent developments, it is suggested that the measurement of quality care by experts and the public's perception of quality care are related, and yet, still diverse issues. For example, as suggested, researchers have begun to achieve an acceptable level of objectivity and accuracy (i.e., validity and reliability) in measuring quality patient care. Nevertheless, in addition to the results reported above, a substantial body of existing research also documents that the public perceives quality (and selects hospital care) contingent upon the type of hospital and services evaluated (Boscarino 1988b; Boscarino and Steiber 1982; Javalgi, Rao, and Thomas 1991; Lane and Lindquist 1988; Smith and Clark 1990). The research indicates that the public's perception of quality is often elementary. Typically, it is not aware of obvious quality differences between facilities, unless they have been extensively reported in the mass media (see Boscarino 1988a). For example, in the case of something as straightforward as government mortality statistics (at least in terms of a simple mortality figure), the public has been found to be uninformed (Gross and Schaffer 1989). However, once aware of this type information, the public does use it to choose a hospital (Gross and Schaffer 1989; Marks and Totten 1990). Another example is the issue of the nursing shortage. In many communities the public perceives the nursing shortage to be a major quality problem and is willing to undertake measures, such as writing public officials, to deal with this perception (Boscarino 1989).

Thus, in the early 1990s the public's understanding of quality hospital care, while becoming more sophisticated, is still limited. If current trends continue, however, the public will become increasingly aware of quality differences, and facilities will most likely resort to promoting the outcome and effectiveness of their services (among other aspects) to attract consumers (MacStravic 1988).

Conclusion

In summary, patient survey data can be used to evaluate the quality of hospital care. However, to do this requires caution. Valid and reliable questionnaire items must be properly administered among a representative group of patients. This means achieving a high rate of participation among patients, which is difficult and expensive. Extensive normative data are also required for comparison purposes to properly evaluate individual hospital results and control for biases. This approach also requires extreme care to avoid comparison of individual hospital results with noncomparable facilities or patients groups in the normative data base. Regardless of the method used to monitor quality, however, it is realized that the provision of quality care is an ongoing process. As a result, it is expected that any patient survey system evaluating this would be designed for ongoing administration and evaluation.

The critical philosophical decision for health care executives at this point in the evolution of the health care industry, is whether to directly address the medical outcome issue within the context of monitoring and providing quality care at their institutions. The least difficult choice at this time would be to simply implement (or maintain) a good patient satisfaction monitoring system together with strong guest relations and quality assurance programs. However, the question hospital administrators must ask is, Do I expect health care consumers (e.g., patients, third party payers, etc.) to endure the high cost of care indefinitely (including quality-of-life costs) without documented efficacy? If the answer to this question is no, then a strategic decision must be made to allocate significant resources to document quality care, including medical outcomes.[9] While controlled clinical trials have historically been the preferred scientific method to evaluate medical outcomes, it is ethical issues, lower costs, and advances in research methods that have made patient surveys a viable alternative. Clearly, more research needs to be done. Nevertheless, if patient surveys are used properly, they can provide a means to monitor quality care in the future.

Footnotes

1. Hospitals from the following states were included in this study: Colorado, Illinois, Indiana, Iowa, Maryland, Massachusetts, Michigan, Missouri, Montana, New Hampshire, New Jersey, Nevada, New York, North Carolina, Ohio, Oklahoma, Pennsylvania, Rhode Island, South Carolina, and Texas. The hospital sample has the following profile: *geographic region*—North = 34 percent, South = 19 percent, Midwest = 44 percent, West = 3 percent; *location*—rural = 21 percent, suburban = 54 percent, urban = 25 percent; *bed size*—200 or less = 29 percent, 201–400 = 42 percent, 401 or more = 29 percent; *teaching status*—nonteaching = 78 percent, teaching = 22 percent; *religious affiliation*—secular = 72 percent, nonsecular = 28 percent. As this profile indicates, the sample tends to underrepresent hospitals from the West and smaller hospitals. For the purposes of the analyses presented, it is assumed, however, that the data are representative of hospitals in the United States. Given the sample coverage, it is believed that the sample biases are acceptable.

2. Each hospital's rating used in these analyses represented a composite score. This score is the arithmetic average of the individual ratings provided by adults in the

292

service area where the hospital is located. Not all adults rated their local hospitals, especially if they were completely unfamiliar with them. In this case, they refused to provide a rating or responded with a "don't know." To base this study on reliable data, no hospital rating was used that was based on fewer than 100 individual ratings.

3. Variables are coded as follows: SES (socioeconomic status) INDEX, percent BLACK, and percent HISPANIC are taken from *The 1985 Sourcebook of Demographics* (CACI 1986) and represent the demographic composition of a hospital's immediate service area. BEDS, CENSUS, CARE LEVEL, TEACHING, EMPL/BED, AFFILIATION, COST/ADM, and AVG. SALARY are derived (for the appropriate year) from the American Hospital Association's *Guide* (1989). CARE LEVEL is a score based on the number of tertiary services offered by a facility. An earlier version of this score is described elsewhere in more detail (Boscarino 1988b). EMPL/BED represents the number of employees per occupied bed. AFFILIATION is based on whether there is a direct facility association with a religious group. COST/ADM represents the average cost per admission. AVG. SALARY represents the average annual salary per employee for the hospital. MORTALITY is based on the 1986 Health Care Financing Administration (HCFA) report of overall Medicare patient mortality (Center for Study of Services 1988). CASE-MIX is based on data provided by HCFA (1986). REGION is based on standard U.S. Census Department categories. Finally, STATE BED AVG. is based on American Hospital Association (1989) data and represents the average hospital bed size in a given state.

4. The definition of a teaching hospital in this report is based on the American Hospital Association's (1989) criteria, which includes more than just academic teaching hospitals. If the latter were only included, the coefficient pattern would probably reflect the "classic" (typically inner-city), academically-affiliated teaching center.

5. There are other methodological issues (such as sampling and data collection methods) that can affect the accuracy of patient survey data. However, the three discussed—reliability, validity, and nonresponse—are normally the most problematic for patient surveys. Unlike household surveys, master computer files typically exist from which "perfect" random samples of patients can be drawn. Sampling, however, is one of the most difficult methodological issues in general community surveys (see Fowler 1988).

6. Although patients would have more specific information with regard to their recent hospitalization experience, it is suggested that they may be far from unbiased, as suggested by Frank (1974) in his classic study of psychotherapy patients. The approach suggested (using a normative data base) recommends a method that can potentially control for biases in patient perception, as well as other factors, such as severity of illness. The latter can also be a serious confounding factor when comparing different facilities. Sicker patients should not only have poorer medical outcomes, but should be more likely to have negative perceptions of the hospital experience. A normative data base can control for this bias as well. Of course, the "pure" scientific method controls for biases (confounding factors) by use of random assignment, the "double blind," placebos, etc. (see Campbell and Stanley 1963).

7. There are numerous studies that have documented key features of perceived quality care (see U.S. Congress 1988). It is believed that the most important can be reduced to the six basic data areas identified. The list provided is not intended to be exhaustive, but only illustrative of the quality areas that have been identified in previous research. Technical, physical plant, and information quality, as well as convenience issues, could also be added to the quality list, although many of these can probably be subsumed under the general categories suggested.

8. By necessity, developing a proper norm data base requires resources beyond the means of most individual hospitals. As a result, facilities would need to pool resources or work with outside organizations to have access to this information.

9. The policy of the U.S. Government in the area of outcome assessment is unequivocal. Many major medical procedures are currently being evaluated by researchers across a variety of health care settings. Both Medicare and non-Medicare patients are being studied in this effort. The plan is to widely disseminate results to a broad range of audiences (see Salive, Mayfield, and Weissman 1990).

References

American Hospital Association. *Guide to the Health Care Field.* Chicago: American Hospital Publishing, 1989.

Arnwine, Don. "Buyers Are Smarter, Looking for Quality." *Modern Healthcare* 17, no. 5 (February 1987): 32.

Boscarino, Joseph A. "Measuring the Impact of Negative Publicity and Repairing the Damage." *Health Care Strategic Management* 6, no. 10 (October 1988a): 10–11.

———. "Predicting Drug Abuse from Social Demographic Factors: A Discriminant Function Approach." *Addictive Behaviors* 6, no. 2 (1981): 177–82.

———. "The Public's Rating of Hospitals." *Hospital & Health Services Administration* 33, no. 2 (Summer 1988b): 189–99.

———. "Speaking Up for Nurses: Concerted Political Action Garners Some Relief for Personnel Shortage." *Health Progress* 70, no. 4 (May 1989): 64–67.

Boscarino, Joseph A., and Steven R. Steiber. "Hospital Shopping and Consumer Choice." *Journal of Health Care Marketing* 2, no. 2 (Spring 1982): 15–23.

Bradburn, Norman M., and Seymour Sudman. *Polls and Surveys: Understanding What They Tell Us.* San Francisco: Jossey-Bass Publishers, 1988.

CACI. *The Sourcebook of Demographics and Buying Power for Every Zip Code in the USA.* Arlington, VA: CACI Publications, 1986.

Campbell, Donald T., and Julian C. Stanley. *Experimental and Quasi-Experimental Designs for Research.* Chicago: Rand McNally Publishing, 1963.

Centers for Disease Control. "Health Status of Vietnam Veterans." *Journal of the American Medical Association* 259, no. 18 (May 1988): 2701–19.

Center for Study of Services. *Consumers' Guide to Hospitals.* Washington, DC: The Center, 1988.

Cleary, Paul D., and Barbara J. McNeil. "Patient Satisfaction as an Indicator of Quality." *Inquiry* 25, no. 1 (Spring 1988): 25–36.

Cohen, Jacob, and Patricia Cohen. *Applied Multiple Regression/Correlation Analysis for the Behavioral Sciences,* 2d ed. Hillsdale, NJ: Lawrence Erlbaum Associates, 1983.

Cooley, William W., and Paul R. Lohnes. *Multivariate Data Analysis.* New York: John Wiley & Sons, 1971.

Davies, Allyson Ross, and John E. Ware, Jr. "Involving Consumers in Quality of Care Assessment." *Health Affairs* 7, no. 1 (Spring 1988): 33–48.

Fisk, Trevor A., Carmhiel J. Brown, Kathleen Cannizzaro, and Barbara Naftal. "Creating Patient Satisfaction and Loyalty." *Journal of Health Care Marketing* 10, no. 2 (June 1990): 5–15.

Fowler, Floyd J., Jr., ed. *Health Survey Research Methods. Proceedings of the 5th Conference on Health Survey Methods*. Washington, DC: National Center of Health Services Research, U.S. Government Printing Office, 1989.

Fowler, Floyd J., Jr. *Survey Research Methods,* rev. ed. Newbury Park, CA: Sage Publications, 1988.

Frank, Jerome D. *Persuasion and Healing.* New York: Schocken Books, 1974.

Frey, James H. *Survey Research by Telephone,* 2d ed. Newbury Park, CA: Sage Publications, 1989.

Gallagher, Jack. "Invalid Patient Surveys: Not a Bargain at Any Price." *Journal of Health Care Marketing* 9, no. 1 (March 1989): 69–71.

Graham, Judith. "Quality Gets a Closer Look." *Modern Healthcare* 17, no. 5 (February 1987): 20–31.

Gregory, Douglas D. "Building on Your Hospital's Competitive Image." *Trustee* 39, no. 3 (March 1986): 16–19.

Gross, Paul A., and William A. Schaffer. "Consumer Awareness of Hospital Mortality Data." *Journal of Health Care Marketing* 9, no. 4 (December 1989): 52–55.

Hays, Michael D. "Consumers Base Quality Perceptions on Patient Relations, Staff Qualifications." *Modern Healthcare* 17, no. 5 (February 1987): 33.

Health Care Financing Administration. "Medicare Program; Changes to the Inpatient Hospital Prospective Payment System and Fiscal Year 1987 Rates." *Federal Register* 51, no. 170 (3 September 1986): 31454–603.

Inguanzo, Joe, and Mark Harju. "Consumer Satisfaction with Hospitalization." *Hospitals* 59, no. 9 (May 1985): 81–83.

Javalgi, Rajshekhar G., S. R. Rao, and Edward G. Thomas. "Choosing a Hospital: Analysis of Consumer Tradeoffs." *Journal of Health Care Marketing* 11, no. 1 (March 1991): 12–22.

Jensen, Joyce. "Choosing a Hospital." *American Demographics* 9, no. 6 (June 1987): 45–47.

Lanning, Joyce A., and Stephen J. O'Connor. "The Health Care Quality Quagmire: Some Signposts." *Hospital & Health Services Administration* 35, no. 1 (Spring 1990): 39–54.

Lane, Paul M., and Jay D. Lindquist. "Hospital Choice: A Summary of the Key Empirical and Hypothetical Findings of the 1980s." *Journal of Health Care Marketing* 8, no. 4 (December 1988): 5–20.

Ley, Philip. *Quantitative Aspects of Psychological Assessment.* New York: Harper & Row Publishers, 1973.

Lohr, Kathleen N., Karl D. Yordy, and Samuel O. Thier. "Current Issues in Quality Care." *Health Affairs* 7, no. 1 (Spring 1988): 5–18.

MacStravic, Robin Scott. "Outcome Marketing in Health Care." *Health Care Management Review* 13, no. 2 (Spring 1988): 53–59.

Marks, Ronald B., and Jeff W. Totten. "The Effects of Mortality Cues on Consumers' Ratings of Hospital Attributes." *Journal of Health Care Marketing* 10, no. 3 (September 1990): 4–12.

Nelson, Eugene C., Ron D. Hays, Celia Larson, and Paul B. Batalden. "The Patient Judgment System: Reliability and Validity." *Quality Review Bulletin* 15, no. 6 (June 1989): 185–91.

Oppenheim, A. N. *Questionnaire Design and Attitude Measurement.* New York: Basic Books, 1966.

Robinson, Michele L. "Sneak Preview: JCAHO's Quality Indicators." *Hospitals* 62, no. 13 (July 1988): 38–43.

Salive, Marcel E., Jennifer A. Mayfield, and Norman W. Weissman. "Patient Outcome Research Teams and the Agency for Health Care Policy and Research." *Health Services Research* 25, no. 5 (December 1990): 697–708.

Smith, Scott M., and Marta Clark. "Hospital Image and the Positioning of Service Centers: An Application in Market Analysis and Strategy Development." *Journal of Health Care Marketing* 10, no. 3 (September 1990): 13–22.

Steiber, Steven R. "Making Use of Patient Survey Data." *Health Care Strategic Management* 7, no. 3 (March 1989): 12–14.

Steiber, Steven R., and Joseph A. Boscarino. "Hospital Marketing, the Concept Is Spreading." In *Health Care Marketing: Issues and Trends,* 2d ed., edited by Philip Cooper. Rockville, MD: Aspen Publications, 1985.

Steiber, Steven R., and William J. Krowinski. *Measuring and Managing Patient Satisfaction*. Chicago: American Hospital Publishing, 1990.

Stewart, Anita L., John E. Ware, Jr., Robert H. Brook, and Allyson Davies-Avery. *Conceptualization and Measurement of Health for Adults in the Health Insurance Study: Vol. II, Physical Health in Terms of Functioning*. Santa Monica, CA: The RAND Corporation, 1978.

Stewart, Anita L., Ron D. Hays, and John E. Ware, Jr. "The MOS Short-Form General Health Survey: Reliability and Validity in a Patient Population." *Medical Care* 26, no. 7 (July 1988): 724–35.

Stewart, Anita L., Sheldon Greenfield, Ron D. Hays, Kenneth Wells, William H. Rogers, Sandra D. Berry, Elizabeth A. McGlynn, and John E. Ware, Jr. "Functional Status and Well-Being of Patients with Chronic Conditions: Results from the Medical Outcomes Study." *Journal of the American Medical Association* 262, no. 7 (August 1989): 907–13.

Tarlov, Alvin R., John E. Ware, Jr., Sheldon Greenfield, Eugene C. Nelson, Edward Perrin, and Michael Zubkoff. "The Medical Outcomes Study: An Application of Methods for Monitoring the Results of Medical Care." *Journal of the American Medical Association* 262, no. 7 (August 1989): 925–30.

U.S. Congress. Office of Technology Assessment. *The Quality of Medical Care: Information for Consumers*. Washington, DC: U.S. Government Printing Office (OTA-H-386), June 1988.

Ware, John E., Jr., Mary K. Snyder, W. Russell Wright, and Allyson R. Davies. "Defining and Measuring Patient Satisfaction with Medical Care." *Evaluation and Program Planning* 6 (1983): 247–63.

Chapter 18

Outcomes Measurement in Hospitals: Can the System Change the Organization?

Jane C. Linder

Jane C. Linder is Assistant Professor, Harvard University, School of Business Administration, Boston, Massachusetts.

This article was published in *Hospital & Health Services Administration* 37, no. 2 (Summer 1992).

The U.S. health care industry is in crisis—a crisis of accountability (Relman 1988). The nation spends more than 12 percent of its gross national product on health care, and these costs show no sign of abating. Despite escalating costs, consumers and purchasers are increasingly concerned about the quality of medical care (Faltermayer 1988; Chambliss and Reier 1990). Our traditional control mechanisms—market forces, regulatory sanctions, and medical professionalism—have all been ineffective in guaranteeing high-quality, cost-effective health care. The state of the industry can be cynically described as "punitive, witch-hunting regulators vainly attempting to inspect an entrenched clan of autonomous peers who protect, but do not discipline each other in spite of delivering inadequate or inappropriate services to customers who cannot tell what they are getting for ever-increasing prices" (Linder 1991).

The problem has been characterized as a failure of information (Ginsburg and Hammons 1988; Arnould and DeBrock 1986; Iglehart 1988). Many believe that improved information, especially outcomes information, is at least part of the solution (Vladeck 1988; Wennberg 1988). With objective information about exactly how their performance compares with that of other professions, physicians could refine their norms of practice. Giving the same kind of information to those in authority positions—regulators, boards of trustees, and administrators—might enable them to manage clinical quality actively.

If this assessment is accurate, outcomes measurement would appear to offer a powerful opportunity to help change our dysfunctional health care delivery machinery into an effective infrastructure—one in which costs and quality are measured and continuously improved. This article examines the experiences of 31 hospitals that implemented MedisGroupsII®, the market-leading outcomes measurement system, to understand whether it had that effect. Data for this study were gathered during late 1989 and early 1990, and the MedisGroups system has been enhanced since that time. The study is intended to focus on management issues in executing organizational change rather than on the current state of the system's technical development.

The next section of the article describes the system and explains why it appears to have the potential to precipitate fundamental change. This is followed by an analysis of why hospitals did not, in fact, report that result.

MedisGroups: The Potential to Drive Change

MedisGroups is a clinical outcomes measurement system designed for the health care industry and used predominantly by hospitals. (Thomas and Longo (1990) present an excellent comparison of MedisGroups and the systems that compete directly with it.) The system helps a hospital assess the effectiveness of its medical care by measuring outcomes. When a patient enters the hospital, MedisGroups determines the disease state by classifying the severity of illness based on clinical instability leading to the risk of organ failure.[2] Cases are assigned a severity score of 0 to 4 by using key clinical findings—about 260 well-defined, objective clinical results obtained from diagnostic tests and physical examinations. Subjectively determined information such as diagnosis is not used to determine severity. MedisGroups also tracks medical services rendered and evaluates a patient's clinical instability after treatment. The system compares the results—both in patient health and charges—with a data base of similar procedures that has been accumulated from all MedisGroups users. This comparison indicates whether the rate of in-hospital mortality and morbidity are statistically different from the current, empirical MedisGroups norm for similar cases.

MedisGroups has flexible reporting capabilities but produces three standard reports for evaluating performance. *Appropriateness reports* focus on low severity and "no findings" cases that may have had treatments not actually required. *Efficiency reports* compare the hospital's procedures and charges to those of other hospitals and compare individual physicians' practice patterns. *Effectiveness reports* compare medical outcomes by disease to those achieved by other hospitals. (Lanning and O'Connor (1990) link these three types of assessment neatly into a comprehensive definition of health care quality.)

MedisGroups data is drawn from medical charts after patients have been discharged from the hospital. Before the charts are permanently stored in medical records files, they are abstracted by a trained reviewer, often a nurse. This individual selects information from the chart based on extremely specific criteria contained in the MedisGroups glossary. For example, a clinical finding is ignored if it is termed "possible," but taken into account if called "probable." A trained abstractor requires about 15 minutes to code an average chart. Abstractors are not allowed to submit data to the MedisGroups national data base until they have been certified as 95 percent accurate. After being certified, abstractors are periodically checked for compliance with the MedisGroups quality standards. (Iezzoni and Moskowitz (1988) provide an excellent description of the abstracting process.)

At the present time, MedisGroups is used by over 500 hospitals in the United States and Canada—more than any other clinical outcomes information system. Pennsylvania has mandated that all of its hospitals generate and report MedisGroups severity and clinical outcome data to the state's central health information commission. Iowa has adopted a similar regulation.

MedisGroups technology is well within the financial and information technology reach of most organizations,[3] and the implications for hospital care are potentially significant. MedisGroups purports to make measures of clinical effectiveness available for the first time. In the past, this kind of information has been fragmented and anecdotal when it has been available at all. Autonomous physicians have controlled clinical decision making without the benefit of comprehensive effectiveness metrics; separately, administrators have managed the fiscal health of the institution. Accurate, reliable outcomes measures should make it possible to assign and execute these responsibilities quite differently. For example, hospital leaders could use outcomes data to consider both the cost and effectiveness of alternative courses of treatment to make prudent clinical decisions. In theory, then, MedisGroups holds the potential to compel important changes in hospital practice that would translate into significant and durable improvements in performance.

Realistic Possibility or Flight of Fancy?

MedisGroups is only an information system. Is it likely to have a dramatic impact on the way hospitals deliver care? The answer to this question hinges on two others: Is the system functional, and if so, is that functionality influential? For the system to be functional, it must be usable and provide information that is accurate, reliable, and valid. Some evidence is available to indicate that MedisGroups meets this test. It is the market leader among severity-adjusted outcomes measurement systems, suggesting an acceptable level of usability. Independent research has shown that its severity measures correlate well with probability of death, although not as well with resource utilization (Iezzoni and Moskowitz 1988). Stringent data collection controls are in place to ensure that data accuracy remains high, both at the hospital level and for the national comparative data base. Finally, because MedisGroups relies primarily on objective clinical findings, its measures and results are relatively immune to the inconsistency and bias of diagnosis-dependent assessment. Some questions have been raised about the validity of MedisGroups data for widespread quality measurement (Iezzoni and Moskowitz 1988), but its use as a screening tool to suggest areas for potential quality improvement is well accepted.

MedisGroups appears to be functional; does that functionality compel change? We know that it is possible for an information system to be instrumental in organizational change (Barley 1986; Leonard-Barton 1988). Prior research has demonstrated clearly that information systems alone do not guarantee change (Kling 1980; Bariff and Galbraith, 1978). The innovative use of information technology does not create change unilaterally, but it appears to be a driving force in some cases (Linder 1989).

MedisGroups would seem to have the potential to compel changes in hospital practice because it enables performance to be measured in a way that was previously impossible. New information might cause procedures that had been accepted as the norm to be revealed as ineffective or inappropriate. Hospital leaders would be provided with objective evidence to instigate changes in practice patterns. However, their ability to use outcomes measurement in this way would depend on their ability to link outcomes with the processes of care that produce them (Vladeck 1988).

To play an influential role, MedisGroups must be adopted, implemented, and actually used (Mohr 1987; Rowe and Boise 1974). This presents a dilemma. A system that compels changes in the way processes work is, by definition, incompatible with existing practices. Yet, this incompatibility tends to inhibit the system's adoption (Rogers and Shoemaker 1971) and threatens implementation (Keen 1981; Bariff and Galbraith 1978). In other words, systems that are likely to be implemented are unlikely to change the way business is conducted, and vice versa.

The system's ability to compel changes in practice, then, depends on whether hospital leaders can accomplish a difficult implementation. (For our purposes, we will define implementation as the ability of the organization to reach the point at which the system is used for a desired purpose.) Several factors are known to be important contributors to success. The involvement of a powerful, respected leader is critical in giving revolutionary change enough momentum to overcome naysayers (Nord and Tucker 1987; Nutt 1986). If this kind of support is not forthcoming, information technology is more likely to be molded to the organization rather than the other way around (Kling 1980; Leifer 1988). Effective leaders sustain their involvement long enough for the change to take a life of its own: the organization becomes convinced that the system's benefits outweigh the financial, political, and attentional costs of change (Rogers and Shoemaker 1971; Markus 1981, 1983; Keen and Gerson 1977; Robey 1987).

While Damanpour and Evan (1984) found that low-technology libraries were likely to undertake administrative innovations before associated technical ones, they argue that effective high-technology firms such as hospitals would reverse this order. They advise a hospital to begin organizational innovation with the technology, then allow the organizational adjustments to follow.

Leonard-Barton (1988) finds that "wringing value" out of innovations also entails managing a process of mutual adaptation between the technology and the organization—of incrementally resolving misalignments between business practices and technology features. This is a kind of give and take in which both the system and the organization adjust over time in a series of adaptive cycles. These vary in disruption, depending on the magnitude of the changes to be made.

Based on prior research, then, we would expect MedisGroups to be influential in changing hospital practices and improving performance if it is championed by powerful hospital leaders who create a perception of its benefits, install the system technically, then help to organize through a process of mutual adaptation to exploit the value of the innovation.

Methodology

To understand how hospitals implement, use, and benefit from MedisGroups, I conducted 103 interviews with 31 MedisGroups users during late 1989 and early 1990. (Nine other hospitals were contacted, but declined to participate.[4]) The hospitals represented a cross-section of MedisGroups users in terms of geography, teaching affiliation, size, and system experience. Each participating hospital had leased the system for at least one year, and the average term of use was more than three years.

In each hospital, I asked to speak with at least three members of the organization involved with outcomes measurement: the quality assurance director, a physician involved in quality management, and a senior executive responsible for outcomes information. Nineteen of 31 participating hospitals agreed to all of these interviews, and I was also able to interview a member of the board of trustees and the information systems manager in several cases. One subsequently became the subject of a case study on total quality management. My access in the remaining hospitals was more limited. Additionally, I interviewed the management of the software vendor, Mediqual Systems, Inc., to get an understanding of the product itself.

The interviews were tape-recorded, resulting in more than 3,000 pages of transcript, which were content-analyzed. These self-report data are subject to the usual caveats about bias; however, they are qualitatively richer than survey information and, I argue, appropriate for an exploratory study such as this one. One-third of the hospitals were willing to share organization charts and recent financial results with me. I used published Health Care Financing Administration statistics for demographic information about the participating hospitals. Table 1 shows that the participating hospitals ranged from small community institutions to large teaching hospitals. They were located in all regions of the country, although more concentrated in the New England and Middle Atlantic states.

Findings: Little Evidence of Change

Despite its potential, the MedisGroups system failed to *compel* important changes in hospital practices that led to performance improvements. Only four hospitals of 31 agreed that the quality of care they delivered had improved as a direct result of using the system. The remainder believed that medical

Table 1
Descriptive Statistics about the Participating Hospitals

	n	Average	Median	Minimum	Maximum
Teaching programs	31	38.7%			
Number of beds	31	434.7	433	116	815
Active M.D.'s per bed	31	.72	.68	.28	1.59
Percent Medicare admissions	23	44.1	45	18	65
1989 capacity utilization	28	73	75	45	92
1988 capacity utilization	28	73	74.5	49	87
Operating profit/revenue	21	.022	.026	−.174	.119
Months on the system	32	38	36	12	78
Number of interviews	32	3.4	3	1	7
Geographic region					
Northeast	8				
Middle Atlantic	5				
Southeast	2				
Central	9				
Midwest	5				
West	3				

quality had not changed or that outcomes measurement was not responsible for changes they had seen. Although more than one-half agreed that the system had helped them cut resource utilization, they claimed they did not achieve this result through changed practices, but through administrative cost-cutting—business as usual. These hospitals received enough benefits to convince most of them to continue to pay an average of $100,000 per year to lease the software and staff the organization; the impact simply was not transforming. The most common view was consistent with this administrator's statement: "We cannot demonstrate any quality improvements from outcomes measurement. Some things may have changed, but they have no relationship to the system."

These results can be explained in terms of three management issues: intention to change, implementation difficulties, and the ability to capture value from the system. The following three sections describe these issues. Figure 1 arrays the hospitals by these management issues, and the appendix defines the variables that are used in this analysis and describes how they were coded.

Intention to Change

Twelve hospitals (37.5 percent) reported no significant organizational changes after implementing MedisGroups because they did not intend such change to occur. Their reasons for purchasing the system and the ways they intended to use it were qualitatively different from those of the other institutions. They

Figure 1
Did the Information System Compel Change?

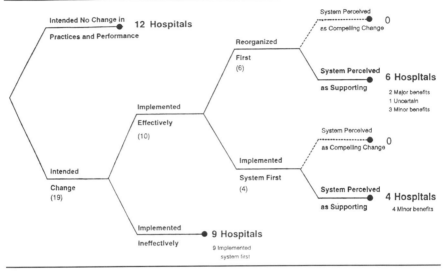

implemented the system as a technical tool but disavowed its organizational potential. These hospitals might be called "pseudo-adopters."

Why did these hospitals install MedisGroups if not to help change their practices, drive performance improvements, or alter their competitive positions, as other institutions reported? Their reasons fell into three categories. Four hospitals intended the system to automate their existing information flows. The director of medical affairs from one said, "We looked for a program that did exactly what we were attempting to do manually. We decided Medis-Groups was the best fit, and we could introduce it without disrupting the medical staff organization as it existed." None of these hospitals used the system to hold medical professionals accountable for their quality or resource utilization. Instead, the system was used to mechanize existing quality assurance functions. In this way, a potential innovation was converted to a safe, ordinary investment.

Four institutions installed the system explicitly to protect themselves from the demands of external constituents. They implemented the system to manage the *image* of quality and effectiveness they presented to their customers and to the regulators who inspected them. MedisGroups reports were used as evidence that 100 percent of hospital admissions were screened for quality problems, as required by the Joint Commission on the Accreditation of Health

Care Organizations (JCAHO). As one medical director remarked, "When we implemented the system, quality was good. We just wanted to be able to show that to people."

The other four hospitals in this category were forced to implement the system by legislative mandate in their state. This use of MedisGroups was an especially ineffective mechanism for encouraging hospitals to change their internal practices. Mandated hospitals kept the system in an organizational closet and managed it for damage control. Its information was not used within the hospital. Administrators tended the system merely to make sure it was coded optimally and accurately.[5] One hospital's chief operating officer said, "How do we use it today? It's an overhead expense. We send in our monthly report [to the state]. When it comes to determining quality of care, it is of no value."

Clearly, introducing MedisGroups did not necessitate change. Despite the system's potential for measuring clinical effectiveness and encouraging professional accountability, it did not, in and of itself, require hospitals to adopt new attitudes or behaviors. This finding corroborates prior research that information systems do not deterministically compel change.

Table 2 compares the hospitals that stated they intended to change the way they delivered care with those that did not. The two groups of hospitals are largely indistinguishable. Hospitals that intended no change have, on average, fewer active physician's per hospital bed. This is not a particularly strong result, however, as it is significant at only the .09 level, but it could indicate that this group of institutions is less specialist-oriented. Pseudo-adopters also tended to have installed the system more recently than their opposite numbers, but when the hospitals that implemented the system because of regulatory mandates are excluded, this distinction disappears.

Implementation Difficulties

Nineteen hospitals (61 percent of 31 study participants) adopted MedisGroups in conjunction with an initiative to make significant changes in their operations and performance. As predicted, implementation was a much more difficult experience for these hospitals than for those that intended no organizational change. Table 3, Panel A, shows that hospitals that intended organizational change were significantly more likely to fail at implementation, defined as achieving system use for a desired purpose.

The two groups described the process of implementation quite differently. Pseudo-adopters complained of technical and resource issues such as coder turnover and the availability of funds for hardware upgrades. These were temporary set-backs that were handled by middle management. Physicians

Table 2
Hospitals That Intended Change Compared to Those That Did Not

	n	Intended Change	Intended No Change	Significance
Proportion with teaching programs*	31	33.3%	50.0%	.3993
Average number of beds*†	31	436.9	430.4	.9400
Active physicians/bed*†	31	.7932	.5702	.0899
Profits/revenues*	20	.0312	.0092	.4276
Percent Medicare admissions*	23	42.8%	46.6%	.5196
1989 capacity utilization*	28	73.4%	72.3%	.8402
1988 capacity utilization†	28	74.8%	69.6%	.1295
Percent of physicians board-certified†	28	77.7%	77.5%	.9600
Average months since system adoption*	31	42.2	27.6	.0597
Average months from adoption to first system output*	22	19.1	11.6	.3188

*Interview data.
†Health Care Finance Administration data.

and administrators in change-intending hospitals, on the other hand, described intense resistance, political battles over who would control the data, and the requirement for board-level involvement in the effort. Three kinds of implementation problems plagued these projects: hospitals experienced difficulty in establishing the system's credibility, in managing project momentum, and in structuring the system's use.

Establishing System Credibility

Attacks on the system's validity, especially by physicians, inhibited its acceptance. MedisGroups' severity scoring algorithm had been kept proprietary to protect it from being copied by competitors. Because physicians were unable to examine and verify the system's logic, they had difficulty accepting its results. Even nonresistant users reflected this discomfort. Additionally, MedisGroups' rigid data-gathering rules that enabled cross-hospital comparisons and kept the system objective forced important, subjective information to be ignored. For example, abstractors were instructed to accept findings described as "probable" and ignore those termed "possible." Physicians frequently disagreed with a case's assigned severity score, which they had no ability to change. Inevitable coding errors exacerbated this issue and threatened the system's credibility.

Table 3
Hospital Characteristics and Implementation Effectiveness

Panel A		Effective Implementation		Ineffective Implementation
Hospitals that intended organizational change associated with system implementation		10 (52.6%)		9 (47.4%)
Hospitals that intended no organizational change		11 (91.7%)		1 (8.3%)
	Chi-square with yates	5.1285	significance	.0254
	correction	3.4977	significance	.0615
	Kendall's Tau B	− .4067	significance	.0259

Panel B		Effective Implementation		Ineffective Implementation
Hospitals that reorganized before implementing the system		7 (100%)		0 (0%)
Hospitals that implemented the system first		4 (30.8%)		9 (69.2%)
	Chi-square with Yates	8.8112	significance	.0030
	correction	6.2360	significance	.0125
	Kendall's Tau B	.6638	significance	.0038

For some hospitals, the way work was structured helped create invalid results. If critical hospital tests were performed on an outpatient basis, the results would not be taken into account in computing a patient's admission severity. These cases would then be reported as having unnecessary or inappropriate medical treatment. Even though a careful analyst would review patient records before drawing conclusions from the system's reports, physicians were enraged that the data could be so potentially misleading. They were concerned that the computer reports would outlast the detailed explanations.

Sustaining Project Momentum

Hospital leaders had difficulty maintaining their interest and commitment throughout the process of implementation. They were frustrated: "It took a long time to get started." This is at least partially due to the nature of the system. Data entry clerks had to be hired, trained, and certified as reliable. The ideal candidates for these jobs were familiar with medical terminology but willing to set aside their own judgment to follow the system's rules explicitly.

Because the system was designed to provide a rigorous, integrated information infrastructure for performance management, it required six to nine months of concerted data entry before the first statistically valid report could be produced.[6]

Many hospitals experienced problems that delayed their first useful outputs even further. For example, one hospital's medical records and quality assurance departments held an internecine war over who would be responsible for abstracting. Other institutions complained of turnover among quality assurance personnel and the press of JCAHO surveys that detracted from their MedisGroups efforts. On average, 17 months elapsed between the time the system contract was signed and information was available for analysis. By this time, initial excitement surrounding the system had faded, sponsors and champions had often moved to other jobs, and the project foundered for lack of interest. One physician commented:

> You don't learn anything in a year except how to go about the process. You certainly don't have any answers. All the initial excitement has died down because nothing seem to be happening. It's hard to maintain the momentum and the level of energy required. The frustratingly slow progress is one reason that the chair of our Medis-Groups committee just quit.

Resistance stalled progress and stretched the time required to implement the system and demonstrate its benefits. When the system was viewed as part of an organizational-change initiative, threatened physicians and administrators recited a litany of "logical" reasons for avoiding adoption. As one doctor said, "The data is suspect because we don't really want to have a quality assurance system, so if we can show it's bad data, we're done with it."

The regulatory environment increased the stakes in this issue because the system reported on the performance of individual physicians. One quality assurance director noted, "Our doctors have a constant fear that the data will be misused. They are paranoid about even members of our own in-house staff having information about them. They don't want these data to exist."

This concern can be explained partially as the threat of accountability. Professionals who have never been subject to performance measurement might well fear scrutiny. However, the regulatory environment of medical care gives physicians some basis for their paranoia. Information that is used for quality assurance is theoretically immune from legal discovery in a malpractice claim. MedisGroups information was secure, but only if handled confidentially[7] *and* if its immunity remained intact in spite of lawyers' efforts to circumvent the protective regulations.

Sustained resistance, either in active or passive form, delayed the system's implementation and inhibited its use. MedisGroups did not gain the credibility of an accepted performance measurement system with predictable consequences. It continued to absorb the time and energy of a nucleus of committed champions even though its benefits materialized slowly at best. Sooner or later, many tired of the struggle. As one administrator said, "It never gained a life of its own; it never became impersonal."

Structuring System Use

As a measurement system, MedisGroups did not impose a structure of use; management had to design and build this. The point at which output first appeared—when interest was often at low ebb—was the time when this structure had to be established. The system's extensive capabilities provided so much latitude to its users that many could not overlay an adequate order on it.

MedisGroups did not come with packaged prescriptions about what reports should be produced, who should see them, how they should be interpreted, or how their results should be linked to processes of care.[8] An enormous amount of information was available without guidelines for action.

For the system to be beneficial, dedicated analysts had to invest time in the system to understand its content, to explore its results, and to draw valid, useful inferences about clinical practice. These analysts required different skills from the data collection organization previously described. The former succeeded by drawing innovative insights from complex statistics; the latter by processing mountains of data with rote, machinelike consistency. Yet, most hospitals asked their quality assurance staffs to do both jobs. One administrator explained:

> The people who want one-page, presynthesized management reports are naive. Evaluating medical care is a complicated process and hard, analytical work. There are not many quality assurance staffs in hospitals today who are qualified to do what we are asking them to do. You need operations research people with a background in organizational theory.

The task of educating physicians and administrators to interpret and use the information was difficult even when they were willing to attend to it. One medical director explained, "We assumed that once we had the data, it would be usable. We collected data for nine months to get to that point, but when we looked at the reports, we discovered they had little meaning. We had not spent time educating ourselves about how to interpret or use the data. It's like learning a foreign language."

311

Hospitals could not rely on assumptions embedded in the system to establish quality measurement. As one administrator explained, "We made the questionable assumption that the system would provide a structure for our quality assurance activities." Instead, they had to make deliberate management decisions about how MedisGroups information would be used in their organizations. This proved to be beyond the capabilities of many hospitals. Without this structure of use, the benefits of outcomes measurement were elusive. As one cynical quality assurance director who described herself "the captain of the Titanic" remarked, "I read the [MedisGroups] reports for entertainment; I can't do anything else with them."

The results were unsatisfactory for many institutions. Some hospitals searched for a less expensive means for severity scoring that would match their costs more appropriately to their perceived benefits. Others continued gathering data in spite of partial or minimal interest in the output. For many hospitals, the system remained operational in that netherworld of half-done initiatives that are too embarrassing to stop and too threatening to push to conclusion.

Achieving Effective Implementation

Ten (52 percent of 19 change-seeking) hospitals were able to implement Medis-Groups effectively in spite of these challenges—that is, they reached a point at which the system was actually used for a desired purpose. Effective implementers captured data, produced reports, evaluated results, and took appropriate action. In contrast, ineffective implementers said things such as, "We can't get our doctors to look at the reports," "We have no ability to discern meaning from the data," and "Our system is on the back burner."

Effective implementers achieved system use through three primary mechanisms. They *changed the organization structure* before implementing the system and found powerful, respected system advocates who helped create a *perception of a proximate threat or opportunity* that the system could address, and they used *staged implementation* to manage project momentum.

Restructure the Organization

Six of the ten effective implementers (60 percent) restructured their organizations before installing MedisGroups. In contrast, all nine of the institutions that implemented ineffectively had installed the system before making changes in the organizational structure. This finding runs directly counter to Damanpour and Evan's (1984) hypothesis that the technical aspects of innovation should precede the administrative ones in a high-technology organization. (Table 3, Panel B, shows the relationship between this organizational structure choice and implementation effectiveness.)

Six effective implementers formally allocated responsibility for an aggressive quality initiative to senior members of the hospital leadership. In five out of six cases, these moves entailed asking physicians to take authority for both administrative and clinical aspects of quality management. They chose MedisGroups as one of the tools they would use to execute their new agenda. As a result, the system had a credible owner, a defined role in the hospital's agenda, and benefits it was intended to achieve. One administrator remarked, "MedisGroups is revolutionary. To keep the system above water until we do the necessary (organizational) redesign requires energy, and more importantly, authority." Effective implementers found a way to bring this kind of authority to bear.

When hospitals failed to make structural changes before implementing MedisGroups, the effort was more likely to languish. Thirteen hospitals made no structural changes before implementing the system; only four of these (31 percent) succeeded in implementation. While these four did not assign formal, structural responsibility for the quality initiative, they were able to secure well-placed, influential advocates for the system. Whether through formal structure or informal advocacy, effective implementers found system champions. These individuals were boundary-spanners, bridging departments and specialties within the hospital. They were tough and relentless in their pursuit of quality and in their insistence on measurement. Through their backgrounds, relationships, or personal styles, they crossed factional barriers and enabled the hospital to move beyond parochial disputes.

The MedisGroups champions at hospitals that had effective implementation remained in leadership positions throughout the implementation process. The opposite was true for ineffective implementers. Ineffective implementers placed responsibility for MedisGroups well down in the organizations, either from the start or as a result of having lost advocacy.[9] When these hospitals did identify influential MedisGroups champions, these individuals left the hospital, rotated out of contact, or lost interest in the system before the implementation process was complete. Consequently, the system was ignored by hospital leaders and never achieved acceptance and use.

These findings support prior research that demonstrates the importance of a persistent champion in change-making projects (Nord and Tucker 1987; Tichy and Devanna 1986). They also suggest that formally allocating responsibility to that individual through organizational structure changes improves the probability of sustained leadership.

Perceived Threat or Opportunity

Effective implementers created a perception of a significant, visible threat or opportunity and positioned the system as an important part of the hospital's response. One hospital had a "bad actor" to deal with—a physician who practiced in a way that endangered patients. Another hospital was working toward earning an award for total quality management. A third built the belief that the hospital had to make significant changes to deal with prospective payment. A fourth was criticized on the evening news for its high costs. Each of these change-triggers was ambiguous enough to give hospital leadership latitude in deciding how to address it, but compelling enough to stimulate progress.

The mandated installation of MedisGroups did not have the same positive impact as these internally acknowledged threats and opportunities. Each of the four hospitals that implemented MedisGroups in response to a state mandate saw it as oppressive rather than beneficial. This perception inhibited their ability to exploit its potential. As a chief operating officer said, "One of our administrators tried to champion the system, but he couldn't maintain the facade that it was good for us." A medical director commented, "Mandating the system removes your commitment to understand how it works and, therefore, your ability to use it."

Staged Implementation

Effective implementers used a staged approach for putting the system in place. They did not try to implement MedisGroups for an entire hospital, but started with more limited objectives. Most began with a particular specialty or set of diagnosis-related groups (DRGs), others with a targeted study of a particular quality problem in the hospital. This enabled them to focus the system's use and demonstrate its benefits explicitly. It also gave them an opportunity to begin to design the ways the system would be used. Staged implementation did not completely counterweigh the long, resource-intensive infrastructure building effort that MedisGroups use demanded, but it did help generate a series of benefits and small successes that system advocates could use to create momentum.

System Impact

Despite achieving system use, the ten effective implementers did not characterize MedisGroups as the change lever postulated at the beginning of this article. These hospitals fell into two groups: two enthusiastic advocates for the system's use as a supporting tool in achieving their strategic aims, and eight that found little value in the system's output (plus one hospital that had high expectations but could not yet assess the system's impact).

In the first group, hospitals extolled the virtues of MedisGroups and, in fact, contradicted some of the criticisms expressed by other institutions. For example, one CEO remarked that MedisGroups was *the* structure for his retrospective quality assurance program. Another claimed that the information system had reached the point where it was an impersonal substitute for hierarchical authority to increase control over physician behavior. However, both of these hospitals emphasized that major structural changes in their quality management programs were made *before* implementing MedisGroups. MedisGroups was seen as a necessary supporting player, but not a change-driver.

After having faced and overcome the implementation issues described above, the eight remaining hospitals (four that reorganized before adopting MedisGroups and four that implemented the system first) found the system's output unsurprising. One medical director said, "It took lots of resources and told us nothing new." Another explained, "Our results were all good. There was no point to it." Others claimed benefits in improving documentation of good care rather than the quality of care itself. The self-reported impact of Medis-Groups on quality was statistically indistinguishable for the effective imple-menters that intended to change and those that sought significant operating improvements.[10]

What accounts for the difference between low-impact and enthusiastic users? Low-impact hospital managers disagreed fundamentally with enthusi-astic users about the system's flexibility. A hospital administrator who claimed the system offered little benefit stated, "MedisGroups is a very canned, rigid standardized product. Maybe it has to be to be valid." An administrator with a similar view cut back on system use before discovering that it was flexible enough to be integrated with the hospital's cost accounting system. In con-trast, an enthusiastic user remarked, "The most critical element of Medis-Groups is that it can evolve. It is structured so that it can improve as we learn." Enthusiastic users continued the adaptive process—adjusting both the organ-ization and the technology to capture additional value—long after low impact users lost interest.

The intricate organizational machinery required to make the system work may well have presented a barrier to learning. To get the system functioning, with its trained data analysts, reporting structures and data flows, security measures, and linkages with quality assurance and utilization review func-tions, the hospital had to construct a tightly managed, fairly mechanistic MedisGroups unit around the system. While this was necessary to implement the system, it tended to freeze the hospital's perception of what the system was and how it could be used. In other words, the burden of building a reliable, consistent data-gathering infrastructure may have inhibited adaptation; yet the system's deep benefits were gained only through continuing, postimple-mentation learning. For example, one enthusiastic MedisGroups user had added employer data to the system and was beginning to feed health care quality information back to benefits officers. This hospital's stated intent was to use this service to create a customer preference for the institution.

A second, counterintuitive explanation for the unspectacular impact of MedisGroups was offered by a hospital administrator. He had the advantage of having managed the system's implementation in two independent hospitals. About the first, he said, "Because quality assurance was considered irrelevant, putting this system in was not threatening to the physicians. As a result, we did not get the resistance we should have gotten for a system of this sort. We didn't fight out the issues, and we didn't learn. Maybe if we had, we would have been able to exploit the system more fully." The physicians in the second were threatened by the system and, as a result, became involved in understanding the content and use of MedisGroups information. Through the process of resistance—questioning and arguing about what the information meant and how it would be used—they were converted from adversaries to advocates. This interesting example suggests that both too little and too much resistance impede change-making information systems. Too much resistance hobbles implementation, too little hobbles the learning that enables the organization to adapt continuously. This is consistent with Keen's (1981) advice to systems developers that they "seek out resistance and treat it as a signal to be responded to."

Both explanations for MedisGroups' modest impact revolve around foreshortened organizational learning. While low-impact hospitals achieved system use, they did not describe the continuing process of adaptation that Leonard-Barton (1988) suggests is necessary for innovations to be institutionalized and exploited.

Conclusions

Despite its apparent potential to compel important changes in hospital performance, MedisGroups failed to fulfill this role. This result reminds us that information technology is not deterministic. It does not structure an organization's behavior without the interest, initiative, and involvement of at least some influential members of the group. Organizational choice—taking responsibility for the decision to change—is an absolutely critical element in achieving results.

This research also points out that implementing change-oriented systems is risky and focuses our attention on the factors that contribute to success. Hospitals implemented the system effectively through sustained leadership by respected advocates who applied their energy and authority to three implementation challenges. They established the system's credibility, and therefore its promise of benefits. They managed the project's momentum to build the perception that benefits were realistic and achievable. And they structured the organization's use of the system to attempt to bridge the gap between information potential and behavioral change. In contrast to Damanpour and Evan's (1984) hypothesis, hospitals did not succeed by implementing the technical aspects of the system first, then allowing organizational adjustments to follow. The opposite was true.

If the MedisGroups experience holds true for other innovative measurement systems, managers are advised to implement by changing organizational structure first, then use the information system to support the new dynamic. They should pay particular attention to the process of mutual adaptation. When it is foreshortened, the organization does not capture full value from system. Rather than something to be avoided or overcome, a certain amount of resistance to change appears to improve the organization's ability to master and benefit from the system.

For the health care industry, the conclusion is basic. MedisGroups may help hospitals attack the "information problem" that stands in the way of effective delivery of care. However, it is neither a quick solution nor a panacea, and the technology certainly does not substitute for responsible, imaginative leadership that is required to make important improvements in hospital performance.

Acknowledgments

My thanks to Amar Bhide, Dorothy Leonard-Barton, Nancy Balaguer, Robert Eccles, James Cash, and four anonymous reviewers for their insightful comments on earlier drafts of the article, and to the Division of Research at Harvard Business School for financial support.

Notes

1.   This article was written with the cooperation of MediQual Systems, Inc., but its conclusions are solely those of the author.

2.   Clinical instability is the likelihood of poor and/or deteriorating health.

3.   The annual costs for labor and the software license vary with hospital admissions. For the group of hospitals in this study, it averaged $100,000. The software is a package that runs on an IBM or compatible personal computer.

4.   The hospitals that declined to participate were no different than the study participants in average size, capacity utilization, proportion that were teaching institutions, percentage of physicians who were board certified, and mortality rates for common diseases as reported by the Health Care Finance Administration.

5.   Where coding choices existed, the hospital wanted to make sure it made the choice that served its own interest.

6.   The system had to accumulate enough cases for each category of disease (diagnosis-related group) to have a statistically meaningful sample.

7.   For MedisGroups information to be legally undiscoverable, it must never be left in an in-basket or on a desk in anything but an envelope marked "Confidential." It must be filed in locked cabinets or stored in a room that itself has controlled access.

8.   Pennsylvania's Health Care Cost Containment Council prescribed the data that had to be submitted to the state and decided how that data would be represented and reported to the public. It did not dictate how hospitals should use MedisGroups information internally.

9.   Depending on strategy, some hospitals considered clinicians most influential, others saw management as dominant, and a third group had struck a collaborative balance. In an administratively oriented hospital, a system with clinical ownership would be poorly positioned in the organization, and vice versa.

10.   With impact of MedisGroups on hospital quality coded as minor or major, the chi-square statistic was .8914, significant at the .3451 level.

References

Arnould, R. J., and L. M. DeBrock. "Competition and Market Failure in the Hospital Industry: A Review of the Evidence." *Medical Care Review* 43, no. 2 (1986): 253–92.

Bariff, Martin, and Jay Galbraith. "Interorganizational Power Considerations for Designing Information Systems." *Accounting Organizations and Society* 3, no. 1 (1978): 15–27.

Barley, Stephen. "Technology as an Occasion for Structuring: Evidence from Observations of CT Scanners and the Social Order of Radiology Departments." *Administrative Science Quarterly* 31 (1986): 78–108.

Chambliss, L., and S. Reier. "How Doctors Have Ruined Health Care." *Financial World* (9 January 1990): 46–52.

Damanpour, Farborz, and William M. Evan. "Organizational Innovation and Performance: The Problem of 'Organizational Lag.'" *Administrative Science Quarterly* 29 (1984): 392–409.

Faltermayer, E. "Medical Care's Next Revolution." *Fortune* (10 October 1988): 126–33.

Ginsburg, P. B., and G. T. Hammons. "Competition and the Quality of Care: The Importance of Information." *Inquiry* 25 (Spring 1988): 108–15.

Iezzoni, Lisa I., and Mark A. Moskowitz. "A Clinical Assessment of MedisGroups." *Journal of the American Medical Association* 260, no. 1 (2 December 1988): 3159–63.

Iezzoni, Lisa I., Mark A. Moskowitz, and A. S. Ash. "The Ability of MedisGroups and Its Clinical Variables to Predict Cost and In-Hospital Death." Boston, MA: Research Report of the Health Care Research Unit, Section of General Internal Medicine, University Hospital, Boston University School of Medicine, 1 July 1988.

Iglehart, J. K. "Competition and the Pursuit of Quality: A Conversation with Walter McClure." *Health Affairs* (Spring 1988): 79–90.

Keen, Peter N. "Information Systems and Organizational Change." *Communications of the ACM* 24, no. 1 (January 1981): 24–33.

Keen, Peter, and Elihu Gerson. "The Politics of Software Systems Design." *Datamation* (November 1977): 80–84.

Kling, Robert. "Social Analyses of Computing: Theoretical Perspectives in Recent Empirical Research." *Computing Surveys* 12, no. 1 (March 1980): 61–110.

Lanning, Joyce A., and Stephen J. O'Connor. "The Health Care Quality Quagmire: Some Signposts." *Hospital & Health Services Administration* 35, no. 1 (Spring 1990): 39–54.

Leifer, R. "Matching Computer-Based Information Systems with Organizational Structures." *MIS Quarterly* 12, no. 1 (March 1988): 63–73.

Leonard-Barton, Dorothy. "Implementation as Mutual Adaptation of Technology and Organization." *Research Policy* 17 (1988): 251–67.

Linder, Jane. "Integrating Organizations Where Information Technology Matters." D.B.A. thesis. Boston: Harvard Business School, 1989.

———. "Outcomes Measurement: Compliance Tool or Strategic Initiative." *Health Care Management Review* 16, no. 4 (Fall 1991): 21–31.

Markus, M. Lynne. "Implementation Politics: Top Management Support and User Involvement." *Systems, Objectives, Solutions* 1 (1981): 203–15.

———. "Power, Politics, and MIS Implementation." *Communication of the ACM* 26, no. 6 (June 1983): 430–44.

Mohr, Lawrence. "Innovation Theory and New Technology." In *New Technology as Organizational Innovation*, edited by J. Pennings and A. Buitendam. Cambridge, MA: Ballinger Publishing Company, 1987.

Nord, Walker, and Sharon Tucker. *Implementing Routine and Radical Innovations.* Lexington, MA: Lexington Books, 1987.

Nutt, Paul. "Tactics of Implementation." *Academy of Management Journal* 29, no. 2 (1986): 230–61.

Relman, Arnold. "Assessment and Accountability: The Third Revolution in Medical Care." *New England Journal of Medicine* 319, no. 18 (3 November 1988): 1220–22.

Robey, Daniel. "Implementing and Organizational Impacts of Information Systems." *Interfaces* 17, no. 3 (May–June 1987): 72–84.

319

Rogers, Everett, and F. Shoemaker. *Communication of Innovations: A Cross-Cultural Approach.* New York: The Free Press, 1971.

Rowe, Lloyd A., and William B. Boise. "Organizational Innovation: Current Research and Evolving Concepts." *Public Administration Review* 34 (1974): 284–93.

Thomas, J. William, and Daniel L. Longo. "Application of Severity Measurement Systems for Hospital Quality Management." *Hospital & Health Services Administration* 35, no. 2 (Summer 1990): 221–43.

Tichy, Noel M., and Mary Anne Devanna. *The Transformational Leader.* New York: John Wiley & Sons, 1986.

Vladeck, Bruce C. "Quality Assurance Through External Controls." *Inquiry* 25, no. 1 (Spring 1988): 100–7.

Wennberg, John E. "Improving the Medical Decision-Making Process." *Health Affairs* 7, no. 1 (Spring 1988): 99–106.

Appendix
Defining and Coding the Variables

Intention to Change:	Hospital leaders explicitly stated an intention to make significant changes in hospital practices or levels of performance.
Examples Coded YES:	"The board wanted to know how we stacked up against our competitors....plus management wanted to get a handle on QA for the medical staff. Our medical director wanted timely information on medical practice so we could use it for reappointment."
	"We want to use the system to identify problems and to get the various departments of the medical staff to focus on those problems, so it's a way to set priorities for the medical staff structure."
	"The health planning folks appeared on a nightly TV series for a week showing four area hospitals' utilization rates.... The data was a public embarrassment for us.... We decided to buy MedisGroups to help us achieve state average rates on length of stay. We held a press conference and put ourselves out there publicly, so we could not go back to business as usual."

continued

Appendix (continued)
Defining and Coding the Variables

Examples Coded NO:	"MedisGroups has a local objective—to support QA activities more cheaply."
	"We can't let [MedisGroups] change the way we operate."
	"When we considered managed care contracts, we always used the argument that they would have to come to us because our hospitals handled the severe cases. We could never prove that, but we believed it. We purchased MedisGroups to demonstrate our quality."
Effective Implementation	**The hospitals reaches a point at which the system is used for a desired purpose.**
Examples Coded YES:	"MedisGroups data now flows to the utilization review committee and to the all-physician subset which is our peer review committee. It also goes to the professional affairs committee of the board. Chiefs get profiles of each of the doctors in their sections."
	"The comparative outcome and research evaluation reports go to the UR committee to compare with the national data base. Other reports go to division heads. They do their own physician QA. The canned reports are not very useful—we've had to get involved in ad hoc reporting to answer our own questions. The division heads ask us, 'Can you get data on this or that?'"
Examples Coded NO:	[After 5 years of experience with the system] "We don't use the MedisGroups data in the individual divisions and the individual doctors don't use it for peer review. We are just beginning to get the data to them.... We want them to decide what information they want from the system."
	[After 2 years of experience with the system] "We have not been able to get our physicians to look at the aggregate data, so they pick apart the individual case codings."
	[After 3 years of experience with the system] "I give presentations to the medical executive committee and everyone wants the data, but it's been difficult to disseminate the information. People say they don't have the resources to do the analysis, so let's just educate people rather than distributing the data. As soon as we get a schedule

continued

321

Appendix (continued)
Defining and Coding the Variables

	together on how we will implement, someone else will interpose, saying we can't do it that way."
Change System or Organization First	Were organizational changes put in place before the system was implemented, or not?
Exampled Coded SYSTEM FIRST:	"When MedisGroups was introduced, we hired a few people in the QA department to do data entry and abstracting. We tried to get a physician MedisGroups committee, but that never happened until four years later."
	"We needed broad commitment [to solve our performance problems], so we formed a committee with representation from the board and handpicked medical opinion leaders.... The committee decided to purchase MedisGroups."
	"We changed the staff and committee structure about two years after we got MedisGroups."
Examples Coded ORGANIZATION FIRST:	When we wanted to increase the emphasis on quality, we hired [Dr. X] as our first Medical Director for Quality Assurance.... She decided to implement MedisGroups."
	"After researching total quality management for a year, we appointed a vice president for quality and began to build that organization.... One of our philosophies was, if you can't measure it, you can't tell whether you're improving it. That led us to MedisGroups."
System Impact	The effect attributed to MedisGroups on the hospital's quality or cost performance.
Examples Coded MINOR BENEFITS:	"We have sanctioned physicians, but not as a result of MedisGroups."
	"Quality problems have been uncovered during the past two years, but not through the formal QA process. The meeting process has pointed out some things that seem to be recurring."
	"MedisGroups is icing on the cake. We are already taking care of our quality problems in other ways. This is merely confirmation."
Examples Coded MAJOR BENEFITS:	"There is some evidence that the doctors move to the norm simply by displaying the data. The data forces movement.... Our care is better. We can probably show that with data."
	"MedisGroups has breathed life into our QA process.... Quality has undoubtedly improved."

322

Part V

Human Resources Management

Human resources management is both a philosophy and area of work. The philosophy of human resources highlights the belief that individuals are the primary force in organizations; that the difference between failure and success can ultimately be traced to the quality of the people within the organization; and that the development and management of individuals and groups is one of the most important issues for organizational leaders. As an area of work, human resources management comprises the tasks, duties, and functions required to support personnel-related assignments: recruitment, selection, job analysis, compensation, performance appraisal, training, development, safety, pension, retirement, and termination.

In Chapter 19, Myron D. Fottler et al. present a framework that challenges health care executives to manage human resources strategically as an integral part of the strategic planning process. Health care executives should consciously formulate human resource strategies and practices that are linked to and reinforce the broader strategic posture of the organization. The article provides a framework for (1) determining and focusing on desired strategic outcomes, (2) identifying and implementing essential human resource management actions, and (3) maintaining or enhancing competitive advantage.

Scott MacStravic (Chapter 20) argues that the health care organization's employees are among its most important assets. The growth of human resources management as a profession and its elevation in the organization demonstrates that the value of these assets is being recognized. By using a customer relations strategy, the organization can increase the value it derives from its human resource assets through increasing the value it delivers. A five-step process is presented for applying the concepts and techniques of customer relations to the challenge of managing these assets.

John Kalafat, Michael L. Siman, and Lee Walsh (Chapter 21) examine a systemic quality service program implemented by a community hospital as the first step in a total quality approach. Based on consumer research, the program is organized around six principles that are effective in producing organizational change and enhancing worker performance. Evaluative data is presented, indicating enhanced performance in problem resolution and reduced response time to problems.

Chapter 19

Achieving Competitive Advantage through Strategic Human Resource Management

Myron D. Fottler
Robert L. Phillips
John D. Blair
Catherine A. Duran

Myron D. Fottler is Professor and Director, Ph.D. Program in Administration—Health Services, University of Alabama, Birmingham. He is a Faculty Associate of the College. Robert L. Phillips is Director, Institute for Management and Leadership Research, and Associate Dean, College of Business Administration, Texas Tech University, Lubbock. He is a Member of the College. John D. Blair is Professor of Management and Director, Graduate Program in Health Organization Management (College of Business Administration); Associate Chair, Department of Health Organization Management (School of Medicine); and Director of the Research Program in Health Organization Management, Institute for Management and Leadership Research, Texas Tech University, Lubbock. He is a Faculty Associate of the College. Catherine A. Duran is Research Associate, Institute for Management and Leadership Research.

This article was published in *Hospital & Health Services Administration* 35, no. 3 (Fall 1990).

Among the major environmental trends affecting health institutions are the changing financing mechanisms, the emergence of new competitors, declining hospital occupancy rates, changes in physician–health care organizational relationships, changes in work-force demographics, and capital shortages. The result has been increased competition, the need for higher levels of performance, and concern with institutional survival (Coddington, Palmquist, and Trollinger 1985; Smith and Reid 1986; Coddington and Moore 1987). Many health care organizations are closing facilities, undergoing corporate reorganization, cancelling major construction projects, instituting staffing freezes and/or reductions in work forces, providing services with fewer resources, changing their organizational structure from one with a traditional, functional nature to a holding company concept, and developing leaner management structures with fewer levels and wider spans of control.

A variety of major competitive strategies are being pursued to respond to the current turbulent environment, including becoming the low-cost provider of traditional health services, providing the highest-quality patient services through extrahigh-technical quality or customer service, specialization into a few key clinical areas (i.e., centers of excellence), or diversification within health care or outside of it (Coddington and Moore 1987; Wilson 1986). Regardless of which particular strategies are being pursued, all health care organizations are experiencing a decrease in staffing levels in many traditional service areas and a growing staff in new ventures, specialized clinical areas, and related support functions (Wilson 1986). Hence, staffing profiles are increasingly characterized by a limited number of highly skilled and well-compensated professionals. Health care organizations are no longer "employers of last resort" for the unskilled. At the same time, most are experiencing shortages of nursing and various allied health personnel.

Developing appropriate responses to the changing external environment received much attention in the past decade so that strategic planning is now well accepted in health care organizations. Zalloro, Joseph, and Furey (1984) report that 60 percent of midwestern hospitals used a formal strategic planning process in 1984. Most of those employed an individual or a department with planning responsibility and had planning cycles of three years or less. However, these authors also reported that *implementation* of the strategic plan was often problematic. The process often ends with goals and objectives development, but without strategies or methods of implementation or performance monitoring. Yet, it is implementation that appears to be the major difficulty in the overall strategy process (Porter 1980).

Perhaps the implementation problem is due to the tendency for strategic planning to be a top-level administration function with the exclusion of middle-level management or staff representatives. Without participation from those whom it would potentially benefit most, strategic planning is not likely to develop into an ongoing process. For example, if the human resource manager is not actively involved, then planning, recruitment, selection, development, appraisal, and compensation of the human resources necessary for plan implementation is not likely to occur effectively. Gerald McManis (1987) has noted: "While many hospitals have elegant and elaborate strategic plans, they often do not have supporting human resource strategies to ensure that the overall corporate plan can be implemented. But strategies don't fail, people do." A major reason for this situation may be the fact the health care industry spends less than half the amount other industries are spending in human resource administration (*Hospitals* 1989).

Human resources as a key competitive factor has not yet received much attention in the health care literature. Rather, the emphasis in this decade has been on marketing (e.g., Kotler and Clarke 1987), information systems (e.g., Austin 1988), and better control of costs via effective health care financial management (e.g., Cleverley 1987). However, Buller (1988) has studied the integration of strategic planning with human resource functions in several nonhealth care firms. He identified three environmental forces that tended to stimulate better integration: increased competition, technological change, and changing labor market demographics. All of these factors apply to the health care industry in the 1990s. Several of the firms studied had recently moved from a regulated environment to one of open competition, causing top management to question the utility of historically paternalistic employment situations. Such firms may be a bellwether for executives in health organizations. Aside from the above environmental forces, there is increasing recognition in the generic human resource management literature of the importance of linking business and human resource management strategies (Tichy, Fombrun, and Devanna 1982; Schuler and MacMillan 1984; Fombrun, Tichy, and Devanna 1984; Dyer 1983, 1985; Lengnick-Hall and Lengnick-Hall 1988; Schuler and Jackson 1987). A key requirement for human resource professionals to gain a foothold on linkages with business strategies is the recognition by top management that improved human resource programs and practices may result in a better bottom line (Cornwall 1980).

In health care, this perspective has only very recently begun to appear (e.g., Eisenberg 1986; Cerne 1988; Fottler, Hernandez, and Joiner 1988). This article reconceptualizes and extends that emerging literature and demonstrates that the actual linkage of strategic management and human resource management can be either mutually reinforcing or counteracting; describes the strategic human resource process and the steps involved in its implementation; discusses the linkage of business strategy and human resource management practices in more detail using examples of health care organizations derived from interviews; and discusses how health care executives can gain competitive advantage for their organizations through strategic human resource management. No previous publication systematically develops these topics either in the generic or the health care management literature. The information in this article is based on a review and reconceptualization of the literature on the above topics as well as ten in-depth, qualitative interviews with practicing health care executives who provided detailed examples of strategic human resource management in action.

Linking Strategy and Human Resources: Mutually Reinforcing or Counteracting?

In most health care organizations, human resource management has been unrelated to the process of strategy formulation and implementation. Managing a health care organization's human resources should not be an isolated act that is independent of the organization's management of its overall strategic approach. Given that the people in the organization are essential to the formulation and implementation of any fundamental decisions and actions the organization may make, strategies for managing these resources need to be connected to the organization's overall business strategy. With respect to the relationship between human resource strategy and strategic (business) planning, there are basically four possible linkages: administrative, one-way, two-way, and integrative (Golden and Ramanujam 1985).

Buller (1988) used these four categories and provided characterizations of four CEO orientations to correspond to each.

- *Administrative.* "We are primarily concerned about the product, the market, and the bottom line. We can always get the right people when we need them. That's personnel's job."

- *One-way.* "Once we have established the business strategy, we make sure that the human resources people understand our needs. It's up to them to respond to those needs with the appropriate programs and services."

- *Two-way.* "We work closely with the human resources function in exploring the human resources implications of various business strategies. Our human resources experts point out some possible blind spots, and show us how we can strategically attract, position, and develop our people."

- *Integrative.* "We don't make financial, marketing, technical, or human resources decisions, we make business decisions. We routinely involve all the functions, including human resources, in important decisions. [Human resources] is just as much a part of the team as anybody else."

In this article, the four possible human resource strategy and strategic planning linkages, as well as probable human resource strategy outcomes and competitive impact, are considered simultaneously and shown in Figure 1. Our model focuses on the implications of different types of linkages for reinforcing or counteracting business strategy and gaining or losing competitive advantage.

Where there is no involvement of human resource strategy with strategic planning, as in the administrative linkage, one cannot expect any outcome other than human resource strategy to be *unrelated* to the competitive strategy at best, or *counteracting*, at worst. It could be a case, with respect to employee behavior, of "hoping for A while rewarding B" (Kerr 1975). The expected impact would be to lose competitive advantage to other health organizations that are doing a better job of linking business strategy to human resource strategies. For example, a hospital seeking a qualitative differential based on consumer service might add valet parking as part of its business

Figure 1
Probable Outcomes of Different Types of Human Resource Strategy/Strategic Planning Linkages on Business Strategy and Competitive Advantage

| | Types of Linkage between Human Resources Strategy and Strategic Planning | | | |
	Administrative	One-Way	Two-Way	Integrative
Probable outcome of human resource practices on business strategy	Counteracting or unrelated	Partially reinforcing	High degree of reinforcement	Constant reinforcement
Probable impact of human resource practices on competitive advantage	Human resource practices decrease competitive advantage	Little impact of human resource practices on competitive advantage	Improved use of human resource practices to gain competitive advantage	Maximized use of human resource practices to improve competitive advantage

strategy implementation. However, if the selection, compensation, training, and appraisal practices are not harmonized with the business strategy, employees dealing with arriving patients or visitors could well act impolitely or inefficiently, resulting in long waits and angry "customers." The hospital might have been better off by not having a valet parking service. This service could end up counteracting rather than reinforcing its business strategy as a result of poorly integrated human resource practices that may have focused, for example, on recruiting minimum wage employees with minimal training to keep costs low.

With one-way involvement, human resource strategy could be expected to be at least partially reinforcing to the competitive strategy. Two-way linkage is better but still short of optimal. We obviously advocate the fourth relationship—integration with full participation in which human resource strategy and strategic planning are mutually reinforcing. Lengnick-Hall and Lengnick-Hall (1988) point out that integration is desirable for two reasons: It provides a broader base from which to draw in solving organizational problems, and it allows all resources, including human, financial, and technological to be considered in goal setting and assessment of implementation capabilities. We suggest that the more members of the top management team are involved in the consideration of human resource issues (and vice versa), the more likely they are to support reinforcing human resource strategies with resources and policies. As a result, there would be a greater degree of human resource reinforcement of the business strategy.

It is important to emphasize that organizational strategies may manifest themselves in several ways. Dyer (1983) has classified formulation of strategies into two categories. One is the formal process of strategic planning. The second is through strategic adaptation that takes place on an ad hoc basis and is usually preceded by a perceived opportunity or crisis. A truly integrative system would involve human resource considerations in both the formal and ad hoc processes of business strategy formulation.

Given a desire to fully integrate human resource strategy with strategic planning, the question arises as to methods of integration. To adopt the standard designation of organizational levels, we need to specify whether we are discussing the corporate level or the strategic business unit level. Further, it would help to differentiate strategic planning from implementation. The human resource management department could be involved in both strategy formulation and strategy implementation at both the corporate level and the strategic business unit level. The human resource unit is involved in strategy implementation at each level (almost by definition), but rarely are human resource considerations explicitly planned at the time the strategy is formulated and implementation is planned. For optimal results, the human resource function should be involved in both the strategy formulation and strategy implementation processes at both the corporate and the strategic business unit levels—the "integrative" linkage shown in Figure 1.

The benefits of linking the organization's strategy formulation and implementation to human resource management has been demonstrated in other industries. During the 1981–82 recession, employers who had linked human resource planning to strategy were able to minimize employee layoffs through hiring freezes, attrition, and other types of advanced action (Mills 1985). Almost three-quarters of these companies were also certain that it improved their profitability. In a study of 300 firms, Gomez-Mejia (1988) found a strong connection between strategic human resource management and exporting.

In the health care industry, there is already limited evidence that the linkage of strategy and human resources fosters organizational survival (Eisenberg 1986). Health care organizations tend to develop a linkage between strategy and human resources when new strategies significantly affect the way work is done, staffing problems inhibit productivity or growth, changes in the organization's structure influence job requirements, and/or significant turnover is occurring (or about to occur) in key positions (Wilson 1986). For example, one HMO in the Southeast became concerned when it discovered that a lack of qualified middle-management personnel was inhibiting its growth and that potential turnover in key positions would have put the whole organization at risk. The strategic human resource management process resulted in a plan for staffing various middle-management positions over a three-year period through both external hiring and developing various management training programs.

The Strategic Human Resource Management Process for Gaining Competitive Advantage

What is strategic human resource management?

> The strategic management of human resources is ensuring that qualified personnel are available to staff the portfolio of business units that will be operated by the organization. . . . To manage human resources strategically, health care executives must understand the relationships that exist among the important organizational components and the human resources functions so that appropriate methods can be selected to accomplish the objectives in

331

service delivery desired by the organization. (Fottler, Hernandez, and Joiner 1988)

In Figure 2, we go beyond definition to provide a model detailing how a health care organization can implement the strategic human resource management process to gain competitive advantage. The first step is to formulate the business strategy through an environmental analysis consisting of external and internal assessment and consideration of the organization's mission. The external assessment process focuses on external environmental opportunities and threats while internal assessment considers the organization's strengths and weaknesses. Among the possible strengths and weaknesses are those related to human resources.

Next, the feasibility and desirability of the possible business strategies are assessed with human resource involvement; that is, feasibility and desirability of each possible business strategy is examined from the human resource viewpoint as well as financial, marketing, and other functional viewpoints. The human resources representative will perform an informal, quick, mental "mini-gap analysis" to assess the organization's human resource strengths, weaknesses, and constraints before providing input into this strategy formulation process. Possible business strategies might include diversification (within health care or outside of it), technical quality leadership, functional quality leadership, cost leadership, or focus on a limited market segment.

Once the business strategy is formulated, the organization needs to determine what human resources gaps (if any) would exist if and when the particular business strategy selected were implemented. The existence of such a gap is determined by comparing the new human resource requirements (in terms of numbers, characteristics, and practices) to the existing human resource numbers, characteristics, and practices. The identified gaps, in turn, drive the formulation of a new human resource strategy that is implemented through modified human resource practices geared to reinforce the business strategy. While all the human resource functions are listed in Figure 2, not all are equally important in the successful implementation of a given business strategy. The key human resource systems that are significant in terms of successful strategy implementation need to be identified. Such mutual reinforcement between the business strategy and the human resource strategy should result in improved individual and organizational outcomes, including enhanced competitive advantage.

Figure 2 provides a framework for determining and focusing on desired outcomes and anticipating essential human resource management actions required for successful implementation of this business strategy. This process should stretch management thinking about human resources and influence

Figure 2
Gaining Competitive Advantage through Strategic Human Resource Management

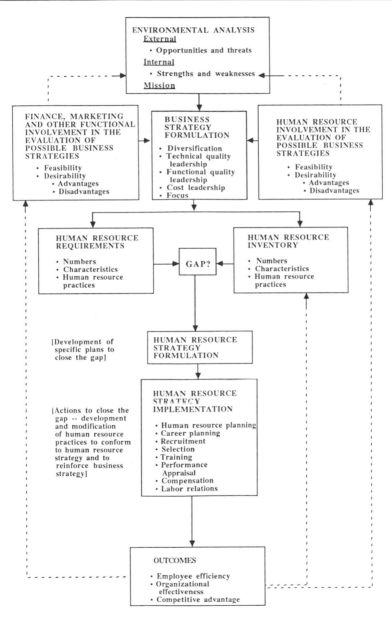

decisions affecting people. In summary, the strategic approach to human resource management includes:

- Assessing the organization's environment and mission
- Formulating the organization's business strategy
- Assessing the human resources requirements based on the intended strategy
- Comparing the current inventory of human resources in terms of numbers, characteristics, and human resource management practices with respect to the strategic requirements of the organization and its services or product lines
- Formulating the human resource strategy based on the differences between the new requirements and an assessment of the current inventory
- Implementing the appropriate human resource practices to reinforce the strategy and achieve competitive advantage.

The final two steps, which are key in the integrative relationship between human resource participation and strategic planning, will be examined in more detail below.

Linking Business Strategy to Human Resource Practices

To enhance and fine-tune our reconceptualization and integration of the existing research literature, we supplemented the theory-building aspects of our research with an initial look at empirical reality through a set of qualitative interviews. These interviews were designed to further understand how particular human resource practices in specific organizations relate to their chosen business strategies. In-depth, semistructured qualitative interviews were conducted with health care executives (chief executive officers (CEOs), chief operating officers (COOs), associate administrators, assistant administrators, personnel directors, and vice presidents for human resources) in ten health care organizations in southwestern and southeastern United States. These interviews represented two academic medical centers, two religious hospitals, two for-profit hospitals, two nonprofit community hospitals, one health maintenance organization (HMO), and one health insurance company. All of these institutions had diversified to some degree, and four of the hospitals were part of a multi-institutional system. An average of two interviews per institution were conducted. This limited, qualitative study was intended to provide insights into the range of actual organizational practices and strategic linkages, not to provide precise estimates of behavioral parameters.

Interviews helped to determine what generic business strategies an organization was pursuing and why, the organization's implementation emphases, the degree to which human resource practices were integrated with business strategy, and the specific human resource practices that were being implemented to reinforce the strategy. All of the organizations studied were pursuing more than one generic strategy, sometimes in different subunits and sometimes within a given subunit. In terms of the four possible linkages in Figure 1, most of the organizations are best described as "one-way" or "partially reinforcing." Two of the organizations used the "two-way" approach, which features a high degree of mutual reinforcement between business strategy and human resource practices. None of the organizations provided an example of an "integrative" approach wherein there is constant reinforcement between the two.

Table 1 shows the pattern of relationships between commonly used, generic business strategies and human resource management practices. The linkages among generic strategies, strategy implementation emphases, and key human resource practices are displayed. The pattern presented in Table 1 indicates practices that are currently being implemented as well as those that the respondents felt *should* be implemented to further reinforce the strategy.

The table reveals that not all human resource practices are equally important for the successful implementation of a given strategy. Table 1 further clarifies and specifies the earlier strategic human resource management literature cited above—most of which has as its fundamental premise that linking organizational strategy and human resource practices would result in superior outcomes but does not specify which human resource practices are relevant for which strategies. Table 1 is not necessarily prescriptive for any organization pursuing a particular generic strategy since there is limited evidence as to which specific human resource practices have the most significant positive impact on the implementation of particular strategies.

Diversification

Health care organizations that desire to gain competitive advantage through the development of new services and new markets will engage in extensive diversification efforts into both health-related and nonhealth-related businesses. The implementation emphasis in the diversified units is the successful development of new products and services with an entrepreneurial orientation. Implementation of the diversification strategy necessitates recruiting and

335

Table 1

The Linkage of Strategies, Implementation Emphasis, and Key Human Resource
Management Practices

Generic Strategy	Implementation Emphasis	Key Human Resource Practices
1. *Diversification into new health-related or nonhealth-related markets*: achieve competitive advantage through service/market development	1. New product/service development; entrepreneurship	1. Recruit/select experienced clinical and executive personnel; reward both based on incentive compensation and/or indirect compensation
2. *Technical quality leadership*: achieve competitive advantage through clinical and technological sophistication	2. Clinical quality; technological sophistication; clinical research evaluating new protocols	2. Recruit/select and retain top physicians and medical researchers; design compensation packages to attract and retain "superstars"; provide high staffing levels
3. *Functional quality leadership*: achieve competitive advantage through responsiveness to patient needs/demands	3. Patient service	3. Provide above-average staffing; implement sophisticated career counseling/promotion career system; monitor employee attitudes; train all staff in guest relations; appraise and reward based on interpersonal skills and responsiveness to patients
4. *Cost leadership*: achieve competitive advantage through being the low-cost provider	4. Economies of scale; cost control; productivity	4. Provide lean staffing related to patient acuity levels; develop measurable performance standards for all positions; appraise based on performance standards; compensate for good attendance and money-saving innovations; redesign jobs for maximum utilization and productivity
5. *Focus (i.e., specialization)*: achieve competitive advantage through dominance of a limited market	5. Varies by specific market niche	5. Recruit/select specialist physicians and other professionals to serve specific market niche; supplemental use of non-employee professionals; other practices depend on how the organization intends to pursue the specialized market (i.e., cost leadership, etc.)

336

selecting clinical and executive personnel who are experienced in the new areas into which the organization is diversifying. Since there is a high degree of risk involved in these new ventures, compensation packages are often based on incentives for successful performance of the venture.

An academic medical center made a decision to diversify in terms of both services and geography by developing an individual practice association–form HMO. Plans were made initially to develop a base of affiliated physicians and patients within the state. Over time, that base would be extended to the regional and national levels. Since no one in the institution had previous experience in either establishing or managing an HMO, the most critical issue was the recruitment and selection of the CEO. The various candidates for the position included individuals with HMO experience but no entrepreneurial experience or entrepreneurs with no HMO experience. The board selected an entrepreneur with no previous HMO experience but significant success in starting several new ventures. An incentive compensation package was developed contingent on the success of the HMO. An individual with significant HMO experience was then hired as medical staff director with major responsibilities for physician recruiting and liaison to the affiliated physicians. This new medical staff director also negotiated an incentive compensation package based on the HMO's future physician base, patient enrollment, revenues, and profits. Once these key personnel were in place, other executives and professional personnel were hired on a salary basis.

Diversification is often primarily pursued in an effort not to spread risk but to permit further vertical integration and to more fully "capture" a patient through making all services available throughout the course of the patient's illness—and to do it in a way that maximizes reimbursement. As a result, many hospitals are diversifying into rehabilitation centers, skilled nursing facilities, and home health care (Giardina et al. 1990). However, significantly expanding the hospital's services or product lines requires not only additional personnel but often new types of personnel, and many of these positions are very difficult to staff because of local labor market shortages. Thus, recruitment away from competitors and retention of personnel from competitors also attempting to diversify become major managerial challenges in implementing the diversification strategy.

One large, tertiary care hospital, following this strategy and faced with recruitment and retention problems, decided to "diversify" further to solve the problem. Prime land across from the hospital was bought not for revenue-producing purposes, but to enhance human resource practices by building a day care center for employees' well and sick children. The hospital has since expanded the facility twice. Not only have recruitment and retention of key personnel needed for their diversification strategy (i.e., those with preschool children) been enhanced, but another human resource problem—absenteeism—has been successfully addressed. The section of the center specifically designed for sick babies, with a full-time nurse and its own medical director from the hospital staff, tends to sick children from infant to 12 years old. These older children would normally be in school and cause parental absence from work when they are ill. This is a service not available at any other local day care center. In addition, the center permits lunch hour (or other employee break) visits by parents, and its hours allow for most shift changes. Parents pay only the marginal costs of paying for the state-certified teachers and nurses, not for the fixed costs of the expensive land and building nor its alternative income-producing uses. This indirect compensation approach has a significant strategy implementation pay-off given the labor-intensive nature of the new services provided.

Technical Quality Leadership

Academic medical centers are a classic case of an organization that strives to achieve competitive advantage through clinical and technological sophistication. Such organizations typically follow a "technical quality leadership" strategy with an emphasis on clinical quality of tertiary care services, technological sophistication, and clinical research evaluating new protocols. Porter (1985) stresses that organizations pursuing a quality leadership or differentiation strategy cannot ignore their cost positions, as the price premium for being unique must be greater than the cost of differentiating. These organizations should monitor costs carefully and possibly reduce costs in areas that do not reflect their particular quality leadership (Porter 1985).

The key human resource practices in institutions that follow a "technical quality leadership" strategy are to recruit/select and retain top physicians and medical researchers, to design compensation packages to attract and retain such "superstars," and to provide enough support services for them in the form of other professionals and support staff. Such institutions tend to have a higher-than-average ratio of personnel to beds and a higher skill level (and higher average wages) than other hospitals.

The academic medical center discussed earlier has always given a top priority to the recruitment, selection, and retention of top physicians and medical researchers. It has established a medical foundation to channel revenues from patient care services back to the physicians through various "in-kind" and tax-advantaged goods and services. It has a total employee staffing level ratio of 7:1 (personnel to beds), which is extremely high.

The individual practice association–form HMO, which is affiliated with the academic medical center, is also trying to take advantage of that affiliation by pursuing a technical quality leadership strategy. Only physicians who are recommended for membership in the HMO by a selection committee are accepted. Criteria include reputation for quality service among their peers in the specialty. Again, the human resource practice of physician recruitment and selection supports the strategic emphasis on an elite group of physicians providing state-of-the-art service within their communities and linked to the latest research at the medical center.

Functional Quality Leadership

Some health care organizations attempt to achieve competitive advantage by responsiveness to patient needs, demands, and preferences. This may mean offering patient amenities that are valued such as valet parking in crowded inner-city hospital locations or a responsive, caring staff that excels in interpersonal relations with patients. Institutions that provide patient amenities and/or interpersonal relations are attempting to implement a functional quality leadership strategy with an emphasis on patient service. They provide above average staffing to better meet patient expectations and emphasize maximizing the job satisfaction of staff members since dissatisfied employees usually cause high turnover and dissatisfied patients (Linn et al. 1985). To maintain and enhance employee satisfaction, these institutions often develop career counseling and formalized promotion systems and monitor employee attitudes on a regular basis. Of even greater importance to these institutions, however, is training *all* staff members in guest relations; one single negative experience could offset otherwise excellent staff-patient relations.

One large nonprofit religious hospital has tied its guest or customer relations implementation of the generic strategy explicitly to its performance appraisal system. The performance appraisal heavily emphasizes interpersonal skills and responsiveness to patients—so much so that relating to patients very effectively is not considered above average performance, but an absolute requirement. Any employee who is not evaluated positively on this aspect of performance is automatically not available for merit increases and will be disciplined. This is not true for other aspects of performance that are evaluated in terms of relative merit. Singling out this most relevant employee behavior illustrates how much the human resource management system is intimately tied to and enhances the implementation of the broad business strategy.

Another nonprofit religious hospital implements a functional quality leadership strategy through a policy of "living the mission." The mission emphasizes Christian values and service to others and is posted throughout the institution. The meaning of "living the mission" is reinforced through training programs in guest relations for all staff members; a call-line for both employees and patients for complaints and suggestions; periodic employee attitude surveys and patient satisfaction surveys; a professional opportunities program that offers staff career counseling and support for further education and training; and special rewards for employees who are nominated by others for providing compassionate care for patients.

The pursuit of a functional quality leadership strategy requires a total commitment at all levels in the organization. One nonprofit community hospital instituted valet parking as an amenity for patients and their families. Unfortunately, the administration did not train the individuals hired as valet parkers in common courtesy, interpersonal relations, or basic information concerning the hospital. When the patient or patient families arrived at the front door, their basic questions were often not answered or not answered with courtesy. These initial negative impressions colored the patient's views of the entire institution. This problem was identified fairly early through the patient satisfaction survey and has subsequently been remedied.

Cost Leadership

Achieving cost leadership is an attempt by a health care provider to become the low-cost provider for a particular geographical area or a particular market segment. If a provider is able to provide services at a lower cost than its competitors and yet obtain reimbursement at prices that are comparable, then it will receive above average returns. Alternatively, a low-cost provider may become a preferred provider of particular services for particular subgroups by virtue of being a low bidder on providing such services. The result is enhanced market share. The implementation emphases in institutions pursuing a cost leadership strategy are economies of scale, cost control, and productivity.

Typical human resource practices in these institutions are lean staffing based on patient acuity levels, measurable performance standards for all positions, performance appraisal based on these standards, compensation related to good attendance and money-saving innovations, and job redesign to enhance productivity and utilization of personnel. For example, some investor-owned hospitals attempt to achieve cost leadership through management systems geared to control resource consumption (e.g., close monitoring of full-time employees per occupied bed). Staffing practices in such organizations tend to reinforce such goals.

One nonprofit community hospital has been forced to pursue a cost-leadership strategy due to a significant decline in patient days over the past five years. Other strategies were viewed as more long term, and the hospital needed immediate relief from the financial pressures associated with declining occupancy. The hospital instituted nurse staffing related to the number and acuity levels of patients based on the Medicus Staffing System. It also began to employ more part-time employees to reduce fringe benefit costs and instituted an incentive program for good attendance, which allows for earned time off. An "extra-special person" award was developed to give credit to employees for money-saving innovations. The credit could be cashed for merchandise at local stores and restaurants. This gainsharing program produced estimated savings of $1.8 million in the first three months. Finally, a job design committee was established to redesign jobs to maximize human resource utilization. For example, clerical and less-technical tasks are now performed by nonlicensed personnel, and multiskilled health technicians have been hired to increase productivity through reduced "downtime."

Focus

Some health care institutions attempt to achieve competitive advantage through focus on or specialization in a given market segment. Examples include women's health care, health care for the elderly, and psychiatric or substance abuse services. The implementation emphases obviously vary by the specific market niche that is chosen. Most focus strategies are developed in combination with other strategies already discussed such as diversification, technical quality leadership, or cost leadership.

The key human resource practice required for successful implementation of the focus strategy is the recruitment and selection of appropriate specialist physicians and other professionals qualified to service the specific market niche selected for specialization. One investor-owned hospital has identified women's health care as its major area of specialization. New physician specialists in obstetrics-gynecology were recruited to complement the existing specialist group. Nurse practitioners with previous work experience in women's health issues were also recruited and selected. The recruitment and retention of these professionals was facilitated by a "beneflex" program of flexible benefits, including pay for dependent care in the hospital's day care center.

Another investor-owned hospital is completely focused on psychiatric care, including substance abuse. It is further focused on segments of the psychiatric market with carefully tailored product lines—for example, eating disorders or adolescent substance abuse. This has placed a very high emphasis on staffing these units with very specialized professionals in addition to having specialized physicians on staff and as unit medical directors.

Since the hospital's focus strategy also emphasizes technical quality and a multidisciplinary approach, expensive and rare specialists in eating disorders and adolescence must be found among many professional groups such as psychologists, clinical social workers, registered dieticians, activity therapists, nurses, and certified alcohol and drug abuse counselors (CADACs). In addition, because of using the Alcoholics Anonymous (AA) program in treating substance abuse, there is pressure to find recovering (formerly addicted but successfully treated) personnel to fill these specialized roles.

Effective human resource management is essential to the success of this focus strategy. Such success includes allowing hospital facilities and resources to be used to supplement the incomes of lead physicians and other professionals through private practice–billed services and supplemental contract services, and keeping the nonemployee professionals actually in the hospital on employee-like schedules, which is necessary for the multidisciplinary team approach to work. Also, hiring expensive professionals and managers into what are often clerical roles elsewhere is part of strategy implementation. For example, the head of admissions does not come from a clerical background and is not part of the business office. Because of the large number of self-referrals and call-ins by family members, admissions is part of the marketing effort and is managed by an individual with a master's degree in business administration and a sales background.

In this and many other cases, adaptations to wage scales and job descriptions must be made to have suitable personnel in key clinical and administrative positions so that the organization can compete effectively using its focus strategy. Large, tertiary care hospitals seeking to diversify into new product lines such as psychiatric care often underestimate the unique human resource issues they will face and are not prepared for effective strategy implementation.

Conclusions

Especially in the current environment, a health care organization's growth, prosperity, and survival is dependent on gaining and retaining competitive advantage. Although there are many paths toward that end, one that is frequently not recognized is capitalizing on superior human resource management. This article specifically applies the concept of strategic human resource management to health care organizations with a focus on reinforcing linkages to delineating the process in some detail and providing illustrations of how certain health care organizations have used human resources to reinforce their business strategy.

While there is little empirical evidence that demonstrates that strategic human resource management directly influences organizational performance and competitive advantage, there is much anecdotal evidence elsewhere

(Lengnick-Hall and Lengnick-Hall 1988) and in this article to suggest that such a relationship does exist. If an organization elects not to adopt a strategic human resource perspective, it necessarily limits its ability to maximize competitive advantage. Human resources will remain a low-level, unsophisticated function that will continue to constrain the successful implementation of business strategy.

While more health care organizations recognize the growing importance of their human resources, few are conceptualizing it in strategic terms. As a result, most forego the opportunity to improve the impact of their organizational strategy through human resource practice initiatives. This neglect of strategic human resource considerations is particularly surprising in a labor-intensive service industry requiring the right people in the right jobs at the right time, currently undergoing severe shortages in some occupations (Cerne 1988). There is fairly strong evidence outside of health care that organizations utilizing more progressive (i.e., strategically linked) human resource approaches do achieve significantly better financial results than comparable (but less progressive) organizations (Gomez-Mejia 1988; Kravetz 1988).

Most of the health care organizations studied here (and probably typically in the United States) are pursuing more than one generic business strategy, which seems appropriate since an exclusive focus on one strategy could hurt an organization in terms of various environmental incentives and constraints. In certain medical specialties, an organization might indeed pursue a technical quality position, whereas in other areas, it may lack the staffing to make such a position credible; thus, it may attempt to be the low-cost producer. In any case, health care organizations must attend to costs, regardless of the strategy selected.

The health care organizations studied here tended to demonstrate a "one-way" linkage between business strategy and human resources. Strategy was developed first with little or no involvement of the human resource department. Later, some human resource strategies and practices were implemented in a partially reinforcing manner. The impact on competitive advantage was slight. However, two of the organizations did consider their human resource strengths and weaknesses during the strategy formulation phase. In these "two-way" linkages, there was a high degree of reinforcement between the formulated strategy and human resource management. Nevertheless, even in those cases, the day-to-day implementation of strategy does not typically consider the human resource implications. Most high-level decisions are not made with input from managers of the human resource function. The potential positive impact of integrative human resources for achieving competitive advantage has not yet been fully attained.

The framework presented here challenges health care executives to manage human resources as an integral part of strategic management. More high-quality, strategically relevant output from the human resource function is needed if a competitive advantage is to be achieved. In the future, the human resource department should be seen as more than just an operational or staff function. Rather, it should be seen as a facilitator of strategic change. Executives should consciously formulate human resource strategies that are linked to the broader strategic posture of the organization and that facilitate the management of its strategy. For example, the five discrete organizational strategies are discussed in terms of the key human resource implications of each (see Table 1).

If the senior human resource executive and ultimately the human resource function is to be included in the strategic planning process, certain conditions must be met. The senior human resource executive must be included in all phases of the strategic planning process. However, the executive needs to be competent and sensitive to the problems, needs, and concerns of line managers. Human resource managers must continuously strive to understand the nature of both strategic planning and the various businesses that make up the typical health care organization today. Human resource activities need to be prioritized based on which practices are most critical at a given point in time. Then those practices need to be implemented well so that the strategic goals are attained. Communication of the successes experienced by the human resource system in helping to implement the strategy is also important in building credibility. In sum, the human resource executive must understand and communicate how the human resource system relates to the other functional activities in the organization as well as how it contributes to managerial and organizational effectiveness (see Figure 2).

The time horizons of managers may be the most significant barrier to implementation of a strategic human resource approach. Skinner (1981) estimates that it may take as much as seven years for managers to install, adjust to, and reap the benefits of major changes in human resource management systems and practices. It may take employees equally long to accept the changes. Yet many health care managers are rewarded for short-term performance. Once the integration of strategy and human resources is accomplished, and the benefits begin to be realized, it is very difficult for competitors to develop a short-term competitive response due to the time and human resource investments required.

Underlying all of the recommendations and discussion of human resource activities and practices is the theme of competitive advantage. Human resource executives should *continually* ask how their human resource practices affect the competitive position of the organization. Some practices may have little direct relevance for competitiveness; others may actually counteract and undermine the organizational goals. Such practices may need to be modified or terminated. Other practices may dramatically increase the health care organization's competitiveness. As health care organizations use present and future business strategies as a screen for existing and new human resource practices, the result should be enhanced competitive advantage.

Research is needed that more systematically relates specific human resource strategies and practices to specific business strategies under various conditions and evaluates the effect of different levels of integration. Determining the relative effectiveness of such linkages would allow scholars and managers to be more prescriptive regarding these linkages. At present it is difficult to conclude that the "integrative" linkage in Figure 1 is superior to the "two-way" linkage. We lack hard evidence because examples of organizations using the "integrative" approach are difficult to find. Yet as the application of strategic human resource management theory is applied in more and more organizations, the empirical evidence will emerge to validate the basic approach and suggest modifications to our prescriptions.

Acknowledgments

We thank Tonia Treat and Karen Long of the Institute of Management and Leadership Research for their tireless work on multiple drafts of this manuscript.

References

Austin, C. J. *Information Systems for Hospital Administration*, 3d ed. Ann Arbor, MI: Health Administration Press, 1988.

Buller, P. F. "Successful Partnerships: HR and Strategic Planning at Eight Top Firms." *Organizational Dynamics* 17 (Autumn 1988): 27–43.

Cerne, F. "Human Resources: Plan Today for Tomorrow's Workforce Needs." *Hospitals* 62 (5 July 1988): 68.

Cleverley, W. O. *Essentials of Health Care Finance*, 2d ed. Rockville, MD: Aspen Publishers, 1987.

Coddington, D., and K. Moore. *Market-Driven Strategies in Health Care.* San Francisco, CA: Jossey-Bass, 1987.

Coddington, D. C., L. E. Palmquist, and W. B. Trollinger. "Strategies for Survival in the Hospital Industry." *Harvard Business Review* 63 (May–June 1985): 137–44.

Cornwall, D. J. "Human Resource Programs: Blue Sky or Operating Priority?" *Business Horizons* 23 (April 1980): 49–55.

Dyer, L. "Bringing Human Resources into the Strategy Formulation Process." *Human Resource Management* 22 (Fall 1983): 257–71.

————. "Strategic Human Resources Management and Planning." In *Research in Personnel and Human Resources Management*, edited by K. M. Rowland and G. R. Ferris, 1–30. Greenwich, CT: JAI Press, 1985.

Eisenberg, B. "Strategic Human Resources Plans Helps Providers Survive Changing Conditions." *Modern Healthcare* 16, no. 6 (29 March 1986): 154–56.

Fombrun, C., H. M. Tichy, and M. A. Devanna, eds. *Strategic Human Resource Management.* New York: John Wiley & Sons, 1984.

Fottler, M. D., S. R. Hernandez, and C. L. Joiner, eds. *Strategic Management of Human Resources in Health Services Organizations.* New York: John Wiley & Sons, 1988.

Giardina, C. W., M. D. Fottler, R. M. Shewchuk, and D. B. Hill. "The Case for Hospital Diversification into Long-Term Care." *Health Care Management Review* 15 (Winter 1990): 71–82.

Golden, K. A., and C. Ramanujam. "Between a Dream and a Nightmare: On the Integration of the Human Resource Management and Strategic Business Planning Processes." *Human Resource Management* 24, no. 4 (1985): 429–52.

Gomez-Mejia, L. R. "The Role of Human Resources Strategy in Export Performance: A Longitudinal Study." *Strategic Management Journal* 9, no. 4 (1988): 493–505.

Hospitals. "Human Resources." 63 (20 February 1989): 46–47.

Kerr, S. "On the Folly of Rewarding A While Hoping for B." *Academy of Management Journal* 18 (1975): 769–83.

Kotler, P., and R. N. Clark. *Marketing for Health Care Organizations.* Englewood Cliffs, NJ: Prentice-Hall, 1987.

Kravetz, D. J. *The Human Resources Revolution: Implementing Progressive Management Practices for Bottom-Line Success.* San Francisco, CA: Jossey-Bass, 1988.

Lengnick-Hall, C. A., and M. L. Lengnick-Hall. "Strategic Human Resource Management: A Review of the Literature and a Proposed Typology." *Academy of Management Review* 13, no. 3 (1988): 454–70.

Linn, L. S., R. H. Brook, V. A. Clark, A. R. Daves, A. Trink, and J. Koseoff. "Physician and Patient Satisfaction as Factors Related to the Organization of Internal Medical Group Practice." *Medical Care* 23, no. 10 (1985): 1171–78.

McManis, G. L. "Managing Competitively: The Human Factor." *Healthcare Executive* 2, no. 6 (1987): 18–23.

Mills, D. Q. "Planning With People in Mind." *Harvard Business Review* 63, no. 4 (1985): 97–105.

Porter, M. E. *Competitive Advantage: Creating and Sustaining Superior Performance.* New York: Free Press, 1985.

———. *Competitive Strategy.* New York: Free Press, 1980.

Schuler, R. S., and I. C. MacMillan. "Gaining Competitive Advantage Through Human Resource Management Practices." *Human Resource Management* 23, no. 3 (Fall 1984): 241–55.

Schuler, R. S., and S. E. Jackson. "Linking Competitive Strategies with Human Resource Management Practices." *Academy of Management Executive* 1 (August 1987): 207–19.

Skinner, W. "Big Hat, No Cattle: Managing Human Resources." *Harvard Business Review* 59 (September–October 1981): 107–18.

Smith, H., and R. Reid. *Competitive Hospitals.* Rockville, MD: Aspen, 1986.

Tichy, N. M., C. J. Fombrun, and M. A. Devanna. "Strategic Human Resource Management." *Sloan Management Review* 23, no. 2 (1982): 47–61.

Wilson, T. B. *A Guide to Strategic Human Resources Planning For The Health Care Industry.* Chicago: American Society for Health Care Human Resources Administration of the American Hospital Association, 1986.

Zalloro, R., B. Joseph, and N. Furey. "Do Hospitals Practice Strategic Planning: An Empirical Study." *Health Care Strategic Management* 2, no. 2 (1984): 16–20.

Chapter 20

A Customer Relations Strategy for Health Care Employee Relations

Scott MacStravic

Scott MacStravic is Vice President, Marketing/Strategy for Provenant Health Partners, Denver, Colorado.

This article was published in the *Hospital & Health Services Administration* 34, no. 3 (Fall 1989).

The importance of good employee relations has long been recognized relative to producing good quality and high efficiency. It is increasingly recognized as key to good customer service relations as well. The concept and practice of internal marketing addresses the need to include customer-contact employee relations as a vital part of marketing strategy and tactics. Unless employees are satisfied, enthusiastic partners in pleasing customers, all the guest relations training in the world may be a waste of time.

The use of internal marketing in health care is less well established than in other service industries. Human resources management has a longer history and a clearer mandate with respect to employee relations in virtually all health care organizations. Marketing is used primarily for health care customers— patients, physicians, and increasingly, purchasers.

With a growing shortage among some key health care employee categories—especially nurses, physical therapists, and medical technologists— there is a growing need to develop more effective approaches to recruiting and retaining employees. Given the essential similarities between attracting *and* satisfying customers and between recruiting *and* retaining employees, there is good reason to consider the application of marketing concepts and techniques to the challenge. This article will examine how a marketing approach can be used to promote employee satisfaction and retention.

Employees as Customers

It is no great challenge to think of employees as customers of the health care organization even though they *are* the health care organization to most of its other customers. Employees are clearly vital to the organization's success and survival. They have competing choices as to whether to work in the health care field at all, or if so, which organization to work for. They daily exchange their labor for whatever mix of positive and negative experiences and benefits the organization offers. Their satisfaction is reflected not only in whether they return to work each day, but also in the levels of quality, productivity, efficiency, and customer satisfaction they contribute.

If thought of as customers, employees are logical targets for customer relations techniques. Because their experiences with the organization occur daily, in contrast to the unpredictable and infrequent experiences of patients, it is sensible to employ techniques geared to loyal frequent customers in managing employee experiences and their relations with the organization. (The same techniques are useful in managing relations with medical staff physicians, volunteers, and long-term patients such as those in renal dialysis and nursing homes.)

350

The Basic Model

The suggested model for planning and managing such relations includes five basic steps. First, *identify* key employee categories and determine the value of their current and potential contribution to the organization. Second, *survey* employees to discover how they define and *judge* value in their experience with the organization. Third, systematically *obtain and monitor* their judgments about their experience and the bases for them. Fourth, *develop and implement* meaningful responses to such feedback. Fifth, *monitor* the effect of such responses on employee judgments, attitudes, and behavior. This fifth step is essentially a repeat of the second and creates a repeating sequence of steps for long-term employee relations management.

Determining Customer Value

It is a common practice in marketing to identify high-leverage customers (Albrecht and Zemke 1985). In health care, physicians are high-leverage customers. If they become and remain satisfied, loyal customers of a hospital, for example, they can contribute hundreds of admissions and hundreds of thousands of dollars in revenue each year over a multidecade customer lifetime (Koska 1988). Discharge planners might represent dozens of referrals a year to a nursing home or home health care organization.

The lifetime potential contribution of high-leverage customers is often measured in millions of dollars in health care. Such a contribution represents the potential value of effective relationship management. Increasingly the focus of marketing efforts is shifting more toward selecting and managing lasting relations with high-leverage customers rather than devoting most attention to indiscriminant attraction of new customers (Paul 1988). The cost of attracting any new customer tends to be great, typically estimated at five to six times the cost of keeping current customers. Unless the contribution of customers is greater than the cost of attracting and keeping them, marketing is inefficient.

In employee relations, there are equally good reasons for being selective about where to focus marketing effort. Some employees make a greater contribution to the organization's success than others. Some may be in far shorter supply, costing far more to replace than others. On such grounds, some would clearly warrant greater marketing concern and effort than others.

On the other hand, both organizational policies and operational realities may preclude overt discrimination among employees by category. Employees themselves are likely to recognize and resent any obvious discrimination, and the entire effort may fail if only some are targeted for attention. Even those who are its beneficiaries may resent such discrimination or become the targets of negative feelings by their coworkers, for example. This does not mean that discrimination is impossible: organizations already discriminate in wage levels, for example. There will frequently be the need to discriminate in the particulars of what is done to satisfy different groups of employees, even different individuals, just as this is true for physicians, patients, purchasers, and other customers. What is unlikely to be acceptable is discrimination in terms of who is targeted for employer relations attention in the first place.

In employee relations, the value of employees in general may be more important to consider. How much would the organization gain if it were able to reduce turnover by 50 percent, for example? How much would it gain if employees significantly improved their technical quality, productivity, or contributions to customer satisfaction? How much more valuable is a loyal, enthusiastic contributor to the organization's mission and survival compared to someone who merely puts in time each day?

In contrast to most customers, it is not easy to quantify the financial contribution potential for employees in general, or any category thereof. Nevertheless, it is essential that the organization develop a reasonable estimate of the value difference that might be achieved through a more effective employee relations effort. This estimate provides the basis for considering the cost effectiveness of the effort as a whole and of any specific tactics to be undertaken. The organization that cannot estimate such a value difference has no basis for allocating resources to the effort, or for allocating resources differentially among employee categories. The organization that does not feel that there is a value difference has no reason to undertake the effort.

Surveying Judgment Dimensions

The second step is to find out what customers think makes a good product and what they determine to be the value of all available options. In employee relations, this means finding out what represents a good employer to employees. How do employees determine whether they work for a good or bad organization, whether it is better or worse than alternative employers? What satisfies and dissatisfies employees?

The literature is full of discussions of factors in employee satisfaction. Nurse satisfaction in particular has been the object of intensive study over the years. While most of the research on the subject is not market research, it offers a substantial contribution to our understanding of what affects retention of employees in general.

To be most effective, however, employee relations efforts should begin with asking what the organization's current employees consider to be the difference between their bad, good, and excellent experiences. This will make efforts more responsive to any idiosyncratic differences between the organization's actual employees and other health care employees as a class. It will also introduce employees to the organization's intention to direct its attention to their expressed concerns, individual and categorical. It also prepares the way for their acceptance of the overall process.

The organization's research into its employees' notions of what makes a good employer can be as simple as asking precisely that question. Focus group discussions are useful in generating ideas on the perceived benefits and costs of working in a particular employment category in a particular organization (Hisrich and Peters 1982). Nominal group discussions are also useful in this regard and are especially suited to differentially rating the importance of selected experience factors (Delbecq, Van de Ven, and Gustafson 1975).

With large numbers of employees, it may be impossible, or at least impractical, to involve everyone in group discussion. At a minimum, every employee should have the opportunity to participate at this stage. A general survey can be used to validate dimensions suggested in group discussion and to suggest additional dimensions as well. Such a survey can be part of the feedback process in step 3, so need not add to the cost of nor delay the process as a whole.

It is to be expected that employees will differ, by category and individually, as to what dimensions determine the quality of their employment experience and which are most important. Categorical differences may be reflected through use of different feedback questions for particular employee categories. In most cases, individual differences will have to be addressed more in terms of responses to feedback. Typical employee experience dimensions are likely to include such factors as wages and fringe benefits; work rules and assignments; relations with supervisors, physicians, and coworkers; opportunities for personal and professional growth; job security, autonomy, and responsibility; perceptions of the organization's quality of care, efficiency, and reputation; and similar factors that make a difference to employees (Blanchard 1987). Which items are on the list, how important they are, and how different employees feel about them, however, should be determined in each organization.

Obtaining Employee Judgments

Once the dimensions that make a difference are identified, how employees perceive the organization and their experience with it in terms of each dimension must be discovered. Just as is the case with other customers, the "truth" is not controlling; it is how the organization is perceived. More important than learning how employees rate the organization and their experience, however, is learning why. Employees should not simply be judges or critics in rating their relationship with the organization, they should be partners in managing and improving that relationship.

Because employees are likely to be concerned that their candid ratings and comments might be used against them, employee feedback is almost always obtained through confidential questionnaires. There are occasions where personal and phone interviews are used, but these are difficult to keep confidential and increase the risk that employees will not be candid. Moreover, with large numbers of employees, mailed or otherwise-distributed questionnaires are likely to be the only practical way to obtain feedback from most, if not all.

There are any number of ways of scaling employee judgments of key relationship dimensions. Agree-disagree scales are popular, as are poor-to-excellent rating scales. Semantic differential scales can be used where dimensions can be described in terms of polar opposites, such as worst-best, supportive-destructive, friendly-unfriendly, and even disgusted-delighted.

The best rating scales are those that cover a broad range of options, from extremely negative to extremely positive. Scales that have few options offer little opportunity for employees to express differential attitudes and may provide little chance of detecting changes over time. When first undertaking employee surveys, it is helpful to offer wide-ranging scales with seven, nine, or 11 named or numbered options. If results cluster nearer the middle than at either end of the scale, so much the better (*Quirk's Marketing Research Review* 1986). If some named or numbered options are rarely selected by employees, they may be deleted in subsequent surveys.

Where employees are asked to rate their supervisors, upper-level managers, and administrators, many prefer a subjective-feeling scale. Employees may feel better about describing how they feel (e.g., from disgusted to delighted) about superiors as opposed to rating them on some objective rating scale (e.g., terrible to outstanding). Moreover, supervisors, managers, and administrators may resent being formally evaluated by employees, whereas learning how employees feel about them is easier to accept.

The scale ratings themselves are not as important as what the employees describe as the reasons for them. Ratings are useful for stimulating such descriptions and as a way of tracking changes over time. The information employees provide in explaining their ratings, however, offers the organization a basis for maintaining and improving employee perceptions, not just monitoring them.

Each rating question should be followed by probing questions. Two forms of probing questions are often desirable: one that asks the employee to describe the reason behind a rating, and the other to suggest what would cause an improvement in rating. While these may create redundancy in some cases, they often provide different insights into what is causing positive and negative perceptions and into how employee attitudes can be improved.

To illustrate, consider a rating question on a dimension such as the supportiveness of supervisors. Such a rating question might ask: "How do you feel about how supportive and helpful your supervisor is?" (Answer options might be: disgusted, mostly displeased, somewhat displeased, satisfied, somewhat pleased, mostly pleased, and delighted.) One probing question might be: "What does your supervisor do or not do that best illustrates how supportive and helpful he or she is or is not?" Such a probe is intended to produce answers that describe in precise, behavioral terms why employees feel as they do.

Behavioral responses are far more useful than would be subjective judgments. Learning that a highly rated supervisor provides written instructions on critical tasks and frequent feedback on good performance is far more useful than being told that the supervisor is very helpful and informative. Nouns and verbs are generally actionable, whereas adjectives and adverbs are not. Learning that a poorly rated supervisor is never available to answer questions or frequently criticizes employees in public is feedback that can be acted on. Learning that the supervisor is unfair or uncommunicative is not.

The more behavioral the feedback, the more useful it is likely to be. First, it should be easier to figure out what to reinforce and what to change in terms of the employees' experiences. Learning what specific actions of the organization and behavior of supervisors make the difference, positively or negatively, provides fairly actionable feedback. Second, where criticism is involved, behavioral comments are likely to be more acceptable to those criticized in contrast to judgments of personal character traits.

Probing questions can hardly be too precise. Customer feedback consistently shows the tendency of people to talk in terms of subjective dimensions rather than behavior (Danko 1988). Patients are more likely to comment that nurses are kind, helpful, or rude, for example, than to cite exactly what they did, unless asked specifically to do so. By clearly asking for a description of behavior, probing questions are more likely to be successful in this end than would some general open-ended probes like "comments." This critical-incident technique has proven effective with health care consumers (Nyquist and Booms 1987).

The second form of probing question would ask employees, for example, "What could your supervisor do that would cause you to feel significantly better about how supportive he or she is?" This form is ideally suited for employees who are basically satisfied with their supervisor on the dimension concerned and for those who are simply reluctant to criticize. Asking for suggestions for positive change may be the only way to learn of some employees' concerns. Even for employees with critical comments, this type of question offers an opportunity to be constructive, rather than leaving their feedback in a negative vein.

Feedback from employees is communicated up the organizational ladder. Immediate supervisors receive all feedback relating to factors under their control. Next-level managers receive feedback from the supervisors who report to them and their employees and so on up the line through assistant and associate administrator to the CEO. Board members should receive at least a summary of ratings results as part of their monitoring of the organization's general health.

Generally speaking, answers to probes need go up only as far as the next level. Behavioral feedback is intended to be used by the supervisor or other manager directly responsible for responding to it. No other manager need have access to such feedback, although the next-level manager may wish to have such access to counsel and assist the supervisor directly responsible. Ideally, the answers to probing questions will provide responsible supervisors and managers with all the information they need to maintain good ratings or elicit improvements in negative ratings. Answers to probing questions without links to specific managers should be analyzed as a whole. Analysis will suggest negative behavior patterns that all managers should avoid, and positive patterns all might adopt.

Responding to Feedback

There are four components in effective responses to the type of relationship feedback that employees provide: (1) The feedback results themselves should be reported openly and completely to those who provided the feedback; (2) specific responses to the feedback should be developed; (3) these responses should be implemented as soon as is practical and in as visible a manner as possible; and (4) responses and their link to the feedback should be announced to call the employees' attention to them.

While feedback should be published to all employees, it should be done selectively based on different focuses. Where rating questions and feedback relate to particular shifts or departments, they should be reported back to employees on the shift or in the department concerned. There is no need for other employees to know how supervisors other than their own are rated. This practice will also protect the feelings of supervisors and reduce potential resentment of the rating process.

Where ratings and feedback relate to other departments or the organization as a whole, they should be published more widely. Employees should be able to learn how their peers rated the same experiences; this offers a kind of reality check to employees with idiosyncratic opinions and also suggests the degree of positive or negative feelings on specific components or experience and the degree of support for specific changes.

Publishing employee ratings and answers to probing questions is clearly a challenging step. It may be embarrassing for organizations that are surprised by negative feedback or traditionally reluctant to admit to the existence of problems. The best results from using this technique, however, come from open communication about the process and its results. Publishing feedback is one of the ways of enlisting organizationwide support for actions that must be taken on by the organization as a whole or affect the entire organization. It is also a way of enlisting employees as partners in addressing problems or seeking improvements.

Organizations may prefer to keep the survey results quiet and report only the problems they choose to address. While this may work once or twice, it is not likely to build a sense of trust or partnership with employees. In the short run, it may save the face of administration, but in the long run it will significantly subvert the potential of the entire process. Organizations not prepared to respond to employee feedback would be better advised not to solicit any in the first place.

Specific responses to the feedback should be developed as soon as possible. Where appropriate, employees providing feedback can discuss and agree on specific responses in a quality circle or quality team approach, for example (Desatnick 1987). Where feedback is provided in behavioral terms, appropriate responses may be easily identified, although they may not always be feasible. The key is to select some clearly visible and significant responses as quickly as possible.

Ideally, some responses will be selected for implementation simultaneously with publication of feedback, which will demonstrate to employees that the organization is responsive to their concerns and will also build confidence that additional responses are forthcoming. If responses cannot actually be made by the time feedback is published, a plan for the implementation of a response may be an effective substitute, as long as that plan is implemented later and is not merely a substitute for taking action. To maximize positive impact, every response that will be taken should be visibly made or clearly promised at the time feedback is published or soon thereafter.

As each response is implemented at whatever level it is carried out, it should be announced to all those employees affected. This may be done in a group meeting when carried out in a work group or department, or published in a newsletter or other internal publication if carried out at an organizationwide level. However visible the response, public announcements will remind em-

357

ployees of actions that have been taken in response to their feedback and should clearly link those responses to the relevant feedback. Each announcement also provides an opportunity to publicly thank employees.

Effective response to feedback will reward employees for having participated in the feedback process; reinforce the specificity of their comments and suggestions in response to probing questions; demonstrate that the organization values their feedback, thereby building or reinforcing morale; and show that the organization is responsive and action-oriented. Quick, visible, and announced responses will promote enthusiastic participation in the next survey, whereas slow, hidden and unpublished responses, or none at all, will tend to extinguish future participation.

Monitoring Employee Reaction

Once feedback has been published and responses both made and announced, it is important to discover what has been the effect on employee judgments. This may be done immediately after responses are completed or at some preselected interval, or where annual or less-frequent employee surveys are routinely used, the organization may choose to wait for the next regularly scheduled survey. The risk, however, is that the longer the organization waits after it has responded, the lesser an impact it may detect and the less specifically employees may relate their feedback to those responses.

Where employee feedback clearly identifies significant work unit or department problems that require immediate attention, both responses and follow-up monitoring may be assigned special priority. Ideally, the immediate supervisor will be charged with developing and implementing effective responses. Where responses require approval or resources-allocation support higher up, the supervisor may submit a response plan for approval. Where all necessary responses can be implemented by the supervisor or manager concerned, prior submission and approval are optional. By supplying employee feedback and identifying the pattern as a significant problem, the supervisor or manager's own superior may deliver sufficient motivation and leave it up to that supervisor or manager to respond appropriately.

To monitor progress made in addressing a significant problem situation, a special survey may be used rather than waiting for the next-scheduled general employee feedback survey. Rather than repeating all the questions used in the original survey, the special survey may concentrate on the areas where problems were detected. Special questions may be added to obtain feedback on specific responses planned or implemented. Further surveys may be used where the first follow-up survey indicates that a problem has not been solved or attitudes are not improving.

In small work units, especially where mutual trust and partnership working relationships are well established, the feedback mechanism may be much less formal. Periodic group discussions can take the place of formal surveys in physician practices, small clinics, and health care "boutiques," for example. They may also be used in work units and departments of larger organizations. In most organizations, however, surveys are useful, if only to monitor the extent to which mutual trust and partnership working relationships are present. They may also be the only way that relationships between the employees and the organization as a whole can be monitored.

Once follow-up surveys are implemented, step 5 essentially becomes step 2 of the next round. The process is iterative and may be used as frequently as the organization finds useful. Where feedback patterns suggest high levels of employee satisfaction, and objective indicators such as turnover, absenteeism, positions filled, quality, productivity, and customer satisfaction levels reinforce such a suggestion, feedback surveys may be carried out every year or so. Where such patterns or indicators suggest that there are problems present or significant improvement desired, a higher frequency is demanded.

While step 2 should have captured most if not all significant value dimensions affecting employee attitudes, it is worthwhile to validate and update such dimensions from time to time because employees themselves change over time and may begin to feel that important dimensions are being ignored and because effective responses to current concerns may produce a change in those concerns as employees perhaps move up Maslow's (1970) hierarchy of needs once lower-level needs are adequately addressed.

It is an unfortunate but unavoidable fact of marketing that customer needs, wishes, and standards change over time as their experience changes (Nord and Peter 1980). What was a delightful surprise when first encountered, soon becomes a routine expectation as customers repeat the experience. The same is true of employees as customers: their expectations and standards are subject to inflation as their experience improves.

For this reason, it is often a valuable component of the employee relations process to monitor employee attitudes toward other employment options as well as toward the organization itself. Employee ratings of the organization may remain well below the highest level of scales used simply because some are "tough graders" or because their expectations inflate. By monitoring how employees rate similar organizations in the area, or other relevant employment opportunities, the organization can keep track of its relative attraction as an employer.

In some cases, employees may seem quite critical on a number of dimensions, but their ratings for competing options on the same dimensions may show that the organization is ahead of others, in their view. This would place a different light on the meaning of their ratings than if employees rated the organization well below or only equal to its competitors. By the same token, even an apparently positive pattern of ratings may not be as comforting if employee ratings of competitors are even higher.

In asking probing questions after rating questions about competing employment options, the organization may learn what specific things others are doing that attract or repel, satisfy or dissatisfy employees, which may prove useful in supplementing what the literature, personal experience, intuition, and employee suggestions offer in the way of practical advice. It may also prove useful in developing marketing strategies for attracting new employees.

Discussion

The five steps of the suggested employee relations program are intended to be mutually supportive. Asking employees what makes an organization good to work for is an initial expression of interest in them and their opinions, as well as a basis for developing an attitude survey. Asking for employee opinions and especially soliciting their comments and suggestions are clear expressions of the organization's recognition of their importance, as well as a basis of better managing relations with them. Employee participation in the feedback process is a way of giving them a sense of control over their environment, which tends to relieve stress, improve mental health, and promote satisfaction (Bateson and Hui 1987).

Reporting feedback results confirms that the organization is serious about the process. Once published in a written form, employees tend to have higher confidence that something will be done about the feedback, for example. Responding promptly and visibly to feedback demonstrates the value of employee participation and reinforces their sense of partnership and control. Announcing responses reinforces these effects and promotes pride in the organization and their participation in its improvement. The first four steps, when properly executed, promote enthusiastic participation in follow-up feedback surveys and subsequent iterations of the process.

There is clearly a gamble involved for any organization to undertake this customer relations approach. It risks the embarrassment of discovering that it is not as highly regarded as it has been believed; it risks the possibility that employees may be galvanized into higher expectations by the very act of asking for their feedback; and it risks the inability to prove effective at responding to employee complaints and suggestions, thereby having a negative rather than positive effect on morale.

The risk of embarrassment should not be controlling. Any organization should prefer knowing how it is perceived by its employees and why, as by its other stakeholders and customers, rather than clinging to blissful ignorance. While employees may be galvanized into disappointment, they can also be enlisted in a more effective and concerted action through mutual participation in this process. If an organization is not willing or able to respond to employee suggestions, it should not undertake the process. If it is so distant from its employees that it cannot even guess what their suggestions might be, and is therefore unsure as to its capability for responding, it is probably time to obtain feedback in any case.

The five-step process described has been used in a variety of stakeholder relations situations, including student-instructor, administrator-medical staff, and corporate office–operating unit relations, as well as employee-organization relations. It has also proven itself in more straightforward customer relations situations involving hospital inpatients and outpatients, emergency room patients, nursing home residents, and substance abuse clients. Essentially the only difference between its application to employees and its use with customers is that the participation of employees is continuous where patient, resident, and client participants change more over time. The steps of publishing feedback and announcing responses, for example, are only recommended for continuous relationships.

The differences between this process and conventional human resources management approaches are for each organization to judge. The use of formal, probed feedback, publication of results and responses, and frequent repetition enhances the quantity and quality of employee suggestions and stimulates practical responses over time. It should give employees a stronger sense of participating in the development of the organization and in controlling their own work experience. At the least, it may be tested to see whether and to what extent it works in promoting employee satisfaction and retention.

This model also provides an excellent basis for identifying information that can be useful in recruiting needed employees. It supplies the organization with publishable survey results that can show how highly current employees think of the organization and how much they like their work. It suggests specific components of the organization and employee experience that may be useful in recruiting advertisements. To the extent that it promotes morale and retention, it takes a lot of pressure off the recruiting effort and allows the organization to be more selective therein.

The same basic approach is equally applicable to managing relations with any set of stakeholders or customers with whom the organization has or wishes to have a continuing, mutually rewarding relationship. It is well suited

361

and well tested in managing relations with medical staff members, referring physicians, other referral sources, and purchasers, although for these high-leverage customers, personal interviews are more often used in feedback than are formal questionnaires. It is certainly applicable to volunteers, auxiliaries, and donors whose voluntary contributions on a continuing basis are important to the organization.

As employees come to feel more important and are more scarce, the organization that does the best job in retaining and recruiting will have a substantial operating and marketing advantage. As employees become more enthusiastic, productive, experienced, and motivated, they are more likely to deliver quality, efficiency, and customer satisfaction advantages to the organization. The more employees are satisfied and loyal, the less the organization will have to spend on recruiting and obtaining replacements or temporary contract employees, thereby giving the organization a potential cost and price advantage in the competitive purchaser marketplace.

It is widely accepted that the organizations most likely to be successful are those that are customer sensitive and customer driven (Peters and Waterman 1982). This belief seems to hold up even when applied to health care organizations (Cleverley 1985). As a commitment to customers becomes policy and practice in health care organizations, it is likely that effective relations programs with employees will prove to be one of the most significant factors in determining which are the best organizations and which are most likely to survive.

References

Albrecht, K., and R. Zemke. *Service America: Doing Business in the New Economy*. Homewood, IL: Dow Jones-Irwin, 1985.

Bateson, J., and M. Hui. "Perceived Control as a Crucial Dimension of the Service Experience." In *Add Value to Your Service*, edited by C. Surprenant, 187–92. Chicago: American Marketing Association, 1987.

Blanchard, K. "How to Determine What Motivates People." *Health Industry Today* (July 1987): 46–47.

Cleverley, W. "In Search of Excellence: Fact or Fiction?" *Hospital & Health Services Administration* 30 (November–December 1985): 26–47.

Danko, W. "Characterizing Hospital Inpatients: The Importance of Demographics and Attitudes." *Hospital & Health Services Administration* 33 (Fall 1988): 361–70.

Delbecq, A., A. Van de Ven, and D. Gustafson. *Group Techniques for Program Planning*. Glenview, IL: Scott, Foresman, and Co., 1975.

Desatnick, R. *Managing to Keep the Customer*. San Francisco: Jossey-Bass, 1987.

Hisrich, R., and M. Peters. "Focus Groups: An Innovative Marketing Research Technique." *Hospital & Health Services Administration* 27 (July–August 1982): 8–21.

Koska, M. "High-Tech Specialists Generate Top Dollars." *Hospitals* 62 (20 October 1988): 72–73.

Maslow, A. *Motivation and Personality*, 2d ed. New York: Harper & Row, 1970.

Nord, W., and P. Peter. "A Behavior Modification Perspective on Marketing." *Journal of Marketing* 44 (Spring 1980): 36–47.

Nyquist, J., and B. Booms. "Measuring Services Value from the Consumer Perspective." In *Add Value to Your Service*, edited by C. Surprenant, 13–16. Chicago: American Marketing Association, 1987.

Paul, T. "Relationship Marketing for Health Care Providers." *Journal of Health Care Marketing* 8 (September 1988): 20–25.

Peters, T., and R. Waterman. *In Search of Excellence*. New York: Harper & Row, 1982.

Quirk's Marketing Research Review. "Rating Scales Can Influence Results." (October–November 1986): 16–19.

Chapter 21

A Systemic Health Care Quality Service Program

John Kalafat
Michael L. Siman
Lee Walsh

John Kalafat is Visiting Associate Professor at Rutgers Graduate School of Applied and Professional Psychology and an organizational consultant at St. Clares–Riverside Medical Center. Michael Siman is Director of Research and Evaluation at St. Clares–Riverside Medical Center. Lee Walsh is Director of the Department of Volunteers and Patient Relations at St. Clares–Riverside Medical Center.

This article was published in *Hospital & Health Services Administration* 36, no. 4 (Winter 1991).

Positive customer[1] relations has become a critical component of health care service delivery (Zemke 1987; Peterson 1988; Perry 1988). As this trend has matured, it has become clear that effective service strategy must go beyond "guest relations" programs to the establishment of an organizationwide culture of service excellence that permeates administrative priorities and strategic planning, policies and procedures, physical design, and staff attitudes and behaviors (Zemke 1987; Hofmann 1987). Such approaches have been referred to as "total quality management" or "continuous quality improvement."

It is one thing for health care administrators to support the concept of "service excellence," but it is quite another to translate that general concept into practical behaviors and procedures, and still more difficult to ensure that appropriate service procedures are consistently maintained. The behaviors that make up excellent service and the means for maintaining them can be derived from established principles from the fields of consumer research and human performance.

Consumer research indicates that successful service strategies are based on the *customer's* definition of quality service, and thus the program must begin by talking with customers (Lee 1989). Patient opinions about hospitals tend to be based on the care and responsiveness of staff, as they feel more competent to judge this than medical procedures (Leebov 1988).

Consumer research also indicates that personal experience and word-of-mouth advertising account for the lion's share of consumer awareness about hospitals, and that satisfied customers will tell between four and five other people about their satisfaction, while dissatisfied customers will share their experience with between nine and ten other people (Peterson 1988). Thus, it is important to address patient concerns before they leave the hospital, or as soon after the visit as possible.

There is evidence that customers who have been given the opportunity to discuss their concerns or complaints are more likely to return than those who do not complain at all. In fact, there is evidence that responding to a customer's concern, even if the response involves no specific action beyond an apology, yields greater return patronage than among customers who had no complaints (Peters 1988; Albrecht and Zemke 1985). Peters (1988) refers to this phenomenon as "remarkable comebacks."

These data mean that it is important to actively solicit customer feedback—that is, customers need to be given the opportunity to say, in their own words, what they liked or did not like about the care they received. Feedback should be obtained through personal contact if possible, since the opportunity to talk to someone seems to be an important component of the above phenomenon. In addition, personal contact is more likely to convey caring than is a survey, and it provides the opportunity for immediate response.

Research in human performance has demonstrated the efficacy of such interventions as task clarification, performance feedback, and social praise for improving customer service performance (Crowell et al. 1988; Brown et al. 1980). Task clarification involves a precise specification of the behavioral components of positive customer relations—that is, what exactly can staff do (and to a lesser extent, avoid doing) that will have a positive effect on customers. These behaviors can be specified and demonstrated in an initial training program. They can be further shaped and maintained on the job through ongoing feedback on staff responses to customers.

Rewards and recognition have been particularly successful in enhancing quality service performance, and as is consistent with established behavioral principles, such rewards and recognition are most effective when administered on an ongoing, short-interval basis (Zemke 1988). Finally, the provision of timely and accurate feedback requires the careful measurement of customer feedback and staff performance (Zemke 1988; Lee 1989).

The remainder of this article describes the application of these principles in the implementation of a quality service program in a 417-bed suburban community medical center. This program represents one component of a total quality approach. It is a critical component because it is based on one important set of customers' definitions of quality and provides ongoing data to drive continuous quality improvement.

The goal of the program is to consistently maintain and/or enhance the quality of the services provided by the medical center. The program objectives are

- To obtain feedback (positive and negative) from every inpatient through personal contact during the hospital stay.

- To maintain a quality service program that ensures an appropriate response, within 24 hours, to concerns raised by patients and family members. Appropriate responses include resolving current or anticipated concerns raised by patients and family members, correcting conditions contributing to problems experienced by patients and family members, and explicitly conveying the center's concern about problems of patients and family members.

- To maintain a service excellence orientation or culture among medical center employees through performance feedback, recognition, and rewards.

The human performance literature also provides a guide for the action steps that can be followed to successfully implement these service goals and objectives in an organization (Rummler and Brache 1988; Mager and Pipe 1970):

1. Establish the *importance* of the performance (Do staff members know the performance is important and why?)

2. Specify clearly the *expectations for performance* (Do staff members know what is expected of them?)

3. Ensure, through *training* and assessment, that staff members have the ability to carry out the performance (Do they know how to do it?)

4. Produce accurate measures of *performance* (good patient relations and appropriate response to patient concerns) and criterion (customer satisfaction) (Do they know what customers are saying and what they do or do not do that affects customer responses?)

5. Provide *consequences* associated with performance (Do staff receive feedback, reward for effective performance, and negative consequences for ineffective or inappropriate behavior?)

6. Remove organizational or *systemic blocks* to effective performance. (Is there something such as lack of resources or inefficient procedures that impedes performance?)

Each of these steps will be illustrated in discussing the implementation of our quality service program.

Importance

Consumer research has established the importance of quality service in health care (Leebov 1988) as well as in service and manufacturing industries (Perry 1988; Zemke 1987). In addition, the Joint Commission on Accreditation of Healthcare Organizations (JCAHO) will be including standards on customer complaints that call for mechanisms for receiving and rapidly responding to patient and family complaints (Koske 1989).

A critical factor in conveying the importance of quality service is the commitment and active involvement of top management in the process (Zemke 1987; Hofmann 1987). In this medical center, the Administrative Council (vice presidents and chief operating officer (COO)) was the first group to participate in the Patient Relations Seminar, which was provided by the education department, and volunteered extra hours to assist in the piloting of revisions of the seminar. The Council also listed quality customer service as its top priority in the organization's annual goals for the past two years. These goals are shared with all department directors.

Clear Expectations

The COO and Administrative Council (vice presidents and COO) have conveyed the expected quality service performance to management and staff in a variety of ways. In response to a request from the medical center's middle management (Department Head Forum) for a clear mandate, the establishment and maintenance of an effective quality service program was identified as the first mandate. The COO addressed the Forum and spelled out the Administrative Council's view of customer service in the form of an inverted pyramid with the customer on top and management on the bottom, serving the staff who serve patients and their families.

Effective customer and employee/interdepartmental relations were also included in the recently developed written performance standards for all staff and management. In addition to their participation in the customer service seminar, all department heads were participants in a workshop organized around the theme "Beyond Close to the Customer" (Peters 1988). (In the words of the COO, their attendance went "beyond strongly recommended.") The workshop was co-led by the COO and the education department. A task force of the Department Head Forum was organized to generate specific Centerwide projects that resulted from this workshop.

All staff have participated in the customer service seminar, described below. Early in that seminar the active participation of the vice presidents in the first version of the seminar and the placement of quality service at the top of the Center's annual goals and mission statement are emphasized. All new employees now receive a personal message on customer service from the COO during their orientation, and, of course, must participate in the customer service seminar.

Staff who have direct contact with patients and their families also receive continuous feedback through the "Patient Response System" described below.

Training

All staff and management, beginning with the Administrative Council as noted, were required to participate in an interactive customer service seminar sponsored by the education department. This seminar was originally adapted from a patient relations program purchased from another medical center. After subsequent in-house modifications, a small portion of the original program remains in its original form. The seminar consisted of five two-hour sessions offered many times throughout 1987–1988 for the purpose of training all staff. In its current form, the seminar is a three-hour program required for all new staff, with a three-hour advanced session available as part of a core management curriculum that is required of supervisors and managers.

As one-shot training programs are insufficient to maintain effective performance (Camp, Blanchard, and Huszczo 1986), staff most closely associated with patients and other customers receive continuous performance feedback through the "Patient Response System" described below.

Performance Measurement, Consequences, and Systemic Blocks

These three elements are each contained in the "Patient Response System" depicted in Figure 1. The overall system will first be described, then the stages of its development and implementation will be chronicled. Finally, initial evaluative data on the impact of the program will be provided.

The system begins with patient representatives visiting with patients (Figure 1, see upper left side). A group of approximately 15 trained volunteer patient representatives works under the supervision of the Director of Patient Relations. These representatives are assigned to a given area of the hospital and given a list of patients to visit during their shift by the director, who receives a current list of patients from admissions each day.

Patient representatives complete a form for each patient (see Appendix). If more than one problem is identified, a supplementary problem form must be completed. This form has undergone several revisions based on feedback from the patient representatives and refinements in our efforts to obtain data necessary for the systematic tracking of patient responses and the provision of feedback to hospital staff and administration. For example, the top priority of the quality service program is to communicate to the patient or family member regarding the resolution of the problem or expressed concern about problems for which no specific action could be taken. Thus, in the problem resolution section of the form, an item was added that required the person responsible for responding to the problem to check how they communicated to the patient.

While patient representatives must complete these forms, they are not the focus of their contact with patients. Rather, their first priority is to specifically inquire if there is anything that can be done to make the patient's hospital stay more pleasant. Representatives are taught to obtain information through a natural conversation with the patients rather than a formal interview. They work closely with the Directors of Patient Relations, Research & Evaluation, and Education to refine this process through highly participatory regular meetings and occasional shadowing of patient representatives by the Director of Patient Relations or of Research & Evaluation. Analyses of the pattern of complaints obtained by each representative are carried out to check for unusual patterns or evidence of particular biases.

Figure 1
Patient Response System

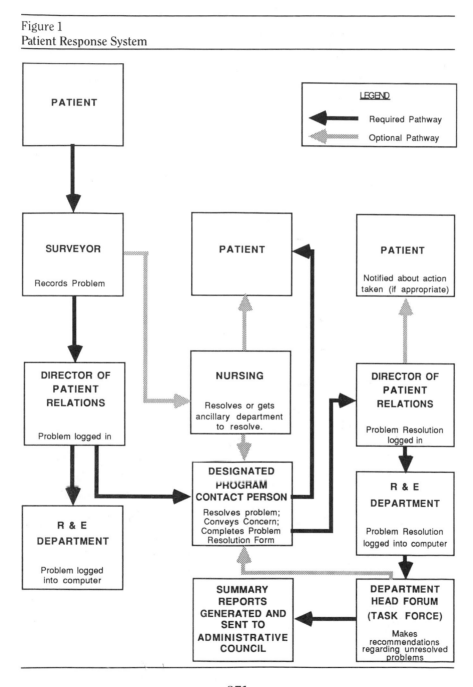

While all feedback gathered by patient representatives must be returned to the Director of Patient Relations to initiate the next steps in the process, another optional procedure depicted in Figure 1 is often carried out. For concerns that require immediate action or could be simply resolved by the nursing staff, the patient representative communicates to the charge nurse, and action is taken at that time. Organizational research in general (Kreps 1986) and a study with nurses and patient representatives in particular (May 1988) indicate that this "horizontal communication" versus hierarchal communication yields superior problem resolution and more positive responses and cooperation from staff involved.

The Director of Patient Relations forwards this data to Research & Evaluation where it is entered into the computer, and also to a contact person designated by each department to respond to patient complaints. To attenuate the impersonal nature of such tracking systems and to ensure rapid response, the complaint forms are preceded by a phone call by the Director of Patient Relations, who alerts the contact persons. These individuals are responsible for completing the problem-resolution section of the patient representative problem form within 24 hours. The contact persons have several options for responding to the complaint: they may be able to resolve it themselves or may decide, in consultation with the Director of Patient Relations, that someone else (including the vice president or COO) may be better able to resolve the complaint. If, however, specific action has been taken or is no longer feasible, they must still convey concern to the patient—preferably in person while the patient is still in the hospital, or by phone or letter if the patient has been discharged .

The Director of Patient Relations then forwards the problem resolution to Research & Evaluation—here a variety of standard reports are generated that permit tracking and follow-up of complaints and compliments, as well as provide overviews of patient feedback and medical center quality service. There are three top priorities in this reporting system for maintaining quality service:

1. *Systematic feedback concerning compliments to medical center staff is provided.* The emphasis in this system is on compliments not only because the compliments-to-complaints ratio is approximately 8:1, but also because positive feedback is critical for the development of appropriate attitudes and behaviors (Zemke 1988). In addition to maintaining horizontal communications with staff as much as possible, the Director of Patient Relations provides specific positive feedback and encourages the department heads and vice presidents to do likewise. The Department of Research & Evaluation provides specific

compliment summaries to each department on a biweekly basis (see Figure 2). These are posted on special bulletin boards purchased for each department. While rewards for compliments are still in the planning stage, this positive feedback (social praise) is already generating results. Evaluation data will be summarized later, but feedback from staff has been very positive as they had not been systematically recognized in the past. In addition, many contact persons have expressed enthusiasm with the opportunity to resolve problems, and they often return forms to the Director of Patient Relations in person so they can discuss the issues and resolutions.

2. *A response is provided to every patient who expresses a concern.* Departments and staff have been told that complaints are information and will not be held against them. Complaints that go unresolved—and resolution always includes communication to the patient—are tracked and remain in the system and its reports until they are resolved.

Figure 2
Patient Compliments Reporting System

Run Date: 3/26/90
Total Number of Hospitalwide Compliments: 100

Department/Program: Urban-III
Reporting Period: February 11 to February 25, 1990

Patient Name	Date of Interview	Room	Compliment Type This Department	Specific Individual Mentioned	Compliment
Rose G.	2/12/90	112A	✔		Peggy on 3rd Flr., everyone
Maureen T.	2/14/90	342A		Jo	Willing to listen
Maureen T.	2/14/90	342A		Maureen	Willing to listen
Maureen T.	2/14/90	342A	✔		Nurses punctual
Helen K.	2/21/90	302A		Regina V	Nurses aid on U-3
Concetta G.	2/21/90	300A	✔		Nursing staff is wonderful
Barbara C.	2/21/90	302B	✔		
Janet H.	2/21/90	318B	✔		Nurses great
Dorothy N.	2/21/90	322A	✔		
Ann C.	2/21/90	330A	✔		Nurses staff was great—very helpful
Richard M.	2/21/90	3344B	✔		Nurses were wonderful and gentle
	Total		8	3	

3. *Systemic problems are identified and resolved at the middle-management (department-head) level if possible.* Many complaints result from systemic problems such as procedures, physical arrangements, or lack of resources. These are addressed by a task force of the Department Head Forum chaired by the Director of Research & Evaluation. They generate recommended solutions that are voted upon by department heads and carried out, or forwarded to the Administrative Council for action. Two examples of systemic problems identified by a pattern of patient complaints may be illustrative. Complaints about the waiting time in the emergency department by patients scheduled to be admitted to hospital floors resulted in enhancing the physical comfort and hospitality of the holding rooms and in meetings with unit receptionists to standardize admitting protocols and thereby speed the admitting process. Also, patient difficulties with completing outside phone calls resulted in the placement of instructional stickers on the phones, training for nurses to answer questions about the phones, and proposals solicited from outside vendors to replace the current phone system with a more "user-friendly" system.

The task force also receives copies of three monthly summary reports of compliments and problems (ratios, totals, responses made or outstanding, and types of problems) broken down by department. Department heads from the Patient Relations Task Force provide follow-up responses to their peers concerning unresolved complaints. In an effort to keep problem resolution at the staff or middle-management (i.e, horizontal) level, one more step is added so that the contact persons are provided an opportunity to respond to unresolved complaints before reports are forwarded to the Administrative Council. Often this involves simply forwarding resolution documentation that had been sitting in an out basket to staff in the Department of Research & Evaluation, who send reports to each department on a monthly basis that list specific patient problems (with date of interview, patient name, room number, and billing number) that have not been returned to the department. The goal of the program is to eliminate the necessity for this report.

In the final stage of this process, vice presidents share with department heads their feedback concerning compliments, systemic problems, or complaints to which there has been no response. The goal of resolving concerns at the staff level rather than hierarchically appears to isolate vice presidents from this patient-response process. Therefore, a policy was recently instituted whereby all vice presidents and department heads personally conduct patient surveys. The active participation of this level of administration also gives a strong message to staff as to the importance of quality service for the institution.

In sum, a combination of high-tech automation and high-touch personal contact with patients and among staff actively solicits ongoing customer feedback, carefully summarizes the feedback for staff, and tracks staff responses to the feedback. Problem resolution is maintained at the lowest level possible, and personal accountability for resolutions is provided for. The feedback system provides consequences, with the emphasis on frequent (short-interval) positive reinforcement and personal action rather than punishment or policing, and also provides ongoing learning and repertoire building for staff.

Specific rewards are planned for, but these will not be instituted until the system has been in place long enough to work the "bugs" out and ensure familiarity and, in fact, the ownership of all involved. This is apparently a common state of affairs in the development of reward systems as most organizations use customer feedback as information for staff, then gradually evolve systems that produce rewards beyond the social praise effect of the feedback (Lee 1989).

Issues in Implementation

A variety of issues must be addressed in the implementation of any quality initiative. A brief overview of some of those associated with the patient response program includes

- *Trust.* Staff must see that the information generated through such a tracking system is used in a supportive, problem-solving manner. Initially, the Director of Patient Relations had to establish trust through a personal, hands-on approach rather than a series of memos and reports. The survey forms employed in this program ensure follow-up and accountability, but they are always preceded and followed up by personal contact with the Director of Patient Relations or a member of the Patient Relations Task Force. Task force members were initially reluctant to approach their peers about patient concerns, but as they have learned to take a "how can we help you address this" approach, their reluctance has dissipated.

- *Positive emphasis.* Related to the issue of trust is the need to apply a basic learning principle—results are more effectively achieved by the recognition and reinforcement of positive behaviors than by punishment of negative performance. When confronted with specific customer complaints, there is a powerful tendency to follow up on these more vigorously than the compliments, and this will sabotage the program at the start. A concerted effort must be made to emphasize recognition of positive performance through such means as the bulletin boards employed in this patient response system.

- *Teamwork.* The necessity for a close working relationship among the Directors of Patient Relations, Research & Evaluation, and Education is clear from the description of this program. Later, this teamwork extended to the Patient Relations Task Force and all staff who are involved in quality service for patients. Again, teamwork is fostered through a supportive, problem-solving approach that emphasizes the goal of quality service rather than specific issues or procedures.

- *Quality data.* There must be a capability for constant data processing and reporting (this is called an "information intensive process"). The system requires an ongoing verification of information and data and generation of reports and reminders. The quality of the data is critical to the efficacy of the program and the maintenance of cooperation and effort from all.

- *Commitment.* Staff, and particularly middle managers (in this case the department heads), required a considerable amount of convincing that the medical center administration was committed to quality service, and that the patient response system was not going to disappear. In fact, middle managers needed several reminders during the first year that the program had started, as they continued to express surprise when reports reached their desks. The main point here is that quality initiatives take time to develop—in this case, three years of continuous feedback and revisions preceded the program described herein. Moreover, it must be recognized that the commitment to quality does not quit at any point, although as specific work groups, and ultimately the entire organization, gel as a team, the effort becomes a natural and gratifying part of the worklife.

Evaluation

The evaluation data currently available will be presented within the framework of the chronology of the implementation of the quality service program.

The first quality service initiative was an in-house patient relations seminar for all emergency room staff in February 1986. In addition to being the largest outpatient department, having interactions with many community caregivers, the emergency room is a major source of inpatient admissions.

The hospitalwide-packaged "Customer Relations Seminar" was begun in April 1987 with vice presidents and department heads trained in the spring, and most of the other medical center employees trained from summer 1987 to summer 1988.

A pilot version of the "Patient Response System" was begun in fall 1988. Department heads were informed of the pilot, but the details of the system were worked out between the team and line staff from the Research & Evaluation, Patient Relations, and Education departments. The formal pilot version of the "Patient Response System" as outlined in Figure 1 was initiated in January 1989 and reviewed in detail with department heads. From January to June 1989, small changes were made in the tracking system and survey form to better capture data for feedback. Reports were shared with department heads but not forwarded to the Administrative Council. During this period, line staff involvement with the system was growing, the importance of the quality service program was emphasized by the COO, and department heads gradually became convinced that this initiative was here to stay. By July 1989 it appeared that the department heads had received sufficient familiarization with the system and feedback as to their roles and appropriate responses to warrant forwarding the formal monthly reports to the Administrative Council.

The implementation process, then, involved a clear commitment from top management (COO and vice presidents) while the actual program procedures were developed at the staff level through task clarification, feedback, and reinforcement. As suggested by Kaluzny (1989), a concerted effort was made to incorporate middle management (department heads) into the decision-making process—particularly through the Forum Task Force.

Patient surveys have been conducted in the medical center since 1984, although differing formats were used and there was no follow-up to the survey information. Keeping in mind, then, some differences in survey procedures and incomplete data sets, it is nevertheless interesting to note the trends presented in Table 1. As noted in the table, the ratio of compliments to problems began to shift after the emergency room and patient/employee relations trainings.

The new patient response survey procedure captured much more patient feedback but not a greater number of problems. This confirmed what staff felt and what a previous survey had indicated concerning the medical center's high-touch reputation: A 1986 mail follow-up survey of 338 randomly selected medical center patients found that 80 percent were very satisfied (top rating on a 5-point patient Likert scale) with the quality of medical care and personal treatment (Ruben, Ruben, and Bowman 1986). More important, the procedure

Table 1
Patient Satisfaction Surveys

Year	Number of Months	Average Number of Surveys/ Month	Average Number of Compliments/ Month	Average Number of Problems/ Month	Ratio of Compliments to Problems
1984	4	142	7	40	1:6
1985*	8	152	12	57	1:5
1986	3	143	44	80	1:2
1987†	2	108	40	75	1:2
1988‡	8	99	74	26	3:1
1989	7	240	260	32	8:1

*E.R. Patient Relations Training completed fall 1985.
†Majority of staff completed Patient/Employee Relations Seminar, fall 1987.
‡Patient representatives trained to employ new patient response format, fall 1988.

provided overwhelmingly positive feedback to staff members and increased their enthusiasm and commitment to seeking out and responding to patient concerns.

The major goal of the patient response program is to ensure rapid response to all identified patient concerns. Figure 3 depicts the increase in percent of documented resolutions as we move toward a goal of 100 percent resolutions. Systemic problems that have been identified, but require more time to resolve, will keep this figure below 100 percent.

Figure 4 depicts the progress toward the goal of rapid resolutions to identified problems. Again, this factor is critical, given the documented impact of response to concerns on customer satisfaction and the role of word-of-mouth advertising in health care services.

The medical center took the risk of devoting significant resources and effort to this project and aggressively seeking customer feedback. Figures 3 and 4 display evidence of a dramatic return on this investment. These data not only help to justify the medical center's commitment, but also document and display positive outcomes in a way that provides clear feedback to staff as to the results of their efforts.

These initial data provide evidence that a carefully grounded and implemented quality service program can enhance staff morale and commitment and significantly improve responses to customers' concerns. The medical center's administrators are convinced that this program has contributed to the current sound fiscal status of the center and the recent commendation

Figure 3
Percent of Problems with Documented Results

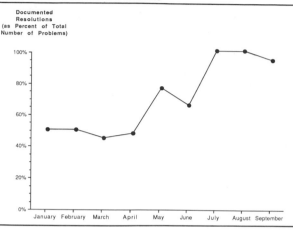

Figure 4
Time Lag between Report of Patient Problems and Problem Resolutions

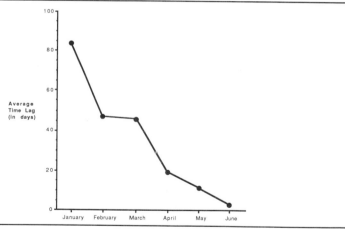

(O'Leary 1990) by the JCAHO that placed this institution in the top tenth percentile of the hospitals it reviews nationally.

As previously mentioned, this program represents but one component of a total quality effort. It illustrates generic strategies that can be replicated throughout the institution in pursuit of ongoing total quality: identifying

379

one's customers (external or internal); obtaining their continuous input and systematically feeding this back to staff; establishing a means of rapidly incorporating continuous improvements into systems and procedures; and carefully monitoring results and providing recognition. The commitment of top administration is essential to the success of any quality effort, but that commitment must be operationalized through procedures that involve staff at all levels if such efforts are to have measurable effects.

Note

1. We use the generic term "customer" rather than "patient" because a service strategy must address interrelationships among patients, family members, doctors, staff, vendors, and community gatekeepers. We also use the term "program" for convenience, while the terms "process" or "philosophy" may also describe customer service strategies.

References

Albrecht, C., and R. Zemke. *Service in America*. Homewood, IL: Dow Jones-Irwin, 1985.

Brown, M. G., R. W. Malott, M. J. Dillon, and E. J. Keeps. "Improving Customer Service in a Large Store Through the Use of Training and Feedback." *Journal of Organizational Behavior Management* 2, no. 4 (1980): 251–65.

Camp, R. R., P. N. Blanchard, and G. E. Huszczo. *Toward a More Organizationally Effective Training Strategy and Practice*. Englewood Cliffs, NJ: Prentice-Hall, 1986.

Crowell, C. R., D. C. Anderson, D. M. Abel, and J. P. Sergio. "Task Clarification, Performance Feedback, and Social Praise: Procedures for Improving the Customer Services of Bank Tellers." *Journal of Applied Behavior Analysis* 21 (1988): 65–71.

Hofmann, P. "Patient Advocacy: The Touch Stone of Administration." *Administrative Radiology* 6 (July 1987): 22–24.

Kaluzny, A. D. "Revitalizing Decision Making at the Middle Management Level." *Hospital & Health Services Administration* 34 (Spring 1989): 39–51.

Koske, M. T. "Be Aware, Not Afraid of JCAHO Complaint Standards." *Hospitals* (December 1989) 40.

Kreps, G. L. *Organizational Communication*. New York: Logman, 1986.

Lee, C. "Using Customers Ratings to Reward Employees." *Training* 26, no. 5 (1989): 40–47.

Leebov, W. *Service Excellence: The Customer Relations Strategy for Healthcare*. Chicago: American Hospital Publishing, Inc., 1988.

Mager, R. F., and P. Pipe. *Analyzing Performance Problems*. Belmont, CA: Pitman Learning, Inc., 1970.

May, K. A. "Interhospital Communication of Outpatient Complaints." Unpublished report. Little Rock, Arkansas Children's Hospital, 1988.

O'Leary, D. S. Personal communication with CEO of St. Clares Riverside Medical Center from the Joint Commission on Accreditation of Healthcare Organizations, March 1990.

Perry, L. "The Quality Process." *Modern Healthcare* (April 1988): 30–34.

Peters, T. "Beyond Close to the Customer." Video Publishing House, 1988. Video.

Peterson, K. "Guest Relations: Substance or Fluff?" *Healthcare Forum Journal* (March–April 1988): 23–25.

Ruben, B. D., J. M. Ruben, and J. C. Bowman. "An Analysis of Patient Perceptions of Quality Care." Survey results presented to St. Clares Riverside Medical Center, Denville, NJ, 1986.

Rummler, G. A., and A. P. Brache. "The Systems View of Human Performance." *Training* 25 (1988): 45–55.

Zemke, R. "Health Care Rediscovers Patients." *Training* 24, no. 4 (1987): 40–45.

———. "Rewards and Recognition: Yes, They Really Work." *Training* 25, no. 11 (1988): 49–53.

Patient Representative Survey

Patient Name _____ Admitted Through:
Patient No. _____ Room No. _____ Bed _____ □ Admitting
Interviewer Name _____ □ Emergency Room
Interviewer No. _____ Interview Date _____

COMPLIMENTS
□ General _____

_____

□ Any <u>department</u> in particular you would like us to share a compliment
    with? _____
    What occurred? _____
□ Any <u>employee</u> in particular you would like us to share a compliment
    with? _____
    What occurred? _____
Did you have contact with any of the following services?
  Contact?   Compliment
  □ YES □ NO   Laboratory   _____
  □ YES □ NO   Pastoral Care   _____
  □ YES □ NO   Phone/TV Services _____
  □ YES □ NO   Physical Therapy _____
  □ YES □ NO   Respiratory Therapy _____
  □ YES □ NO   Social Services   _____
  □ YES □ NO   X-Ray   _____

PROBLEM #1
(check one) □ Current? or □ Past?
Hospital Department or Unit _____
Date _____ Time _____ Place _____
Employee Involved _____
What occurred? _____

_____

_____

_____

_____

- -

PROBLEM #1 RESOLUTION (FOR DEPARTMENT USE ONLY)   Communicated to Patient:
                                         In Person   □
Date _____ Person _____ By Telephone □
                                         By Letter   □
Action Taken _____

_____

_____

_____

_____

_____

FOR OFFICE USE ONLY:	TRACKING OF REPORTED PROBLEMS
Surveyor informed nursing of problem □	Date form was sent to contact: _____
Surveyor informed department of problem □	Date form was returned: _____
Director of Patient Relations informed contact person □	Resolution Code: _____

Part VI

Leadership Ethics

In 1975, ten years after Medicare gave further urgency to the issue of economics in health care, Daniel Callahan of the Hastings Institute announced that he had found "no literature on morality and health care management." At the time of his comment, the subject was not regarded as an area worthy of sustained analysis and scholarship; thus, an observer might have concluded that ethical concerns in matters of reimbursement, conflicts of interest, and the allocation of limited resources were considered of less consequence than concerns relating to patients.

Since that time, the literature on health care management ethics has grown quite markedly. To a degree, this change has occurred as a countervailing response to the "corporatization" of health care—a kind of urgent counsel to uphold traditional principles. Owing to the efforts of a handful of concerned individuals, ethical awareness has slowly gathered strength as a topic deserving of serious study. That ethics in health care management is finally receiving its due is suggested by its heightened visibility at conferences and workshops, as well as by the growing number of citations in the *Hospital Literature Index*.

The articles that follow address the clash of business and patient care values in the hospital setting. In Chapter 22, James W. Summers reviews the demands of "doing good" and "doing well," arguing that the administrator should be a leader, "one who inspires, who embodies the ethical ideals, the obligations of the whole institution." Kurt Darr, Beaufort B. Longest, Jr., and Jonathon S. Rakich, Chapter 23, consider five problem areas in health services governance and management: fiduciary duty, conflicts of interest, confidential information, resource allocation, and consent. The authors note that those who govern and manage health services organizations face an ethical imperative: they are moral agents with an independent duty to protect patients and further their interests. This duty is separate from any existing between caregivers—such as physicians—and patients.

Finally, in Chapter 24, Samuel Levey and James Hill use the concept of "advocacy" for health care professionals to frame an argument for recasting the traditional model of patient care along more socially responsible lines.

"Meta-advocacy," their term for this approach, refers to a collective responsibility involving both the patient and the health care team, as well as those less directly involved in patient care, from researchers to policymakers.

The chapters on managerial ethics constitute a fitting conclusion to this volume because they return us to one of the main emphases of the introduction: the imperative for hospital leaders to be accountable in ways that go beyond simply "doing well." To consider the ethics of a situation in a hospital setting is to ask the question "What ought we to do?" which raises more questions of principles, of right and wrong, of duty and obligation in professional conduct. It is through such questioning and self-analysis that fiducial accountability in hospital leadership is best advanced and preserved.

Chapter 22

Doing Good and Doing Well: Ethics, Professionalism, and Success

James W. Summers

James W. Summers is Assistant Professor in the Department of Health Administration, Southwest Texas State University, San Marcos. He is a Member of the College.

This article was published in *Hospital & Health Services Administration* 29, no. 2 (March/April 1984).

Health-services administrators face no shortage of pressures to ensure that their institutions are doing well. Indeed, with all the concern over cuts in reimbursement, prospective payment schemes, rate review, rate regulation, consumer-choice health plans, preferred provider organizations, competition and regulation, it is no wonder if we often see our roles in financial terms. Much of the literature on models for hospital organization or on the meaning of being a professional administrator exhort us to adopt businesslike ways as the solutions to our problems.[1] Graduate training encourages us to see hospitals as analogous to manufacturing facilities where physicians are customers and patients the raw material. We have learned much from study and application of these business skills. We speak now of diversification, mergers, corporate restructuring, financial-maximization strategies and marketing with considerable aplomb. Apparently, we have succeeded too well.

Robert Cunningham (1983) argues that a shift from patient care values to business values will lead to a loss of public confidence.[2] Recent chairpersons of the American Hospital Association (AHA) have stressed the need for retention of humanistic and charitable values. Stuart A. Wesbury, Jr., Ph.D., FACHA, President of the American College of Hospital Administrators (ACHA) [since 1985, the American College of Healthcare Executives (ACHE)], argues that our leadership role forces a consideration of ethics.[3] Peters and Wacker (1982) say that hospital strategic planning must be rooted in values and ethics. Echoing Cunningham, they note that the legitimacy of hospitals in the public eye is tied to perceiving hospitals as "sustenance organizations," with a charitable ethic instead of an exchange ethic. Failure to keep this in mind while considering diversification, divestment, nontraditional revenue sources and the like poses such a threat to public confidence that it may threaten their survival in the traditional forms. Harry Levinson (1979) noted management consultant in organizational theory, motivation, and the management of change, shows that for the administrator to succeed he or she must build a values consensus with the board, the medical staff, and the other employees.[4]

This literature and the concern of our leaders, while overwhelmed by cost and operational issues, is noteworthy. It seems important to achieve two goals relative to this sentiment. First, in terms of leadership as individuals and in terms of professional development as persons in the role of hospital administration, it seems we need to become clear on just what our values are. Part of this article is devoted to doing that and along the way showing why such clarity is needed at this time in the history of our profession. Second, the article addresses techniques by which discussions about values and ethics can be useful in achieving success at leadership. Doing good and doing well are compatible. With these tasks in mind we may begin to question ourselves about our values, why we hold them, and the consequences on our long-term effectiveness.

Why Are We Here?

The quickest way to find out what your values are concerning hospitals is to ask yourself why you are in the field—why you chose it, why you remain. Most express the view that they are in health services administration because they like the idea of involvement in a meaningful way with an organization that helps people when they seem to most need it, what Peters and Wacker (1982) called a "sustenance organization." There is a value in "doing good," which tends to influence our actions whether we are in the investor-owned or non-profit sector.[5] But unlike our colleagues in medicine, nursing, and other health professions, or even nonprofessional employees, this ethical commitment to doing good seldom surfaces. In fact, our training and our ideas about professionalism in management make it appear that we deliberately distance ourselves from such "sentimentality" and "subjectiveness." However, this leads to a conflict.

Administrators face this conflict, not just as individuals with their own values, but as professionals and persons trying to understand or even redefine the hospital's mission. We see management and professionalism in terms of the bottom line results and pride ourselves on these successes. Our skills in translating problems and solutions into quantifiable terms, in being able to transcend management by crisis through planning and implementation of sound policy, are essential and should be matters of pride. Yet the results-oriented, no-nonsense approach is sometimes packaged in a suit of callousness, empire building and ruthlessness, all of it then festooned with an aura of manipulation that we may believe is the attitude of objectivity. But this misguided management style leads to conflict with the values of the boards, the health care workers, and perhaps even the now-suppressed values of administrators. The emphasis on doing well, in terms of a purely business model, is limited by the public image of hospitals, an image enforced by the board.

The Trustee Image of the Hospital

As Johnson (1979) points out so well, trustees consider significant amounts of black ink on the bottom line to be taking advantage of the public.[6] Even if the hospital is owned by a for-profit chain, management is typically careful to present an image of public and social concern for the medical needs of the community, including the indigent. To fail in presenting this image usually means the community perceives the values of the institution as somehow suspect.

The trend toward investor-owned hospitals has probably saved many non-profits by helping to legitimize the need for a reasonable return on investment in the trustee community, thus avoiding bankruptcy, extreme deficits, or take-over by the same for-profits. While days of worry about excessive black ink may be few and far between, this is still a profession where applying management skills prompts us to "do good" along with "doing well." These two values are not in conflict; "doing good" does not mean spilling red ink, although some-times people outside of the health care field tend to impulsively act as if it does.

The public image of hospitals as not just another business, of having a "product" that is something besides a mere economic commodity, leads to problems not just with the board, but with the medical staff. These problems may not be solved unless we more deliberately see our own values commit-ment to doing good brought to the fore in our activities and in our profes-sional identification. Why is this the solution?

The Medical View of Hospitals

Physicians and nurses embody, in their own minds and in the public's concep-tion of them, a dedication to the relief of individual suffering. Their professional identity has been clear about this primary obligation for a long time, both clear to them and to the public. Failure to live up to this obligation to individual patients is not seen as a failure in the formulation of the profes-sional role but as a failure among the practitioners. Trustees, the public, and typically both physicians and nurses see the hospital as a place for them to carry out this role. Johnson (1979) states the problem well. This grouping of role players sees the purpose of the hospital in terms of a cause, not a business. They all identify the hospital as primarily a medical institution. Neither trust-ees, physicians, nor nurses typically see the hospital chief executive as the person who leads and inspires for the sake of this cause. Levinson (1979) puts the problem in a sociological perspective.

Physicians and nurses are socialized to identify with their professional role and its obligations above all. These roles and obligations, in Freudian terms, are super-ego oriented, resulting in conscience-driven or conscience-guided behavior. Further, this orientation is on person-to-person services; the goals of their activities take on strong moral overtones. The mission—the purpose of the institution—is experienced in terms of facilitating their meeting the eth-ical obligations of their cause.

Given such powerful needs to do good, there is a vast problem in living up to the professional role. Obviously those who prevent them from providing "quality patient care" sets themselves up as targets or scapegoats for ventilat-ing a sense of inadequacy or perhaps even sin. Rules, budget constraints, quality assurance, diagnosis-related groups (DRGs)—all these sorts of things pose a threat that doing good will be harder or that inadequacy in doing it will be verified and made public. Small wonder that we find ourselves subject to vociferous attacks on our motives, our values, our roles and that what seem to be obviously beneficial policies or changes are resisted tooth and nail. The response seems to have been to suppress our own doing good values behind a veil of businesslike professionalism, much to our disadvantage.

Board Suspicions Verified

If hospitals are perceived primarily as value-laden, cause-oriented, ethically superior institutions, as places for the practice of skills that fulfill these values, then administrators should not be surprised to find themselves expendable when the medical professions begin to complain that administrative behavior prevents the organization from carrying out its mission. The seeming injustice and arbitrary nature in which boards carry out medical staff wishes stems not just from recognition that physicians control the revenue, but from sharing their views about the purpose of the hospital. Sensitivities to this mission by the board leads them to quickly side with the physicians against an administrator who appears to "stand in the way" of good medical care (Johnson 1979). Cultivation of purely business values does little to let do-gooders feel inspired or motivated. If we are to be leaders, we must plug into the value system in a deliberate way instead of cultivating an image that places us outside it or even an enemy of it.

Careful Redefinition of the Hospital

The current move into diversification and corporate restructuring carries great risks in terms of diluting the goodwill hospitals have enjoyed in the public eye and from the employees. Workers no longer accept low pay and poor working conditions as a just sacrifice to the cause. A variety of factors explain that, but one frequently overlooked is the loss of the ability to identify oneself with a cause through the institution. Self-sacrifice is not expected in a business. The more removed one's task is from the cause of alleviation of suffering and the more it seems bureaucracy, machinery, or bigness inhibits this work, the more likely one will be unwilling to endure unnecessary sacrifices. However, let's examine what we say in the mad dash toward diversification, corporate restructuring, and the business model.

Moving into nontraditional revenue sources (Goldsmith 1982; Kernaghan 1982) such as manufacturing of products, real estate, restaurants, hotels, health spas, or even the new prevention and wellness services requires a restatement of the hospital mission.[7] Mergers, acquisitions, development of

389

multihospital systems, and corporate restructuring in general create, for these super-ego people, a problem regarding the hospital's purpose and their relation to it (Cunningham 1983). To the extent management seems to become more powerful and more able to control their activities, they will be threatened and feel their ability to fulfill the cause is being undermined. The changes prospective reimbursement will require in administrator-physician relations is especially threatening for this reason. However, that topic requires a separate article.

If corporate restructuring is perceived as making medical professionals accountable to a chief executive instead of to the standards of the role, it will be fiercely resisted, with the expectation of administrator demise or a curtailment of authority (Johnson 1979; Cunningham 1983). To the extent management is involved in the heady game of setting up nontraditional services, nontraditional revenue sources, or involved in the multihospital system game, he or she will be perceived as empire building, which is at least suspicious, and perceived as threatening if this may result in power to influence medical decisions. If these actions are justified in terms of institutional survival or progress and no clear and present danger is perceived by the medical staff or the employees, the games will still be seen as empire building or be seen indifferently. In any case, these activities will be seen as tangential or irrelevant to the cause and make it harder to identify the hospital with that cause— a loss of goodwill, conceived internally. But this need not be.

Redefinition Can Confirm Shared Values

The redefinition of the hospital presents a superb opportunity to gain respect, tie into the value system, and get the entire hospital organized psychologically and normatively around a mission that might help overcome resistance, fear of interference, and disparagement of the chief executive. The quickest way to begin is to emphasize how a hospital differs from a business in mission values, types of employees, why employees work there, and so on. School with master's in health administration programs would do well to conside this. Quite frankly, the emphasis on the business model and quantitative methods seems popular because it is easier to teach. Values are somehow soft where bottom lines are hard. Relating to people is far more difficult to teach than management science, finance, marketing, and the like.

When relating is taught in terms of negotiation or motivation or the management of change, it is frequently done in a context of manipulation, conceiving the other as an adversary to be overcome or the mere means to an end.[8] Learning to relate to people in a manipulative way is easily identified by cause-oriented persons who do not subscribe to that view of how to get along.

Certainly it does nothing to inspire confidence as a leader to them, for a leader must share the values of the cause. We are being taught to squander the ingredients that make us leaders in more than title: a shared ethics with our colleagues in medicine, one that emphasizes how hospitals and health professions differ from businesses and business professions (Cunningham 1983; Peters and Wacker 1982; Long 1976).[9]

Regaining Confidence

Being credible to suspicious or hostile physicians or nurses about the fact that you share their commitment, their values, but from a different perspective, begins with the self-analysis noted earlier and is worth emphasizing again. Why did you choose this field? If it was a second or third choice, what relationship did it have to those first choices that led you to select it? Why do you stay? Besides reasons such as prestige, fairly good money, having a position of power, I suspect most will agree we chose hospital work because there is a fundamental, gut-level congruence of the work with our values. We want a role in helping people and that is what hospitals do. Probe the psyche of a dedicated hospital worker, or even a burned-out one, and you find a do-gooder. Why should we hide it behind some sort of model of ourselves as business people? Sure we are in business, but it is what is special about this business that made us choose it. Let us emphasize that specialness and find a way to join hands with doctors and nurses because of it, instead of crossing swords. Our professional identity should build on the value in helping those who need it, as should our hospital mission and any redefinition it may get.[10]

Tremendous opportunities emerge from the decision to flaunt your specialness and your values, opportunities physicians and nurses have used to distance themselves from us. The project of clarifying the hospital's mission should be one that involves all employees, beginning at orientation. Learning what a place is, what it stands for, why it is there, and continually showing it, serves as a tremendous motivation to get people to pull together, put up with adversity, and even to define their role—perhaps even themselves—in terms of that mission.

Diversifications, mergers, corporate restructuring, new services—all of these projects present an opportunity to inquire again into the mission, inquire with the employees and the medical staff in a way that reaffirms the congruence of these changes with the mission and shows that the mission statement is a living document. In a certain sense, this is like zero-based budgeting, but on a value level—why are we here, what are we doing, should it continue, and how much of it? Now, this may be valuable in becoming worthy of leadership in the eyes of medical workers, but it will become more powerful

391

if the role of hospital leadership is seen as part of the proper role of a health services administrator per se and not just as a quality found in a particular administrator. This means doing some hard thinking about professional identity, what it says to the outsider, and what we have to do to get it accepted such that the failure to be a leader is seen as a failure in fulfilling the professional role instead of something that was never expected anyway.

Leadership Is More Than Administration

An extremely important reason the administrator must not only take, but earn, the right to a leadership role is because external pressures are forcing the hospital into a reconsideration of its mission in order to survive. There is no need to belabor this point or the reasons for it (see Wesbury 1980). The point is that physicians no longer embody the mission of the new hospital, and it falls to the chief executive officer to rise to the occasion. Prospective reimbursement will add force to this shift upward in status. And rise it must, for if this analysis is correct we are seen neither by the public, by the medical staff, or by professional or nonprofessional employees as embodying this new mission, which is itself not yet clear. To achieve a consensus on the mission of a health services facility, to seek to exemplify the ethical ideals of that mission in personal conduct, to belong to a profession that encourages and supports these two goals, that is professional development in a sense that properly transcends the mere emphasis on competency at business skills. And this is necessary to become a leader and be followed, or to get beyond the problems of a role-oriented organization in which we are obstacles or enemies and begin molding a task-oriented organization characterized by shared values, trust, and role flexibility so that success for the nurses, for example, is not understood as a victory over physicians and administrators (Levinson 1979). How does one do this? There are three levels of inquiry: What are my reasons for doing hospital work? What does my profession seem to expect of me? What really is the mission of my hospital, or even hospitals in general, and what can I do to get it to meet that function? When these are reasonably clear, then the ongoing effort at achieving consensus and being recognized as the leader may begin.

Building a Values Consensus

The first level, the individual inquiry into values, has already been mentioned. Openness, instead of manipulation, seems to be highly valued as an ingredient in building the confidence base for recognition as a leader (Foster 1982; Wesbury 1980; Parrish 1977; Levinson 1979).[11] Second-level inquiries lead to the profession itself: What do we expect of ourselves as administrators? What are our yardsticks of success? Our values? Our obligations?

The superficial answer is that professional success is evidenced by promotions, increasing responsibility, higher pay, advancement in the American College of Hospital Administrators, holding office in various hospital associations, etc. Success for a hospital, in our eyes, is an extension of those things by which we measure our professional success: strong financial position, latest equipment, good consensus, competent and loyal workforce and medical staff, expansion of services, perhaps corporate restructuring, the institution being the flag ship in a multihospital system, recognition and respect from colleagues that it is a good hospital, as evidenced by referral patterns, and so on. But lacking in any of these indicators of success for the administrator or the hospital is an evidence of dedication to values, to the cause that motivates other health care workers. Does the professional organization for health care administrators provide that sense of identity, mission, obligation?

Essentially, the American College of Hospital Administrators[12] (ACHA) is the only organization claiming to represent administration in general. It states the goals of the profession in its seven objectives—focusing primarily on competence and education—and eight obligations of individual practitioners—which stress integrity and dutifulness along with helping to advance the profession per se, and it provides a fairly detailed Code of Ethics. The ACHA (1982) now in its 50th year, claims to have had as a goal creating a profession where there was none. Our fellow professionals in the cause do not have the problem of creating a professional identity.

Physicians, who could be said to embody the ethical values of individual medical care, at least in an ideal sense, have a well-recognized ethical tradition that has endured thousands of years. Nurses have a much briefer history as a profession but can look to Florence Nightingale as the model of devotion, care, and self-sacrifice. Nurses can even point to their key role as caregivers since the origin of hospitals as pest houses, places people went to die, or places for the impoverished. Again, there is an ethical ideal that nurses are to strive for. Is there such an ethical ideal available for the administrator?

What the American College of Hospital Administrators Says

The ACHA (1976) publications describe our obligation as to the institution. We are urged to identify ourselves with this role of dedication to the institution. It becomes appropriate to then question the function of the institution. The ACHA refers us to the American Hospital Association's (AHA) Hospital Code of Ethics. There we recognize multiple responsibilities—patient care, the community, the employees, the medical staff, and so on. This multiplicity of responsibilities, this conflicting constituency (Bell 1975) includes all the above but also creditors, suppliers, regulatory agencies, third party payers of all kinds, perhaps the other elements in our multihospital system, the various associations, and even shared service oranizations. It is this incredible diversity of conflicting responsibilities that puts the chief executive in a position of authority to be a leader, to pull together a values consensus on how the institution shall represent itself externally and internally to these constituencies. But while the board, physicians, nurses, and other employees may recognize the difficulty of this task, it is not likely that stating it in this way will result in them sensing many shared values with us. Nor is it likely to give rise to such sharing if we appear to be deliberately adopting business values and attitudes, attitudes that will seem less than pure at their best (Levinson 1979).[13]

Perhaps some self-analysis is again useful here. Did we get into hospital management primarily because we like the management of complex organizations or did we get into hospital management because we wanted to help people through management? Use of power—use of management skills to help people in the aggregate—seems no less laudable than direct patient care. Surely we can point, if only statistically, to patients saved, patients getting well quicker, patients avoiding iatrogenic infections, people served better by new services and new equipment, employee or patient or family benefits resulting from shared services, diversification, multihospital systems, and the like. Since the belief is that power corrupts, we must show how we have used it to help in terms they understand—benefits to individuals. Our work may benefit large numbers of people we will never see, but that is no reason for hands-on care providers to consider us as having noncaring, nonhumanistic values.

Indeed, business today is moving to try to show that good business is compatible with such values, not greed, exploitation, empire building, nor ruthless achievement of profits at any moral, human, or environmental cost. Yet we foolishly squander our possibilities for being viewed as leaders by cultivating a business image, an image crusading do-gooders will see in the worst possible light because we often have to control their spare-no-expense approach. It will be tough winning their confidence, but getting them to think about the hospital mission and seeing how your values as a professional mesh with theirs, even if the perspectives differ significantly, is a start. In other words, the professional obligation of the health care administrator is helping people, not just patients, and helping them through the skillful use of management techniques. It gives a point of leverage. Now, how does one go about building this consensus?

Specific Techniques—Professional Development

Administrators are experts at achieving results and discovering things by indirect methods. The following ideas should show that developing a hospital mission that helps us to achieve a sharing of values, a task orientation, is not too different from launching other touchy projects.

A good place to begin to find a commonality of values is with your subordinates or with other administrators over lunch or drinks. One need not appear foolish by asking why someone chose hospital work when other work might have been less stressful and more lucrative. If most of us are closet crusaders, getting that confession out into the open serves as an important basis for values consensus. Probe their thoughts and your own about what it is about hospitals that is special and inspires a bit of dedication. Discuss the value conflicts Levinson (1979) and Johnson (1979) point out among administration and both the board and the medical staff, not to even speak of most of the employees. Note reasons for the conflicts and note places you really share values. Shared values can be a powerful force, and savvy managers will discover them or create them and do their best to make them meaningful. Such a source of goodwill should be looked on as a valuable resource not to be squandered. In terms of management, this phase could be considered professional development. The next stage in getting you in the leadership role is organizational development (Schermerhorn 1979).[14]

Organizational Development

Organizational development must begin indirectly to properly build a credibility base. At appropriately informal times, created if need be, the administrator might begin asking physicians, department heads, key nurses, long-term employees, etc., why they are in medical or hospital work. Assuming patient care values are the typical response, the very fact that you showed concern about values should be a step toward confidence building.

Of course, if the context of the hospital's administrative style is one of reciprocal manipulations, such questions will be suspicious and threatening, leading to second guessing about motives. Consensus building in this area is not like putting together a coalition of self-interested groups for a specific purpose; it is instead the creation of a group by establishing common values.

For these questions to be confidence builders, there must have been a tradition of openness already. Discussion can then lead into comparisons of views about the purpose of hospitals, especially in the changed environment of today. An administrator must be sensitive enough to the professional and ethical obligations of direct care professionals not to become agitated if his or her role is described in support function terms. Being in a support position does not mean being a lackey. Our goal is to help people through the management of a complex organization dedicated itself to helping people.

As confidence builds and these discussions continue, the administrator may discover an awareness of apparent value conflicts between the roles and then find ways to prove the essential convergence of his or hers with theirs. At the same time, the administration may find out the length of the row that must be hoed before these value conflicts are overcome sufficiently enough for him or her to be the leader. It is important here to be sensitive to the fact that they may suspect your values because of the strong business coloring. Further, their values have a much longer tradition and a profoundly greater degree of public respect. It is your values that must be seen as meshing with theirs. Perhaps opportunities will arise to point out how your perspective has long-range usefulness in helping them fulfill their obligations.

After these discussions have been going on for awhile, perhaps even with board members, depending on the situation, some will suggest following up on these questions about values, role conflicts, shared goals, and the hospital mission at staff meetings. These issues will interest them, as indeed they should, if the seeds planted on that row have been tended well.

The progression from staff meetings to departmental meetings should follow, with the administrative staff helping to explore the questions. If the process works, there should be less fighting over turf and more task-oriented behavior. Causing this to happen means breaking down suspicions and encouraging a sense of common goals, resting on a foundation of common values. It means breaking out of the zero-sum game mentality where every department in the hospital tries to maximize its position at the expense of the others. This process will be ongoing, but opportunities to find and use common values will be frequent as hospitals try to find their way in a rapidly changing and often hostile environment.

Merging Ethics and Management

Wesbury (1980) notes that, if we are to fill this new leadership role that circumstance has cast upon us, "our personal values and those of our institutions must rise to the surface and become a part of the decisions that we must make." This involves testing oneself and one's institution, not just developing slogans or developing mission statements that are filed away. As Wesbury (1980) says, "Stimulate in your own mind problem situations. Think through what your role might be in these situations and the possible out-comes...Discuss ethical situations openly with a variety of people on a frequent basis." Discussions of cases at staff meetings or with different departments can bring role conflicts to the surface and present opportunities for everyone to emerge with a sense of a bigger picture. Some examples illustrate the point.

Medical professionals are presumably committed to the ideals of informed consent and protection of individual autonomy. Present a case that shows a conflict between doing good, from their point of view, at the cost of informed consent and autonomy. After a discussion of the medical uses of information point out your own commitment to openness and accuracy in dealings with them, how that ties in with their values and repudiates the view that management, like some paternalistic medical professionals, will be manipulative about information, seeing it as a tool to their own ends. Most medical professionals have probably never thought about how the values of informed consent apply to management. Having reviewed the Codes of Ethics of the professionals with whom you are speaking will bolster your prestige and keep them honest. Most professionals know as little about their Code as you probably do about the ACHA code. Of course, these Codes are not laws from on high, but subject to interpretation or perhaps even rejection. Or maybe the Code does not go far enough. Working these problems through in a group is an effort to reach a consensus on values that transcends mere role identity and is a major element in gaining the consensus you will need to function as a leader.

Discussions about the right to refuse treatment, death with dignity, and euthanasia may get some consensus going about the possibilities of more humane care, respect for persons, and the like. This could be channeled into a desire to open a hospice. Your homework should be done ahead of discussions that might lead to the suggestion of a hospice. If the numbers will not allow it to contribute, be ready to explain it. Many discussions about values may lead to discussion of specific services. This presents an excellent opportunity to bring up questions about resource allocations and the obligations of the professions and the institution, and so on.

Choosing the Right Cases to Discuss

Dilemmas about resource allocations are generally understood by medical personnel as agonizing over which patient gets the life-saving equipment when there is too little of it. This sets up the situation with you being the "fall guy" for why they cannot do their job or leads to talk about rights, government stinginess, the "real world," and so on. Instead of letting this happen, guide discussion to allocation cases that pertain to decisions about opening entirely new services. Here the patients are in the abstract and you can get the direct care people to think more in terms to which you are accustomed.

Use the new service case—perhaps a burn unit, or a pediatric intensive care unit—as an opportunity to discuss the realities of third-party reimbursement and the ideal of highest quality, state-of-the-art, patient care. The impact of giving medical practitioners a virtual blank check to use for the benefit of their patients may have been great for their crusading super-egos and their patients, but certainly turns its back on social responsibility. Getting them to recognize a social responsibility and then to feel the moral dilemmas of a value conflict in their profession may do wonders when you point out your own value conflicts and how they are no less troubling in the administrator's office. Particularly good cases are those that show how extreme emphasis on doing good for an individual patient or perhaps even specific types of patients consumes so many resources that it renders problematic the ability to handle other patients in the future. The issue of inequity will trouble crusaders, and certainly you can show how your job requires balancing and weighing these equity issues in a way that may be more responsible than what they have been doing. Some good things can result from discussion of resource allocations that are a step removed from their ordinary specific patient concerns.

Cases That Support Management Goals

Something as simple as the need to be more reasonable in cooperating with a shared service organization or even group purchasing may suddenly be perceived as having the moral overtones of social responsibility. Representatives of multihospital systems can explain why these forms of organization reflect an effort to be socially responsible in the sense that effectiveness and efficiency help the community and the nation and assist the direct caregiver by enhancing institutional viability. Making all these points may take a series of discussions, but it will be interesting to these crusaders if you continually relate what you are doing back to values they recognize and acknowledge. Diversification into nontraditional revenue sources must be handled the same way.

A hotel can be seen as showing a real interest in the families of the patients. Apartments and real estate firms can show an interest in the employees. Manufacturing can be justified not only in cost terms (if it can be this must be demonstrable) but in terms of quality control. Profits can be seen as not evil but as used to help them help patients. Here openness about how money moves is important.

It can be surprising to discover how little direct care professionals know about the financial side of hospitals. Remember, concern with money is a pejorative in their eyes. Even if it has been previously explained, they may have tuned it out. Relate it to value issues that help them do good by seeing why what you are doing is coherent with those concerns. Explain third-party reimbursement, cross subsidization, costs versus charges, the different sorts of third party payers and what they pay. Just remember their common denominator is not the bottom line, but values, the cause. You cannot go back to values enough.

If you succeed, your difficult job will be respected as one that has values like theirs. Get *them* to emphasize how a hospital is different from a business. Get *them* to recognize that hospitals must change to survive. And get *them* to see how what you must do does not violate that specialness. They may well suggest and then support new services you want. Those who see how to fulfill their values through specific projects can become very enthusiastic crusaders. If their suggestions are financially or politically ill advised, be prepared to explain it to them in value terms.

Retreats, continuing education, seminars, consultants, all the usual educational tools for the management of change are likely to be employed as the process gets rolling, especially at larger institutions or multihospital systems. Bringing out the values involved and their congruence may require the help of people skilled in values analysis. They can serve as coaches to the administrator, help facilitate discussion, provide feedback on how well the discussions met the needs of the administrator and keep the discussions on track. But it is *discussion* not lecture, that is needed.

Success in this project occurs when the administrator is recognized as the leader, the one who inspires, who embodies the ethical ideals, the obligations of the whole institution, a person "of unimpeachable character. . .that will make integrity his way of life (Foster 1982). A tall order indeed, but crusaders require goodness in their leaders, and it will take people who are willing to fill tall orders to keep hospitals on track in the days ahead. Levinson describes the administrator-leader as therapist for the whole institution, whose tools are the abilities to reach consensus on values and effectively use management skills from that base (Levinson 1979). Presenting the administrator as a value therapist is likely to help him or her achieve recognition as a leader, far more than merely presenting him or herself as a business person and the institution as merely a business.

Notes

1. For representative articles, see H. L. Hirsch, "Health-Care Is A Business!" *Medical Trial Technique Quarterly* 25, no. 1 (Summer 1978): 77-83; Richard McQueen, "Hospitals Need Business Instincts Too," *Health Care* 4, no. 10 (October 1979): 58; Alan L. Applebaum, "Hospitals Must Be Businesslike," *Hospitals* 53, no. 21 (1 November 1979): 107–8, 111–12; Richard L. Johnson, "The Wobbly Three-Legged Stool," *Trustee* (May 1976): 9–14.

2.   See also a collection of Cunningham's articles in *The Healing Mission and the Business Ethic*, Chicago: Pluribus Press, 1982.

3.   In his speech, Wesbury argues that technological changes, social changes, and the involvement of third parties has changed the health care system such that administrators are the logical leaders. And leadership involves a clarity about values and mission we seem to have lost in our concerns over the problems management itself presents, a problem he wishes to redress.

4.   This article should be obligatory reading; it points out the root causes of many of our frustrations in a very clear way.

5.   Cunningham notes that 20 years ago the difference in values between these two sorts of ownership belied an underlying philosophic difference. This opinion still breaks out, which perhaps the emergence of the Federation documents, in spite of counsels to the effect that the phrase "not-for-profit" is a mere technical legal term. See also Long 1976.

6.   Long (1976) recognizes this same set of beliefs and urges they be transcended because of the real needs for substantial return on investment in order to survive.

7.   These articles point out some of the sorts of diversifications and the issues to be considered. While both mention the need to be consistent with the hospital mission, the emphasis is on how to do it and make money, requiring administrators to "expand the limits of their vision beyond the traditional hospital role of patient caregiver" (Kernaghan 1982). As noted, such expansion should not risk losing goodwill.

8.   That this is often the way it is does not excuse us for letting it continue or for seminars or other training to try to legitimize it. In a Fall 1978 *Health Care Management Review* article, "The Power Broker—Prototype of the Hospital Chief Executive," Richard L. Johnson (1978) exemplifies to the extreme the values, or manipulation, prompting in the "letters to the editor" criticisms by a physisician (see the Summer 1979 issue) and approval of its accuracy by an administrator (see the Winter 1979 issue). While I totally agree with its accuracy, the long-range consequences will only further alienate us from our values and prevent any likelihood of becoming a leader in the eyes of medical workers. As the sociologists Peter L. Berger and Thomas Luckman, *The Social Construction of Reality* (New York: Doubleday, 1967), point out, "If this phenomenon becomes widely distributed, the institutional order as a whole begins to take on the character of a network of reciprocal manipulations." The ensuing distrust, suspicion, second guessing, and cynicism do little to enchance an environment conducive to leadership or patient care. The accuracy of Johnson's article should be a matter of major concern, not applause. It is also noteworthy that the very good article of his, Johnson (1976) points our that many administrators "say that the fun has been taken out of their profession." Certainly in a network of reciprocal manipulations the sense of working together in a common cause would seem to end. Perhaps it is not just fun we have lost, but a sense of values.

9.   Cunningham (1983) argues that the only difference in the hospital and physician ethic is one of application. Hospitals have collective obligations; physicians have

individual obligations. Peters and Wacker (1982) describe this collective obligation as to the community. Long (1976) makes a similar point for nonprofit hospitals.

10.   The redefinition of the hospital in terms of these values is what Cunningham (1976) and Peters and Wacker (1982) advocate.

11.   Levinson (1979) is emphatic that administrators understand their own values and their conflicts and assess their fitness for the leadership role in terms of the values it requires

12.   The organization was unsuccessful in its 1981 effort to change the name to the American College of Health-Care Administrators, perhaps noteworthy of our own ambivalence about the changes in the mission of the hospital and our role in it.

13.   Levinson notes that direct care medical professionals pride themselves on not dirtying their hands with business and politics, activities a leader must not only do well, but take pride in. My own recent experiences bear out that academics are even more extreme than medical professionals. It is interesting that to those in business, being accused of having dirty hands is a major insult, whereas to these more or less outsiders any activities undertaken primarily for personal or institutional gain are somehow suspect. Levinson points out that recognition of these value differences is a major step toward directing them into a shared set of institutional values, operating under transcendent but meaningful mission.

14.   Schermerhorn uses these terms and provides a checklist for effective change. His analysis is not targeted to values, which presents some different problems in terms of top management commitment.

References

American College of Hospital Administrators. *A Brief Description*. Chicago: The College, 1982.

_____. *Code of Ethics*. Chicago: The College, 1976.

Bell, Daniel. "The Revolution in Rising Entitlements." *Fortune* (April 1975): 99.

Cunningham, Robert M., Jr. "More Than a Business: Are Hospitals Forgetting Their Basic Mission." *Hospitals* 57, no. 2 (16 January 1983): 88–90.

Foster, John T. "A Letter to a Young CEO." *Hospital & Health Services Administration* 27, no. 3 (1982): 57–64.

Goldsmith, Jeff. "Diversification." *Hospitals* 56, no. 23 (1 December 1982): 68–73.

Johnson, Richard L. "The Wobbly Three-Legged Stool." *Trustee* (May 1976): 9–14.

Kernaghan, Salvinija G. "Nontraditional Revenue." *Hospitals* 56, no. 23 (1 December 1982): 75–81.

Levinson, Harry. "The Changing Role of the Hospital Administrator." *Health Care Management Review* 1, no. 1 (Winter 1979): 79–89.

Long, Hugh W. "Valuation as Criterion in Not-for-Profit Decision-Making." *Health Care Management Review* 1, no. 3 (Summer 1976): 34.

Parrish, William C. "Is Fear a Part of Your Management Style?" *Health Care Management Review* 2, no. 3 (Summer 1977): 17–24.

Peters, Joseph P., and Ronald C. Wacker. "Strategic Planning: Hospital Strategic Planning Must Be Rooted in Values and Ethics." *Hospitals* 56, no. 11 (16 June 1982): 90–98.

Schermerhorn, John R., Jr. "The Health Care Manager's Role in Promoting Change." *Health Care Management Review* 4, no. 1 (Winter 1979): 71–84.

Wesbury, Stuart A. "Ethics in Health Services Administration: A Case for Constant Reevaluation." 8th Annual Reverend J. Flanagan, S. J. Lecture in Hospital Administration, Saint Louis University Alumni Association, 19 March 1980.

Chapter 23

The Ethical Imperative in Health Services Governance and Management

Kurt Darr
Beaufort B. Longest, Jr.
Jonathon S. Rakich

Kurt Darr is a professor of hospital administration and of health care sciences, The George Washington University, Washington, DC. He is a Fellow of the College. Beaufort B. Longest, Jr., is a professor of health services administration and of business administration, and Director of the Health Policy Institute, the University of Pittsburgh, Pittsburgh, Pennsylvania. He is a Fellow of the College. Jonathon S. Rakich is a professor of management and of health services administration, The University of Akron, Akron, Ohio. He is a Faculty Associate of the College.

This article was published in *Hospital & Health Services Administration* 31, no. 2 (March/April 1986).

W hat is ethical in this situation? Which interests should be considered? These questions increasingly affect those governing and managing health services organizations. This article suggests a construct in which to consider them.

Some may see a direct correspondence between law and ethics, that is to say, "whatever is legal is also ethical, and vice versa." This need not be the case and is not necessarily true for several reasons. The most important is that law provides only the minimum standard of performance, either positive or negative (but usually the latter), expected from members of society. Professions demand compliance with the law but add other duties and hold members to a higher standard. This means that even when the law does not require a certain activity of any citizen, including a specific group, a profession's code may. This makes an activity legal, but not necessarily ethical. A model showing the relationship of law to ethics has been developed by Verne Henderson (1982). Figure 1 presents a matrix of the possible combinations of legal, illegal, ethical, and unethical.

This article discusses the administrative ethical aspects of issues, all of which have biomedical components as well. Issues analyzed and for which preventive measures or solutions are suggested are fiduciary duty, conflicts of interest, confidential information, resource allocation, and consent. Primarily biomedical ethical issues such as medical experimentation, death and dying, and abortion are not considered.

The technical and complex nature of medical care severely compromises the patient's ability to judge it and effectively interact with caregivers. This highlights the need for everyone in the organization to protect and further the patients' interests, whether affected by biomedical or administrative ethics. Since all are moral agents whose decisions and actions have moral implications, this is the ethical imperative for those who govern and manage health services organizations.

Guidance for Leadership

Personal Ethic

Those in positions of leadership have already developed a personal morality—a *weltanschauung*—to guide their lives. This is their personal ethic, and those leading health services organizations consider this an important part of their professional lives. To effectively identify and understand, but most importantly to solve, ethical problems—whether biomedical or administrative—one must have a well-developed personal ethic. Leaders, as well as followers, in health services organizations apply this ethic in the context of their organization's

Figure 1
A Conceptual Framework

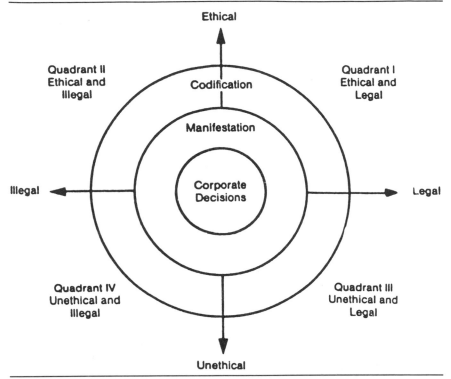

Source: Henderson, Verne E. "The Ethical Side of Enterprise," *Sloan Management Review* 23, no. 3 (Spring 1982) 37–47.

philosophy—that statement of morality developed by the organization. A compatibility between the two is important to developing an effective corporate culture.

Principles

Implicit in any personal ethic adequate to effectively solve ethical problems will be the presence of four basic principles as they affect the patient: autonomy, beneficence, nonmaleficence, and justice (Beauchamp and Childress 1983). It is patients the health services organization serves, and all actions must be measured against the goal of protecting them and furthering their interests.

405

Autonomy means that the wishes of self-legislating (competent) patients are followed, that they are involved in their own care to the extent they choose to be, and that when patients are not self-legislating because they are children or of diminished competence, the organization has special procedures for surrogate decision making or substituted judgments. Autonomous patients are treated with respect; it is unethical to lie to them. The principle of autonomy is especially important in terms of consent and use of confidential patient information.

Beneficence requires a positive duty to contribute to the patient's welfare. This principle has a long and noble tradition in the health professions and is equally applicable to the organization's governance and management. Tom Beauchamp and James Childress (1983) divide beneficence into two components: provision of benefit (including prevention and removal of harm) and balance benefits and harms. The latter can be used only to consider the costs and benefits of a treatment or action, not to override the other principles.

The third principle to be included in a personal ethic is nonmaleficence, a duty that obliges us to refrain from inflicting harm. This harm can be mental as well as physical and is readily extended into an organizational setting to issues such as patient privacy. While beneficence is a positive duty, nonmaleficence is negative—refraining from doing something that harms. Beneficence and nonmaleficence affect governing body members and managers in issues such as fiduciary duty, use of confidential information, and conflicts of interest.

Justice is the final principle important to a personal ethic. A major problem is defining what is just or fair. Egalitarians say that it is just to provide like amounts of services to all with similar needs. Libertarians stress merit and achievement as measures of what is just. Aristotle asserted that "equals" should be treated equally, "unequals" unequally. An interpretation of Aristotle's view means that most medical care should go to those in greatest need, since in terms of health they are situated unequally. There is broad latitude in developing the specific content of the principle of justice, but there are limits nonetheless. Considerations of justice have most apparent application in resource allocation.

These principles are found explicitly or implicitly in codes of ethics propounded by various professional groups. The American College of Healthcare Executives Code of Ethics is among the most comprehensive, but even it is specific and precise *only* on conflicts of interest. Governing body members and managers should look to organizational philosophy and professional codes for assistance, but they can only be effective leaders if they have a well-developed personal ethic that includes attention to the principles of autonomy, beneficence, nonmaleficence, and justice.

Ethical Issues Affecting Governance and Management

Fiduciary Duty

Fiduciary is a concept that arose from Roman jurisprudence and means that certain obligations and duties are present in a relationship. A fiduciary is someone with superior knowledge or position, and neither may be used ethically for personal gain. This requires managers to act only in the organization's best interests, with the caveat that the independent duty of the moral agent toward the patient cannot be ignored.

Governing body members of both for-profit and not-for-profit corporations have a fiduciary duty. The legal standard for meeting this obligation is more demanding when governing body members are true trustees—that is, they hold title to the assets and administer them to further the purposes of the trust.

> Loyalty means that the individuals must put the interest of the corporation above all self-interest, a principle based on the biblical doctrine that no man can serve two masters. Specifically, no trustee is permitted to gain any secret profits for himself, to accept bribes, or to compete with the corporation.
>
> The fiduciary duty of responsibility means that members of the governing board must exercise reasonable care, skill, and diligence proportionate to the circumstances in every activity of the board. In other words, the trustees can be held personally liable for negligence, which can be an affirmative act of commission, or omission (Southwick 1978).

The legal standard sets the tone for ethical guidelines but should be considered only a minimum. Managers are not fiduciaries in the same sense as are governing body members, but they have similar ethical responsibilities in the terms of loyalty and a duty to avoid conflicts of interest. The American College of Healthcare Executives Code recognizes these duties.

Conflicts of Interest

Conflicts of interest are major sources of problems in health services organizations. They occur when someone has sets of obligations and duties that are inconsistent—they are in conflict—and meeting one set means abrogating another. Accepting extravagant gifts is an obvious example. Others are more subtle.

Has the manager who uses a position of influence and power to gain personal aggrandizement of title, position, and salary at the expense of patient care or other organizational activities acted ethically? Is the manager who is lax in implementing a more effective patient consent process behaving ethically? Is it ethical for a governing body member whose physical and mental capacities are diminished to remain on the board? Is the manager who insists that all reports to governance be prepared in a manner that inadequately shows negative results behaving ethically? Is it ethical for a governing body member or manager who suspects there are problems in the department of surgery to fail to prove or disprove this suspicion? While problems of these types may have legal implications, all raise ethical questions.

The difficulty with conflict of interest is that many types are very subtle and it takes continued questioning and self-analysis to identify them. They are likely to increase as competition intensifies. The College's Code and the American Hospital Association's (AHA) statement on conflicts of interest suggest ways of reducing or eliminating the problem. They concentrate on disclosure of real or potential conflicts of interest, divestiture of outside interests that might cause a conflict to arise, seeking guidance from the governing body when questions arise, and not participating in or attempting to influence any matter in which conflicts might exist.

Confidential Information

Any unauthorized use of confidential information about the patient or organization is unethical. The most common misuse occurs when employees and medical staff gossip about patients. Though this may seem innocent, it is not, and discussion of patients should be on a need-to-know basis only.

Careless internal use of patient information is the most common problem regarding confidential information, but misusing it in other ways receives more public attention. This latter abuse occurs when patient- or organization-confidential information is used to benefit an individual or other persons with whom that individual is associated or related. Examples include disclosing information about governing-body decision making so that associates can make advantageous sales or purchases, giving or selling patient medical information to the media or attorneys, and making marketing strategies available to competitors, whether for profit or revenge.

An example with potential for both conflicts of interest and misuse of confidential information is found when the health services manager serves on the governing body of another health services provider or planning agency. Allegiance to one's organization conflicts when another's certificate of need or marketing activity is considered. A more subtle problem arises when those in such a situation become privy to information important for business purposes or planning in their own organization. Regretfully, the importance of that type of confidential information in a competitive environment may necessitate that managers and governing body members avoid all involvement with any potentially competing organization.

The College's Code views misuse of confidential information broadly and prohibits all that are inappropriate. It is immaterial that the organization is unharmed.

Resource Allocation

The process of resource allocation has recently received more attention as an activity raising ethical issues. Whether macro or micro, it necessitates making decisions—literally who gets what, when, and how. This means making judgments about importance, worth, usefulness, merit, need, societal value, and the like. Sometimes when the government is involved, decisions are also based on political motives and ideals.

Like governments, all health services organizations make macro allocation decisions. Micro allocation is usually a function of the physician's willingness to refer, the patient's access to services and technologies, and sometimes, economic considerations. Often, micro decision making is guided (in a sense, prejudged) by policies and procedures of government as well as the organization.

Numerous theories have been developed about making macro allocation decisions. At one extreme are those who argue all technologies must be available to all persons; a corollary of this hyperegalitarian position is that if services or a technology are not available to all, none should receive them. This position is based on the concept that each human being has inherent dignity and thus a right to receive equal health services. Conversely, there are those for whom health services are not a right to be guaranteed by society; rather, they are an earned privilege. This hyperindividualistic position also holds that health services providers have no obligation to those who cannot pay, unless they choose of their own free will and humanitarian instinct to provide care. Between these extremes is a view that society is obligated to develop, encourage, and perhaps even provide health services in limited situations. Medicare and Medicaid are examples where such a position has been adopted.

Theories about allocating exotic life-saving treatments on a micro basis— i.e., to individual patients—have been developed by James Childress (1970) and Nicholas Rescher (1969). These theories aid decision making about which patients get what. Childress (1970) rejects subjective criteria such as future contributions and past record of performance saying that such comparisons demean and run counter to the inherent dignity of the human being. He argues that a system that views as equals all persons needing a certain treatment recognizes human worth, and once medical criteria are used to determine need, opportunities for a scarce treatment should be available first come, first served, or alternatively, on a random selection basis, such as a lottery (1969).

Rescher's (1969) schema is two-tiered: The first is basic screening and includes factors such as constituency served (service area), progress of science (benefit of advancing science), and prospect of success by type of treatment or recipient—for example, denying renal dialysis to the very young or old. The second tier deals with individuals and uses biomedical factors (relative likelihood of success for that patient and life expectancy) and the social aspects such as family role, potential future contributions, and past services rendered. If all actors are equal, a random selection process is used for the final choice. Social aspects are the most difficult. They are heavily dependent on value judgments and cause ethical dilemmas when true scarcity exists. For example, the shortage of donor kidneys raises questions about the appropriateness of foreign nationals on transplantation waiting lists.

Each micro allocation theory has advantages and disadvantages. Yet, it provides guidelines that permit the issues to be addressed in an organized and predictable fashion. This may not result in decisions that satisfy everyone, but it has the advantage of systematizing the frameworks for decision making. Public awareness of how choices are made is an important attribute in a democracy.

Consent

The concept of consent began at law as a recognition of one's right to be free from nonconsensual touching. The ethical relationship expands this right and includes the principle of autonomy—self-determination. It also reflects the special trust and confidence (a fiduciary relationship) between physician and patient, as well as that between those who govern and manage the organization and the patient. Inherent in consent is a view of the equality and dignity of human beings. Its emphasis on patients' rights or sovereignty is an idealized view and contravenes long traditions of medical paternalism that put the physician in the role of authoritarian figure who makes decisions in the patient's best interests (President's Commission for the Study of Ethical Problems in Medicine and Biomedical Behavioral Research 1982). Such a history suggests the difficulties inherent in perfecting the principle of autonomy.

The legal minimum requires full disclosure about the nature of the condition, all significant facts about it, and explanation of likely consequences that might result from treatment or nontreatment. Ethical guidelines build on this base. The principles described above suggest active patient participation. Guidelines developed by the President's Commission for the Study of Ethical Problems in Medicine and Biomedical and Behavioral Research (1982) state that patient sovereignty with complete participation is preferred. The Commission recognized such participation as a goal to be sought rather than a readily achievable relationship.

Organizations generally apply a legally oriented consent process that focuses on self-protection. There is relatively little emphasis on the ethical relationship with the patient. This is legally prudent, but ignores the separate, positive ethical obligation to maximize involvement of patients out of respect for them and recognition of their autonomy.

Solving Administrative Ethical Issues

Organizational Philosophy

A crucial starting point for solving administrative ethical issues is that there be a specific statement of philosophy that defines the organization's reason for existence and the goals it seeks to achieve. Such a philosophy must be sufficiently precise and detailed so performance can be reviewed or, even more preferable, evaluated. Anecdotal information suggests that few health services organizations have an explicitly stated philosophy; fewer have philosophies with components specific enough to measure achievement of them. Nonetheless, an implicit philosophy is identifiable for all organizations.

Decisions and actions of governing body and management have a philosophical basis, even if vague or ill-defined. The lack of a stated philosophy providing a basic point of reference encourages inconsistency and a lack of continuity and may lead to contradictory policies and results. Furthermore, it diminishes the organization's ability to develop an effective corporate culture.

Responsible governing bodies will emphasize in their statements of philosophy and mission, as well as derivative policies, the importance of protecting patients and furthering their interests—an application of the principles of autonomy, beneficence, nonmaleficence, and justice. Accountability will be included as inherent in the independent relationship between organization and patient. This relationship results from the fiduciary duty owed the patient as well as the ethical responsibility to protect patients from harm.

This accountability is broad. Some (Williams and Donnelly 1982) argue it is sufficiently demanding that patients harmed through medical malpractice, but unaware of that harm, should be informed of it by representatives of the organization. A radical view? Perhaps, but one consistent with the high degree of trust the public places in health services organizations and an appropriate measure of the duty that those who govern and manage them should execute in return.

The strategic planning process is also a function of the organization's philosophy, a primary manifestation of which is the mission statement. An organizational philosophy must be articulated before planning objectives can be established. The organization's mission statement reflects ideals—ends thought unattainable—but progress toward which is believed possible (Ackoff 1981). In this respect, perhaps the most difficult aspect is selection of an appropriate balance between social responsibility and economic performance (Webber 1982).

Governance and management are responsible for developing the organization's philosophy and deriving the mission and specific operational plans. In addition, management interprets and implements the plans. The dynamic is clear. The probability of an organization's moral survival is enhanced to the extent there is maximum congruity between its philosophy and expressions of the personal ethic of governance and management. This is not to say professional managers cannot work effectively in an organization where there are variances between personal and organizational ethic. But the duty of loyalty and allegiance to the organization requires governing body members and managers to uphold the organizational philosophy until it is at variance with their personal ethic.

None can disregard their role as moral agents whose actions have consequences for patients and others. If they act unethically even at the behest of organization or superior, it is no defense to argue that they were only following orders.

Institutional Ethics Committees

As conceived, institutional ethics committees considered a terminally ill patient's prognosis and assisted in answering the question about ending life support. This concern with biomedical ethical problems was reflected in their membership and purposes. Here, it is recommended they be used to assist in developing and implementing an organizational philosophy and to assist governance and management in identifying and solving administrative ethical problems.

Robert Veatch (1983) argues ethics committees can and should have various roles, many of them mutually exclusive. Adopting this view, it is apparent that a committee most likely to be effective in administrative ethics will have fewer clinical personnel and more representatives from governance and management. Clinical personnel must be included because research suggesting organizations are most effective when they involve clinicians in management decision making is also likely to apply to solving problems of administrative ethics.

412

A national study conducted by the President's Commission (1983) about the structure, procedures, activities, and effectiveness of biomedical ethics committees in hospitals suggests some useful parallels as well as pitfalls to be avoided in establishing administrative ethics committees. The Commission reported biomedical ethics committees facilitated decision making when they clarified important issues, shaped consistent hospital policies with regard to life support, and provided opportunities for professionals to air disagreements. The committees were not found particularly effective for educating professionals about issues relevant to life-support decisions.

The study also found that only 1 percent of hospitals had committees; on average they reviewed only one case per year. Although specialized ethics committees, specifically infant care review committees, are rapidly growing in number, anecdotal information suggests there are fewer new biomedical ethics committees with general functions than had been predicted.

One President's Commission (1983) finding suggests there are problems with patient autonomy.

> The composition and function of committees identified. . .would not allay many of the concerns of patients' rights advocates about patient representation and control. Committees were clearly dominated by physicians and other health professionals. The majority of committees did not allow patients to attend or request meetings, although family members were more often permitted to do so.

This is a matter affecting resource allocation and consent and should be of vital concern to governance and management.

There is evidence that biomedical ethics committees are most effective when they wait to be consulted rather than interposing themselves. A consultative role means committees make recommendations, not final decisions (Freedman 1981).

Similar limitations may apply in administrative ethics—depending on the specific facts and issues under consideration. Generally, the committee should be proactive in developing and revising the organizational philosophy and in considering macro resource allocation questions. Similarly, it should take the initiative in reviewing and revising the consent process. However, it may choose a more passive role and wait to be consulted in specific instances of conflicts of interest and misuse of confidential information.

The findings of the President's Commission (1983) as to the relative ineffectiveness of biomedical ethics committees in educational activities is puzzling and may be an aberration. The composition and experience of an administrative ethics committee will make it a reservoir of knowledge and expertise, and these resources should be made available to the staff. This will generally add sophistication and improve the quality of ethical decision making. Two recent books provide useful information about establishing institutional ethics committees (Read 1983; Cranford and Doudera 1984).

Ethicists

Many large teaching hospitals, typically those with university affiliations, include ethicists on their staffs. Ethicists are usually doctorally qualified philosophers who are teaching faculty at a university or medical school. Primarily, they participate in solving biomedical ethical issues. There is no reason, however, why their involvement should be limited in that fashion. Ethicists could aid governance and management as well.

Health services organizations interested in obtaining the assistance of an ethicist should not limit their search to medical schools, but should consider all persons with specialized preparation in ethics and its application in the health field. The literature reports that physicians are more likely to ask assistance of an ethicist than an ethics committee. One reason suggested for this is that committees are not seen as cost effective. Similarly, and beyond considerations of efficiency, it may be more palatable for the typical manager to consult with an ethicist to assist in identifying and analyzing the moral obligations and rights and responsibilities bearing on a case than to seek guidance from a committee.

Summary

Organizational philosophies, ethics committees, and ethicists provide assistance to governance and management. But, as with all tools, those who use them must know when there is a problem and when assistance is needed. This requires governing body members and managers to be sophisticated about the presence of ethical problems. Such knowledge comes with education and experience. More important, those who would implement their personal ethic and meet their duties as moral agents must be willing to act. Lacking this, all else is futile.

Conclusion

All decision making and activities of health services organizations contain ethical dimensions, whether administrative or biomedical. In this regard, two problems confront managers and governing bodies. The first is to recognize the presence of administrative ethical issues. The second is to apply analytical and reasoning processes to address them, thereby enhancing the quality of decision making. Applied ethics is an emerging aspect of health services management. Its effective use enhances the purpose for which health services organizations exist.

Economic pressure from cost cutting by third party payers and increased competitiveness affect all health services organizations, but especially hospitals. Governing bodies and managers may be tempted or feel compelled to take actions that negatively affect patients in terms of the principles of autonomy, beneficence, nonmaleficence, and justice. To do so puts them in derogation of their independent moral duty to protect the patient; and, in so doing, they fail to honor the ethical imperative. The potential conflict between economic interests and patient care considerations are not far below the surface in the patient relationship; for those who govern and manage health services organizations, the ethical implications are enormous.

References

Ackoff, Russell L. *Creating the Corporate Future*. New York: John Wiley & Sons, 1981.

Beauchamp, Tom L., and James F. Childress. *Principles of Biomedical Ethics*, 2d ed. New York: Oxford University Press, 1983.

Childress, James F. "Who Shall Live When Not All Can Live?" *Soundings, An Interdisciplinary Journal* 53, no. 4 (Winter 1970).

Cranford, Ronald E., and A. Edward Doudera, eds. *Institutional Ethics Committees and Health Care Decision Making*. Ann Arbor, MI: Health Administration Press, 1984.

Freedman, Benjamin. "One Philosopher's Experience on an Ethics Committee." *Hastings Center Report* 11 (April 1981): 20–22.

Henderson, Verne E. "The Ethical Side of Enterprise." *Sloan Management Review* 23, no. 3 (1982): 41–42.

President's Commission for the Study of Ethical Problems in Medicine and Biomedical and Behavioral Research. *Deciding to Forego Life-Sustaining Treatment*. Washington, DC: U.S. Government Printing Office, March 1983.

———. *Making Health Care Decisions*, Vol. 1. Washington, DC: U.S. Government Printing Office, October 1982.

Read, William. *Ethical Dilemmas in a Changing Health Care Environment: Hospital Ethics Committees*. Chicago: Hospital Research & Educational Trust, 1983.

Rescher, Nicholas. "The Allocation of Exotic Medical Lifesaving Therapy." *Ethics* 79 (April 1969).

Veatch, Robert M. Quoted in "Ethics Committees' Proliferation in Hospitals Predicted." *Hospitals* (1 July 1983): 43–48.

Williams, Kenneth, and Paul Donnelly. *Medical Care Quality and the Public Trust*. Chicago: Pluribus Press, 1982.

Chapter 24

Advocacy Reconsidered: Progress and Prospects

Samuel Levey
James Hill

Samuel Levey is Gerhard Hartman Professor, Graduate Program in Hospital and Health Administration and Center for Health Services Research, College of Medicine and Graduate College, University of Iowa, Iowa City. He is a Fellow of the College. James Hill is Research Associate, Graduate Program in Hospital and Health Administration, University of Iowa, Iowa City.

This article was published in *Hospital & Health Services Administration* 33, no. 4 (Winter 1988).

Dutiful and sustained advocacy in response to a human being made vulnerable by illness is the moral wellspring of the healing professions; it is anticipated in ethical codes from the Hippocratic Oath to the guidelines of the American Medical Association; at its farthest extension, it implies that the health care interests of the patient, once taken up by the advocate, will be pursued until function is restored, pain relieved, or anxiety stilled.

In spite of the flow of ceremonial rhetoric assuring us of its vitality with health care professionals, advocacy exists more in word than in practice. As one observer of the health care culture astutely observes, there has been surprisingly little discussion of what is meant by "patient advocacy," and what specific responsibilities fall to physicians as patient advocates (Watts 1986). This condition of fluidity may be salutary, however, for it presents health providers with the opportunity to review a narrow tradition and to recast the concept of advocacy along more socially responsible lines.

A review of the advocacy literature reveals a major problem to be the conflict of interests experienced by health providers who must dispense care under the burden of institutional and governmental constraints. By its very nature, advocacy cannot abide constraint. As it is commonly understood, advocacy in health care occurs in the one-on-one relationship of a provider supplying all necessary care—even that of marginal benefit—to the individual patient, regardless of cost (Hotchkiss 1987). A patient advocate *cannot* participate in rationing or underutilization of resources and *cannot* weigh society's interest with that of the patient—so goes the oft-cited stricture of the concept. Indeed, advocacy and rationing are antithetical terms.

Swiryn (1986) addresses this opposition of interests and speaks for the community of traditional physician providers in saying, "My advocacy is for my patient, second for her family, third for all patients, and rarely (in cases of certain communicable diseases, for example), for society." Levinsky (1984) states flatly that physicians are "required" to do all that may benefit a patient "without regard to cost or other societal considerations." Abrams (1986) extends this obligation, arguing that the physician who "fails to maintain the primacy of patient advocacy, has failed his profession and his patient." He goes on to say, in support of Swiryn and Levinsky's priority, "In the exhortations to the physician to enlist on the side of society lies the threat to the physician's traditional and essential role."

While we admire the *idea* of a strong, single-minded, and sustained advocacy in response to an individual compromised by injury or illness, we recognize a number of problems that prevent it from achieving the height of its rhetoric. Among these difficulties are

- Economic pressures that may limit physicians' ability to treat their patients

- Battles for control of health care that pit physicians against managers, other physicians, and the representatives of patients and consumers
- The erosion of physician authority caused by the fragmentation of responsibility and the framing of legal requirements such as disclosure and consent
- The public's expectation of a successful outcome to every treatment and its propensity for litigation in the event of failure
- The expanding domain of "health" and health awareness
- The new and difficult ethical choices introduced by sophisticated technologies.

In view of these constraints, we propose that the idea of advocacy as a model of service be examined and evaluated in the context of what providers are now able to do for the patient. Beyond that, we suggest that the focus of advocacy discussion be broadened to include societal implications as well as the individual ones—that a "meta-advocacy" of social concern be more powerfully merged with traditional one-on-one advocacy. This "higher" advocacy and the social vision it implies deserve the attention of all parties in the health care continuum, from researchers to policymakers, to physicians and patients.

Advocacy Defined

In general terms, advocacy is a tripartite arrangement involving an agent who takes the part of a victim (or client) against an adversary to impart protection, rescue, or relief. Historically, wherever the weak have been defended by the strong, advocacy has been practiced. Today, entire organizations are devoted solely to the work of advocacy (e.g., Amnesty International, the American Civil Liberties Union, the Civil Rights Commission). In the realm of contemporary health care, advocacy is often seen as another term for "caring": it suggests a psychosocial dimension, beyond merely scientific and technical expertise, and is exercised on behalf of the patient against distress, disease, or infirmity with a view to relieving pain or restoring wholeness. Some purists would argue that a "full" advocacy is realized only when all necessary care is given, the continuous needs of the patient are met, and the rights of the patient within the health care institution are assured (Levinsky 1984). Other commentators assign a less comprehensive scope (Schoolman 1977).

Traditional advocacy is rooted in physician paternalism, which is to say, control of the clinical encounter by the doctor: the physician is thought to have

419

such "special esoteric knowledge and humanitarian intent that he and he alone should be allowed to decide what is good for the layman" (Freidson 1970). The "age of paternalism," as Siegler (1985) terms this venerable tradition, extends through all of human history and was only recently superseded by the "age of autonomy," in which a shift in the unequal power relationship of physician and patient began to occur. The conjunction of the two "ages," with its problematic interface of physician paternalism and patient autonomy, has been a source of concern for bioethicists for the past 20 years (Thomasma 1983; Vanderpool and Weiss 1984).

Among the various pressures that have served to modify the paternal model are the above-mentioned urgings of egalitarianism, with physician autonomy yielding to demands for disclosure, informed consent, and patient self-determination and cost-containment programs (because of this growing emphasis, Siegler (1985) characterizes the emergent period as the "age of bureaucracy"). The decline of the physician's professional dominance—and with it the liberties of paternalistic behavior—is neatly symbolized by new legal rulings: according to Starr (1982), "Few other developments so well illustrate [this decline] as the increased tendency of the courts to view the doctor-patient relationship as a partnership in decision making rather than a doctor's monopoly." Indeed, the root meaning of advocate, "to speak out," is now overshadowed by the imperative "to discuss." In this participative arrangement, the proper role of the up-to-date advocate is to *inform* the patient and then to give *support* for whatever decision is made (Kohnke 1982).

While "speaking out" may imply listening, sifting, and advising, it may also mean overriding the self-determination of the patient. Because of new limitations, then, traditional paternal advocacy can no longer serve to describe or direct all relationships in health care. These limitations, however, are merely a further burden of constraint on an advocacy principle that has already been compromised.

Advocacy Compromised

In the long history of Western medicine the responsibility of physicians has been a partnership of social accountability and economic incentive, with the structure of professional services and the organization of their lives shaped in varying measures by both. The early physicians who aspired to follow the example of Hippocrates, for example, were motivated largely by an interest in doing well individually, notwithstanding their pledge to "do good," to benefit the patient and do no harm. Over the course of centuries, this tradition merged with the

Judeo-Christian ethos of charity and self-sacrifice, forming the moral foundation of modern medicine (Jonsen 1983). Yet, the conflict inherent in controlling demand for services (the physician is both advisor and supplier) remains. Today, tensions between social and self-interest in health care are vividly present in the conflict of human service and commercial interest—especially notable in the expansion of entrepreneurialism—and serve to fuel an ongoing exchange of impassioned commentary.

Before the appearance of third-party insurance, most physicians gave evidence of this dual interest by providing charity care: "The physician's conscience was the most important health care resource for those who could not afford to pay" (Cassel 1985). With the arrival of "open-ended" reimbursement and the proliferation of medical technology, however, full exercise of the physician's "conscience" ("blank check" advocacy, one unhindered by bottom-line concerns) led to overutilization of resources and, with that, to ever higher medical expenditures.

Only recently has the revolution in health care organization, financing, and delivery—the rise of a corporate ethos—put accountability on a new footing. Solo, fee-for-service practice has steadily given way to alternative modes of delivery in which the provider organization, the corporation, and government cast a critical eye on the physician's use of resources. Quite naturally, this broad responsibility to others besides the patient may conflict with the central principle of advocacy, the obligation to serve the interest of the patient first: with their auditors now attending to the medical transaction, physicians, in the view of Mechanic (1984), are expected to behave more as allocators of resources than patient advocates—those who "balance the patient's wants and needs against the aggregate population and a fixed budget." Americans, says Iglehart (1987), are searching for a new paradigm in their relationship with doctors—one that will mean an evolution of the physician from an advocate with scant concern for medical economics to a resource allocator living on a finite budget.

Not surprisingly, perhaps, the paradigm that the rising cost consciousness and the proliferation of alternative delivery systems appears to be ushering in, is viewed with alarm by many physicians. Reagan (1987), for example, sees a "dilution" of advocacy in the gatekeeping concept, which requires the physician to weigh patient needs against institutional cost-control policy. Relman (1987) adds that a physician "cannot easily serve his patients as trusted counselor and agent when he has economic ties to profit-seeking businesses that regard those patients as customers."

While a fixed budget—diagnosis-related groups (DRGs), capitation, and other cost constraints—and rigorous utilization review may compromise physicians' ability to honor their obligation, even to the point of an early discharge, neither the patient's expectation of comfort or cure, nor the physician's ethical responsibility has decreased; indeed, the complexity of decision making has grown, making a good working knowledge of bioethical issues an important part of physician training.

In addition to economic accountability, other developments have served to weaken the advocacy role of the physician:

- That the great bulk of writing on advocacy is currently found in the nursing literature ought to suggest the centrality of this role in the profession. It was not always so. Traditionally, nurses performed their duties subservient to the physician, acting the part of the good soldier who follows orders without question (Winslow 1984). As the treatment dispensed by the physician has drawn away from extended consultation and toward technical procedures, however, the role of nurses, and other physician extenders, has broadened to take up much of the life-enhancing (i.e., psychosocial) advocacy function and provide continuity of care. Moreover, patient representatives have entered many health care settings with the purpose of assisting the patient toward care that is respectful of that person's rights.

- Advocacy has also been tested by the rise of "defensive" medicine brought on by the malpractice litigation crisis. Professional liability may be the biggest problem currently confronting American medicine and has contributed to a "maximalist" approach to treatment on the part of many physicians—a tendency to do more than is required for the patient so as to reduce the level of uncertainty regarding litigation.

- The AIDS epidemic has generated an acid test of advocacy by introducing an added risk to health care workers in the treatment of this class of patients. Many health care professionals either openly refuse to care for this group of patients or take extraordinary precautions that amount to the same avoidance behavior.

Reviewing this situation from a historical perspective and examining current professional codes, Zuger and Miles (1987) appeal for a new ethic to guide doctors in their care of AIDS patients: a virtue-based medical ethic, they argue, goes beyond the enforceable requirements of law and contract. Pellegrino (1987) supports this view of *obligation* on the part of physicians, arguing that "a medical need constitutes a moral claim on those equipped to help."

Advocacy Enhanced

An ethic that places the well-being of the patient *first* is not limited to scholarly writing, of course. Codes of ethics are invoked with some regularity, and programs intended to preserve the advocacy ethic from the manifold threats to it are frequently proposed. Relman (1987), for example, has presented a four-point set of imperatives that would allow the physician to fend off threats to the advocacy function by minimizing conflicts of interest:

- Limit practice incomes to fees or salaries earned from patient services personally provided or supervised
- Those in independent office practice should avoid any arrangement with a for-profit corporation that rewards them for choosing a particular facility or service for their patients or restricts the choices they can make
- Those practicing in a for-profit setting should be either self-employed or part of a self-managed and self-regulated medical group that contracts with the company
- Physicians should not enter an arrangement with any organization that directly rewards them for withholding services from their patients.

Other commentators see the surest protection of advocacy in maintaining and upgrading quality assurance measures. Some argue for expanding the role of the physician, rather than maintaining purity of motive; Reagan (1987), for example, urges participation by physicians in policy development in various contexts, "both private and public, local and national settings," while Friedman (1986) argues that either physicians will take up the burden of resource allocation, or no one will.

Other commentators favor broadening physician "literacy" skills and knowledge outside of the medical sphere. Hillman et al. (1986) argue that if physicians are to "gain control of the medical-industrial complex," they must acquire business skills and adopt the role of "physician executive." Presumably, these skills will permit the doctor to deal with allocation decisions in a wiser manner; certainly, they will add to their base of power in the decision-making process. May (1986), similarly, suggests that if physicians are to exercise greater control over the health industry—to protect advocacy—they must become "physician entrepreneurs," developers of the new alternative delivery systems. The consequence of inaction, according to May, is a kind of proletarianization of physicians through a passive evolution to a salaried employee—and a dramatic loss of advocacy power.

In Search of a Model Advocacy

Assuming the power base of physicians will change, to what model of medical practice can they appeal when faced with ethical and patient entitlement dilemmas and their multiple obligations to medical staff, governing board, and society if their purpose is to uphold the fundamental value of health care—an advocacy responsible to both the individual and society? What models of behavior are available as means for fostering the most ethical and mutually satisfying type of physician-patient relationship within the framework of constraints and conflicting interests mentioned earlier in the article?

Advocacy and the Individual

Since the 1950s, a host of paradigms, from Szasz and Hollander's (1956) doctor-patient behavior models (activity-passivity, guidance-cooperation, and mutual participation) to May's (1975) "covenant," have been introduced in the health care literature to describe how we ought to structure the clinical encounter.

A *single* model would appear to be inadequate to define and direct the extensive range of physician-patient relationships and the different stages of care, since the physician and patient assume a range of respective roles depending on the disorder. According to Inui and Carpenter (1985), "No single system of description and analysis could hope to capture the full richness and complexity of human communication." Yet the broad ideal of a "shared" relationship has been cited as the normative model for our time—a desirable framework that combines paternalism's forwardness and penchant for decisive action and consumerism's restraint and respect for self-determination, within the limitations set by macroallocation decisions handed down by society and the health care institution.

To be sure, this model is not a visionary construct, but a considered relationship that receives the support of the President's Commission for the Study of Ethical Problems in Medicine (1983). According to this study, ethical decision making in the clinical encounter of physician and patient is a "shared" arrangement "based upon mutual respect and participation [and is] not a ritual to be equated with reciting the contents of a form that details the risks of particular treatments."

"Shared," like advocacy, is a broad concept; it can be linked to such terms as "partnership," "friendship," and "contract"—all models whose distinguishing merits have been discussed in the literature (Clouser 1983). The "covenant" model is theoretically superior to all three inasmuch as it not only unites the equality and respect of partnership, the active benevolence of friendship, and the guarantees of contract, but goes a further step in placing the physician in perpetual "debt" to a patient—a kind of ongoing obligation. Clouser (1983) sees the effort to translate such lofty frameworks to practice as a fruitless endeavor, and he dismisses all such models as "whimsical gestalts." The physician-patient relationship, he argues, would be "better served if we simply listed what we morally ought not to do."

The Social Model: Meta-Advocacy

If "shared" is stretched beyond the physician-patient encounter, the obligations of advocacy become problematic. This is largely because the direct appeal of the "identified individual" is to the advocate far more compelling than the diffuse needs of the abstract body we call society. A graphic personal need is more persuasive than the distant and unfocused moral imperative of the group: "Distance seems to blunt the moral imagination," says Churchill (1987), "and the lack of identified lives to whom to relate the rescue impulse seems to paralyze social ethics altogether." As a result, most discussions of advocacy center on ethical individualism.

When health care is placed in a social context, as it is in a discussion of rationing, the opprobrium of thwarted advocacy is heard. Typical of this view is Angell's (1985) comment that "any role in limiting useful medical care is inconsistent with our role as advocates for the health of our patients." And yet, ironically, physicians have *always* practiced the "anti-advocacy" of rationing: whenever they deny a patient *some* available care or delay a treatment, waiting to see if the person's condition improves or worsens, they allocate care. Inasmuch as money usually guarantees access to health care, its influence brings physicians into a rationing scheme by price.

Although participation in rationing on the part of the provider is seen by skeptics as a species of anti-advocacy, properly conducted it can be regarded as "meta-advocacy": individual advocacy informed by social awareness. Such a dual focus is neither contradiction nor luxury, but a responsibility of all providers of health care. As Churchill (1987) points out, concern for both the identified individual and society is a moral imperative: "The supposed opposition between ethical individualism and [social-mindedness] is finally false. The moral life is irreducibly social, as well as inexhaustibly individual." An example of this coincidence of micro and macro concerns exists in Britain's National Health Service where physicians function as rationing agents within a system of universally accessible primary care, exercising the advocacy of professional judgment under a fixed budget.

But, one must ask if providers in our system of health care would *ever* be able to practice a meta-advocacy of restraint without cost-conscious mechanisms such as the prospective payment system and structures such as health maintenance organizations. The incentive for saying "no" to marginally beneficial treatment for patients at micro levels of care is difficult for reasons already mentioned: for example, a tradition of aggressive advocacy, fear of malpractice litigation, and self-interest on the part of the physician. Realistically, a provider in our health care system can be constrained from overutilization only by a policy of budgeted resources and careful review (Daniels 1986).

On a larger scale, however, meta-advocacy may be more feasible—at the very least, in defining a social agenda. Among the priorities for this agenda are access to infant and prenatal care for the underprivileged, more extensive investment in mental health programs, coming to grips with the AIDS problem, and—perhaps most important—an appreciation of the "medical commons" and the assurance of equitable *access* to its resources (particularly, for the 37 million uninsured).

A more challenging aspect of this agenda is the leveling off of health care expectations. This philosophy of *limits* (a sobering attitude in view of our abundance, our fascination with technology, and our resistance to imposed constraints) applies not only to resources, but also to the ever-expanding purview of both illness and entitlements to care and our culture's insistence on massive expenditures to forestall natural physical decline and death.

As to resources, Califano (1988) reflects a growing consensus in his appeal for cost reductions in health care through limits on hospital admissions, numbers of procedures, malpractice awards, and provider responsibility for consumer health. Regarding rising expectations, Barsky (1988) encourages providers to be aware of the price of a heightened consciousness of health among consumers: the paradox of better health may be a "medicalization" of daily life accompanied by a resultant deterioration in subjective well-being. Related to this paradox is what Callahan (1987) presents as modern medicine's philosophy of denying limits, particularly where aging and attempts to extend life are concerned. The result of this tendency may be, in the view of Churchill (1987), "a medical commons depleted of resources because of physicians who are zealous for all treatments possible and a public clamoring for longevity."

Conclusion

Broad mandates to extend *access* to health care and to impose limits on *costs* have formed, and the paradox they imply must be resolved within the paradigm

426

of meta-advocacy. Under this scheme, individual well-being will come to be viewed, more than at present, as a collective responsibility involving both patient and teams of health care professionals; at the macro level, it will involve all members of the health care continuum, from researchers to policymakers. Perhaps, ultimately, through a broader inquiry into social justice and a clearer definition of mission, we will come to view this inclusive model of individual, organizational, and social interdependence, respect, and responsibility as the ideal form of advocacy—and as a suitable moral end for policy formulation.

References

Abrams, F. R. "Patient Advocate or Secret Agent?" *Journal of the American Medical Association* 256 (3 October 1986): 1784–85.

Angell, M. "Cost Containment and the Physician." *Journal of the American Medical Association* 254 (6 September 1985): 1203–7.

Barsky, A. J. "The Paradox of Health." *New England Journal of Medicine* 318 (18 February 1988): 414–18.

Califano, J. A. "The Health-Care Chaos." *New York Times Magazine* (20 March 1988): 44–46, 56–58.

Callahan, D. *Setting Limits: Medical Goals in An Aging Society.* New York: Simon and Schuster, 1987.

Cassel, C. K. "Doctors and Allocation Decisions: A New Role in the New Medicine." *Journal of Health Politics, Policy and Law* 10 (Fall 1985): 549–64.

Churchill, L. R. *Rationing Health Care in America: Perceptions and Principles of Justice.* Notre Dame: University of Notre Dame Press, 1987.

Clouser, D. K. "Veatch, May, and Models: A Critical Review and a New View." In *The Clinical Encounter: The Moral Fabric of the Patient-Physician Relationship,* edited by E. E. Shelp. Dordrecht, Holland: Reidel, 1983.

Daniels, N. "Why Saying No to Patients in the United States is So Hard." *New England Journal of Medicine* 314 (22 May 1986): 1380–83.

Freidson, E. *Professional Dominance.* New York: Aldine Publishing Co., 1970.

Friedman, E. "Doctors and Rationing: The End of the Honor System." *Primary Care* 13 (June 1986): 349–64.

Hillman, A., D. Nash, W. Kissick, and S. Martin, III. "Managing the Medical-Industrial Complex." *New England Journal of Medicine* 315 (21 August 1986): 511–13.

Hotchkiss, W. S. "Doctor as Patient Advocate." *Journal of the American Medical Association* 258 (21 August 1987): 947–48.

Iglehart, J. K. Speech. Chicago, 8 May 1987.

427

Inui, T. S., and W. B. Carpenter. "Problems and Prospects for Health Services Research on Provider-Patient Communication." *Medical Care* 23 (May 1985): 521–38.

Jonsen, A. R. "Watching the Doctor." *New England Journal of Medicine* 308 (23 June 1983): 1531–35.

Kohnke, M. F. *Advocacy: Risk and Reality.* St. Louis: C. V. Mosby Co., 1982.

Levinsky, N. "The Doctor's Master." *New England Journal of Medicine* 311 (13 December 1984): 1573–75.

May, W. E. "Of Ethics and Advocacy." *Journal of the American Medical Association* 256 (3 October 1986): 1786–87.

May, W. F. "Code, Covenant, or Philanthropy." *Hastings Center Report* 5 (December 1975): 29–38.

Mechanic, D. "The Transformation of Health Providers." *Health Affairs* 3 (Spring 1984): 65–72.

Pellegrino, E. D. "Altruism, Self-Interest, and Medical Ethics." *Journal of the American Medical Association* 258 (9 October 1987): 1939–40.

President's Commission for the Study of Ethical Problems in Medicine. *Summing Up.* Washington, DC: U.S. Government Printing Office, 1983.

Reagan, M. D. "Physicians as Gatekeepers." *New England Journal of Medicine* 317 (31 December 1987): 1731–34.

Relman, A. S. "Practicing Medicine in the New Business Climate." *New England Journal of Medicine* 316 (30 April 1987): 1150–51.

Schoolman, H. M. "The Role of the Physician as a Patient Advocate." *New England Journal of Medicine* 296 (13 January 1977): 103–5.

Siegler, M. "The Progression of Medicine." *Archives of Internal Medicine* 145 (April 1985): 713–15.

Starr, P. *The Social Transformation of American Medicine.* New York: Basic Books, 1982.

Swiryn, S. "The Doctor as Gatekeeper." *Archives of Internal Medicine* 146 (September 1986): 1789.

Szasz, T. S., and M. H. Hollander. "A Contribution to the Philosophy of Medicine: The Basic Models of the Doctor-Patient Relationship." *Archives of Internal Medicine* 97 (May 1956): 585–92.

Thomasma, D. C. "Limitations of the Autonomy Model for the Doctor-Patient Relationship." *Pharos* 46 (Spring 1983): 2–5.

Vanderpool, H. Y., and G. B. Weiss. "Patient Truthfulness: A Test of Models of the Physician-Patient Relationship." *Journal of Medicine and Philosophy* 9 (November 1984): 353–72.

Watts, M. S. "How About Some Affirmative Action for Patient Advocacy?" *Western Journal of Medicine* 144 (April 1986): 458.

Winslow, G. R. "From Loyalty to Advocacy: A New Metaphor for Nursing." *Hastings Center Report* 14 (June 1984): 32–40.

Zuger, A., and S. H. Miles. "Physicians, AIDS, and Occupational Risks." *Journal of the American Medical Association* 258 (9 October 1987): 1924–28.

Index

431

About the Editor

Samuel Levey, Ph.D., FACHE, is Gerhard Hartman Professor and former Head of the Graduate Program in Hospital and Health Administration and Center for Health Services Research, College of Medicine and Graduate College, The University of Iowa. The author and co-author of several books and monographs on health management, he was editor of *Hospital & Health Services Administration*, the official journal of the American College of Healthcare Executives, from 1987 to 1991. His current research interests focus on leadership and behavior of health care organizations.